Ernst Nyström · Gertrud E. B. Berg · Svante K.G. Jansson
Ove Tørring · Stig V. Valdemarsson

Thyroid Disease in Adults

Ernst Nyström · Gertrud E. B. Berg
Svante K.G. Jansson · Ove Tørring
Stig V. Valdemarsson

Thyroid Disease in Adults

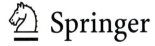

Prof. Ernst Nyström
Sahlgrenska Academy,
University of Gothenburg,
Institute of Endocrinology
41345 Göteborg
Sweden
kerstin.nystrom@ving.se

Gertrud E. B. Berg
Sahlgrenska University Hospital
Department of Oncology
41345 Göteborg
Sweden
gertrud.berg@oncology.gu.se

Svante K.G. Jansson
Sahlgrenska University Hospital
Department of Surgery
41345 Göteborg
Sweden
svante.jansson@vgregion.se

Ove Tørring
Institution for Clinical Science
and Education
Karolinska Institutet
Södersjukhuset
Sjukhusbacken 11
11883 Stockholm
Sweden
Email: ove.torring@ki.se

Stig V. Valdemarsson
Skanes Universitets
Sjukhus/Lund
Dept. of Oncology
22185 Lund
Sweden
stig.valdemarsson@skane.se

ISBN: 978-3-642-13261-2   e-ISBN: 978-3-642-13262-9

DOI: 10.1007/978-3-642-13262-9

Springer-Verlag Heidelberg Dordrecht London New York

© Springer-Verlag Berlin Heidelberg 2011

This work is subject to copyright. All rights are reserved, whether the whole or part of the material is concerned, specifically the rights of translation, reprinting, reuse of illustrations, recitation, broadcasting, reproduction on microfilms or in any other way, and storage in data banks. Duplication of this publication or parts thereof is permitted only under the provisions of the German Copyright Law of September 9, 1965, in its current version, and permission for use must always be obtained from Springer-Verlag. Violations are liable for prosecution under the German Copyright Law.

The use of general descriptive names, registered names, trademarks, etc. in this publication does not imply, even in the absence of a specific statement, that such names are exempt from the relevant protective laws and regulations and therefore free for general use.

Product liability: The publishers cannot guarantee the accuracy of any information about dosage and application contained in this book. In every individual case the user must check such information by consulting the relevant literature.

Cover design: eStudio Calamar, Figueres, Berlin

Printed on acid-free paper

Springer is part of Springer Science+Business Media (www.springer.com)

Foreword

This book is a compilation of updated and expanded editions of two Swedish books previously published by Nycomed AB, *Thyroxine Treatment of Adults* and *Thyrotoxicosis in Adults*.

The aim was to produce a clinical handbook for thyroid disease to be used by general practitioners and internal medicine specialists, but also to be of value for specialists more directly devoted to thyroid disease. To facilitate reading and use in everyday work, we have included numerous illustrations as well as concise summary boxes.

We have invested much time in harmonizing the differences that exist in the practical management of patients with thyroid disease between clinicians and clinics in Sweden. We thereby hope to have reached some form of consensus, which we believe will not only be applicable to Sweden, but also have a more general acceptance.

Bo Ch. Warin at Nycomed AB has provided tremendous support and has been an enthusiastic, patient and faithful motivator. Media Center TVB AB in Linköping, Sweden, has been invaluable in coordinating the work on the book and contributing to text processing, illustrations, diagrams, photos and layout.

We have also received help from our many colleagues who have contributed towards the illustrations and offered good advice and valuable points of view. But most of all, we wish to thank Associate Professor Leif Tallstedt of St. Erik's Eye Hospital, Stockholm, Sweden and Dr. Kerstin Norrsell, Ophthalmology Clinic, Sahlgrenska University Hospital, Mölndal, Sweden, for help with matters relating to ophthalmology, Dr. Johan Mölne, Department of Pathology, Sahlgrenska University Hospital, for contributing to the section on cytological diagnostics, as well as for cytology/PAD images. We thank Dr. Anders Höög, Department of Endocrine Pathology, Karolinska University Hospital, Solna, for cytological images.

In addition, we would like to thank Agneta Lundström, at Medical Physics and Technology, Sahlgrenska University Hospital, for help with photos. Many thanks to Consultant Barbara Bergman, Clinical Radiology, Sahlgrenska University Hospital, for help with ultrasound images, and Consultant Madis Suurküla for pictures from nuclear medical investigations on patients with thyroid cancer. We have also gratefully received photographs from Rolf Hägglund in Mölndal.

Finally we would like to thank Associate Professor Ola Winqvist, Clinical Allergologic Research Unit, Karolinska University Hospital, Solna, for invaluable comments on the section relating to immunology and the thyroid, Professor Robert Eggertsen, Mölnlycke Vårdcentral (primary care), and Regional Medical Officer Anders Ehnberg, Strömsunds Hälsocentral, for the large amount of work they have invested in reviewing and commenting on the book from the perspective of a primary care provider.

Sweden, November 2010   Prof. Ernst Nyström

Contents

Chapter 1
Historical Background

1.1 Goitre and iodine 1
1.2 Hypothyroidism 1
1.3 Hyperthyroidism 3

Chapter 2
Anatomy and Physiology

2.1 The Embryologic Development
 and Anatomy of the Thyroid Gland 5
2.2 Iodine and the Thyroid 9
2.3 TSH and TSH Receptors 11
2.4 Synthesis and Secretion of Thyroid Hormones 12
2.5 Hypothalamus–Pituitary–Thyroid Axis 17
2.6 Deiodinases 18
2.7 Mechanisms of Action of Thyroid Hormones 18
2.8 Biochemical Indicators of the Peripheral
 Effects of Thyroid Hormones 22
2.9 Factors Affecting Thyroid Hormone Homeostasis 24
2.10 Effects of General Illness and Pharmaceuticals (NTI) 25

Chapter 3
Biochemical Investigations

3.1 TSH 29
3.2 TRH-Stimulated TSH Secretion 32
3.3 Thyroid Hormones 32
3.4 Free Thyroid Hormones 33
3.5 Analytical Problems 34
3.6 Reference Ranges (Normal Values) for
 Thyroid-Associated Hormone Analyses 35
3.7 Antibodies Against Thyroperoxidase (TPOAb) 36
3.8 Antibodies Against the TSH Receptor (TRAb) 37
3.9 Thyroglobulin (Tg) 38
3.10 Antibodies Against Thyroglobulin (TgAb) 38

Contents

3.11 Thyroxine-Binding Globulin (TBG) and Transthyretin (Prealbumin) 39
3.12 Calcitonin 39
3.13 Iodine in Urine 39
3.14 Genetic Diagnostics 39
3.15 Analytical Strategy 40

Chapter 4
Other Investigations

4.1 Investigations Using Radionuclides 47
4.2 Positron Emission Tomography (PET) 54
4.3 X-ray, CT, and MR 54
4.4 Ultrasound 55
4.5 Fine-Needle Biopsy 58

Chapter 5
Clinical Investigation of the Thyroid

5.1 Medical History 67
5.2 Physical Examination 67

Chapter 6
Iodine and the Thyroid Gland in Health and Sickness

6.1 Global Aspects of Iodine Intake 72
6.2 Thyroid Dysfunction Caused by Excessive Iodine Intake 73
6.3 Iodine in Foodstuffs and Medical Preparations 74
6.4 Iodine Blocking 75

Chapter 7
Autoimmunity and the Thyroid Gland

7.1 Immunological Background 79
7.2 Autoimmunity 83
7.3 Predisposing Factors 84
7.4 Exogenous Factors 86
7.5 Autoimmune Polyglandular Syndrome 87
7.6 Immunological Markers in Clinical Work 87
7.7 Treatment Strategy 89

Chapter 8
Growth Regulation of the Thyroid Gland

8.1	TSH	92
8.2	Hyperplasia and Goitre	92
8.3	Neoplasms and Tumours	93

Chapter 9
Thyroiditis and Pathogenesis

9.1	Thyroiditis	97
9.2	Autoimmune Thyroiditis	98
9.3	Other Triggering Factors for Thyroiditis	104

Chapter 10
Causes of Hypothyroidism

10.1	Primary Hypothyroidism and Chronic Autoimmune Thyroiditis	107
10.2	Epidemiology	107
10.3	Hypothyroidism After Treatment for Hyperthyroidism	108
10.4	Hypothyroidism After Surgery for Nontoxic Multinodular Goitre	108
10.5	Hypothyroidism After Surgery for Thyroid Cancer	109
10.6	Central Hypothyroidism	109
10.7	Iodine-Induced Hypothyroidism	109
10.8	Iatrogenic (Medicine-Induced) Hypothyroidism	109
10.9	Hypothyroidism After External Radiation of the Head and Neck Regions	110
10.10	Other Causes of Hypothyroidism	110

Chapter 11
Symptoms of Hypothyroidism

11.1	Autoimmune Thyroiditis – Natural Progression	111
11.2	Organ-Related Symptoms	113
11.3	Symptoms and Findings in Hypothyroidism	114
11.4	Central Hypothyroidism	116

Chapter 12
Treatment of Hypothyroidism

12.1	Primary Hypothyroidism.	119
12.2	Laboratory Tests – Special Aspects	121
12.3	Special Problems.	121
12.4	Resorption of Thyroxine	122
12.5	Pharmaceutical Interaction in Thyroxine Treatment	122
12.6	Oestrogens and Hypothyroidism.	122
12.7	Do All Patients Tolerate Thyroxine?.	123
12.8	Treatment with Triiodothyronine.	123
12.9	Parenteral Treatment with Thyroid Hormone	124
12.10	Overdosing with Thyroxine and Triiodothyronine	125
12.11	Compliance	125
12.12	Temporary Treatment with Thyroxine	125
12.13	Central (Secondary) Hypothyroidism	126

Chapter 13
Subclinical Hypothyroidism

13.1	Introduction	127
13.2	Prevalence	127
13.3	Substitution Treatment with Thyroxine in Subclinical Hypothyroidism	128

Chapter 14
Myxoedema Coma

14.1	Symptoms	131
14.2	Diagnostic Tests.	132
14.3	Treatment	132

Chapter 15
Causes of Thyrotoxicosis – an Overview 135

Chapter 16
Symptoms of Thyrotoxicosis

16.1	Weight Loss and Energy Metabolism	139
16.2	Mental Problems	139
16.3	Muscle Weakness	140
16.4	Cardiac Arrhythmia and Cardiac Insufficiency	140
16.5	Sympathetic Nervous System.	141
16.6	Dermatological Symptoms	142

16.7	Reduced Glucose Tolerance and Effects on Blood Lipids	142
16.8	Fertility	142
16.9	Bones and Calcium	142

Chapter 17
Hyperthyroidism Treatment Options – an Overview

17.1	General Considerations	145
17.2	Medical Treatment	146
17.3	Laboratory Checks After Treatment for Hyperthyroidism	154

Chapter 18
Graves' Disease

18.1	Pathophysiology	155
18.2	Symptoms Specific to Graves' Disease	155
18.3	Diagnosis	157
18.4	Treatment	158
18.5	Quality of Life	165

Chapter 19
Thyroid-Associated Ophthalmopathy

19.1	General Eye Symptoms in Thyrotoxicosis	167
19.2	Eye Symptoms Specific to Graves' Disease	167
19.3	Risk Factors and Pathophysiology	168
19.4	Symptoms and Diagnosis	169
19.5	Practical Management	174
19.6	Clinical Activity Score	175
19.7	The ATA Classification	176
19.8	TAO in Autoimmune Chronic Thyroiditis	176
19.9	Euthyroid TAO	176
19.10	Choice of Therapy for Hyperthyroidism in Patients with Ophthalmopathy	177
19.11	Treatment Considerations	177
19.12	Follow-Up	180

Chapter 20
Autonomous Adenoma

20.1	Definition and Prevalence	181
20.2	Pathophysiology	182
20.3	Specific Symptoms	182

20.4 Diagnosis 183
20.5 Treatment – General Considerations 183
20.6 Surgical Treatment 184
20.7 Radioiodine Treatment 185

Chapter 21
Toxic Multinodular Goitre

21.1 Development of Toxic Nodular Goitre 187
21.2 Specific Symptoms and Clinical Picture 188
21.3 Diagnosis 189
21.4 Risk Groups/Risk Situations 191
21.5 Differential Diagnosis: Considerations 191
21.6 Treatment 191

Chapter 22
Subclinical (Mild) Thyrotoxicosis

22.1 Nodular Goitre/Autonomous Adenoma 195
22.2 Graves' Disease/Thyroiditis/hCG 196
22.3 Exogenous Causes 196
22.4 Suppressed TSH After Treatment for Thyrotoxicosis 196
22.5 Symptoms 196
22.6 Cardiac Effects 197
22.7 Effects on Bone 197
22.8 Psychological Effects 198
22.9 Clinical Recommendations 198

Chapter 23
Thyrotoxicosis in the Elderly 199

Chapter 24
Thyrotoxic Crisis/ Thyroid Storm

24.1 Symptoms 201
24.2 Diagnosis 201
24.3 Treatment 202

Chapter 25
Thyroiditis – Clinical Aspects

25.1 Thyroiditis with Autoimmune Mechanism 205
25.2 Thyroiditis from Other Causes 208

Chapter 26
Subacute Thyroiditis (de Quervain´s Disease/Giant-Cell Thyroiditis)

26.1	Etiology	211
26.2	Symptoms	211
26.3	Progression	212
26.4	Diagnosis	212
26.5	Treatment	214

Chapter 27
Other Causes of Thyrotoxicosis

27.1	Central (Secondary) Hyperthyroidism/ TSH-Producing Pituitary Adenoma	215
27.2	hCG-Dependent Hyperthyroidism	216
27.3	Ectopic Production of Thyroid Hormones	216
27.4	Thyrotoxicosis Factitia	217
27.5	Iodine-Induced Hyperthyroidism	217

Chapter 28
Nontoxic Goitre

28.1	Goitre and Its Causes	221
28.2	Goitre Due to Iodine Deficiency	221
28.3	Colloid-Rich Multinodular Goitre	222
28.4	Intrathoracic Goitre	227

Chapter 29
Thyroid Lumps

29.1	Incidence/Prevalence	229
29.2	Classification of Palpable Thyroid Lumps	229
29.3	Diagnosis of Thyroid Lumps	229
29.4	Treatment of Palpable Thyroid Lumps	232
29.5	Investigation Algorithm	234

Chapter 30
Thyroid Cancer

30.1	Classification of Thyroid Tumours	235
30.2	Characteristics of Common Thyroid Tumours	236
30.3	Epidemiology	237
30.4	Risk Factors	238

30.5	Diagnostic Investigation	241
30.6	Prognostic Factors	241
30.7	Prognostic Classification System	243
30.8	Treatment	245
30.9	Follow-Up	248

Chapter 31
The Thyroid and Pregnancy

31.1	Maternal Physiology During Pregnancy	251
31.2	TSH, T4 and T3 During Pregnancy	252
31.3	Maternal/Placental Interaction	254
31.4	Thyroid Function in Mother and Foetus	254
31.5	The Thyroid and Fertility	256
31.6	Hypothyroidism and Pregnancy	257
31.7	Hyperthyroidism and Pregnancy	259
31.8	Goitre and Palpable Lumps in the Thyroid	262
31.9	Development of Thyroid Diseases During the Postnatal Period	263

Chapter 32
Thyroid Disease in Adolescents

32.1	Goitre	267
32.2	Autoimmune Thyroiditis and Hypothyroidism	268
32.3	Hyperthyroidism/Thyrotoxicosis	269
32.4	Palpable Thyroid Lumps	271

Chapter 33
Medicines and Other Medical Preparations

33.1	General	273
33.2	Iodine	273
33.3	Amiodarone	273
33.4	Other Iodine-Containing Preparations	277
33.5	Antithyroid Drugs	278
33.6	Lithium	278
33.7	Oestrogen	279
33.8	Interferon	279
33.9	Carbamazepine/Fenantoin	279
33.10	Miscellaneous	280

Chapter 34
Thyroid Hormone Resistance ... 281

Index ... 285

Presentation of Contributors

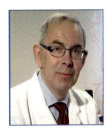

Ernst Nyström: Professor and Senior Consultant at the Endocrinology Section, Sahlgrenska University Hospital in Gothenburg. He is attached to the Thyroid Unit, and his main interests lie within the changes in body composition, metabolism, and mental state, during and after hyper- and hypothyroidism. He is particularly interested in communication of medical information to colleagues and the general public.

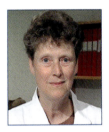

Gertrud Berg: Associate Professor, Senior Consultant and Vice Chancellor in Oncology at Sahlgrenska University Hospital in Gothenburg, where she works in the Thyroid Unit. Her main interests are iodination mechanisms in the thyroid, and therapeutic application of radionuclides in thyroid diseases and cancer.

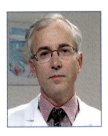

Svante Jansson: Associate Professor and Senior Consultant in Surgery at Sahlgrenska University Hospital in Gothenburg. Fields of special interest in clinical and research areas are cancer of the thyroid, hyperthyroidism, parathyroid diseases and adrenal tumours.

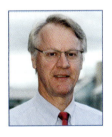

Ove Tørring: Associate Professor and assistant head of the Institution for clinical research and education at the Karolinska Institute, Södersjukhuset, and Senior Consultant in the Endocrinology Section, Department of Internal Medicine, at Södersjukhuset, Stockholm. His main interests are diseases of the thyroid gland, osteoporosis, and calcium metabolic bone diseases. Further interests are thyrotoxicosis, ophthalmopathy and the effects of thyroid and calciotropic hormone on bones and at cellular level.

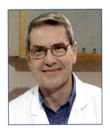

Stig Valdemarsson: Associate Professor and until recently Senior Consultant at the Department for Endocrinology and Diabetes, Lund University Hospital. He has recently moved to the Department for Oncology at Lund University Hospital, with focus on diagnosis and treatment of thyroid diseases. He is primarily interested in classic endocrinology, and has a particular interest in diseases of the thyroid, pituitary and parathyroid, but also in neuroendocrine tumours, osteoporosis and adrenal diseases.

List of Abbreviations and Definitions

General

Adenoma
Benign tumour of glandular tissue.

Autoimmune polyglandular syndrome (*APS*)
Concomitant occurrence of multiple autoimmune diseases.

Basedow's disease
See Graves' disease.

Binding proteins
The proteins to which thyroxine (T4) and triiodothyronine (T3) are extensively bound when the hormones are transported in the blood.

Colloid
The content of the lumen of the follicle, where thyroglobulin, iodine and thyroid hormones are stored.

Deiodinases
Enzymes that catalyse deiodination of the T4/T3/rT3 molecules.
- Type I (D1) primarily converts T4 to T3 and rT3 to T2, but can also convert T4 to rT3 and T3 to T2
- Type II (D2) converts T4 to T3 and rT3 to T2
- Type III (D3) converts T4 to rT3 and T3 to T2

Endocrine ophthalmopathy/thyroid-associated ophthalmopathy
Effects on orbital tissues can be seen in autoimmune thyroid disease, most frequently hyperthyroidism due to autoimmune Graves' disease. The term endocrine ophthalmopathy is synonymous with thyroid-associated ophthalmopathy (TAO). The latter term is now more commonly used and is therefore generally used in this book.

Follicle
The functional unit of the thyroid built up of a single layer of epithelial cells around a lumen in which the colloid is stored.

Graves´ disease/Basedow's disease
These names are used synonymously and describe autoimmune diffuse toxic goitre (hyperthyroidism caused by TSH receptor-stimulating antibodies). The immunological disturbances of this disease can also affect organs other than the thyroid, usually the structures of the orbit (thyroid-associated ophthalmopathy), but also the dermis and periosteum.

Human antimouse antibodies (HAMA) can cause analytical interference.

Hyperthyroidism
Overactivity of the thyroid with increased release of thyroid hormones.

Hypothyroidism
Underactivity of the thyroid gland. Most often a result of disease in the thyroid, primary hypothyroidism. Inadequate TSH secretion can also lead to central (or secondary) hypothyroidism.

Sodium iodide symporter (NIS)
NIS is the common name of the iodide pump and is a membrane protein that is responsible for active transport of the iodine into the follicle cell.

Nodule
Common designation of a palpable lump in the thyroid.

Nonthyroidal illness (NTI)
NTI is also known as euthyroid sickness and is a condition in which organs other than the thyroid affect the release and metabolism of thyroid hormones and TSH. In NTI, thyroid function is often considered to be normal and the patient clinically euthyroid.

Pendred's syndrome
Name of an inherited metabolic condition that leads to hypothyroidism and impaired hearing.

Goitre
Enlarged thyroid gland without reference to function or cause.

Thyroid-associated ophthalmopathy (TAO)
Synonymous with endocrine ophthalmopathy.

Tg
Thyroglobulin. A thyroid-specific protein that is produced in the follicle cell and stored in the follicle lumen. The iodinated thyroglobulin molecule comprises the source for hormone synthesis and is an important depot of thyroid hormone and iodine.

Thyrotoxicosis
Symptoms that occur at excessively high concentrations of thyroid hormones in body tissues, regardless of whether this is due to hyperthyroidism or other causes.

Thyroperoxidase (TPO)
A membrane-bound enzyme present in the thyroid gland. The enzyme is found in the part of the follicle cell that interfaces with the follicle lumen and is important in several stages of thyroid hormone synthesis.

Hormones

Calcitonin
A peptide that is released from the thyroid C cells. Calcitonin is not thought to play any major physiological role in humans. Calcitonin is commonly used as a biochemical marker for medullary thyroid cancer.

Thyroid stimulating hormone (TSH)
Thyroid stimulating hormone, or thyrotropin, is released from the pituitary gland.

TSH receptors
Follicle cell receptors for TSH. When TSH is bound to its receptor, the synthesis and release of thyroid hormone increases.

Thyroid hormone analyses
In current clinical routine, analyses of the free fraction of thyroid hormones (free T4 and free T3) are increasingly used rather than analysis of the total amount of thyroid hormones (T4 and T3).

In sections that discuss biochemical diagnostics we have therefore chosen to mention only the analytical methods for free hormones, well aware of the limitations of these methods and that some clinics prefer analysis of total hormones as the first-line analysis.

T4
Thyroxine (3, 5, 3', 5'-tetraiodothyronine). The numbers denote the position of iodine atoms the thyronin molecule. T4 is the thyroid hormone secreted in largest quantities from the thyroid. T4 exhibits low metabolic activity and is a prohormone, which is deiodinated peripherally to the active hormone T3. T4 is present in the blood, to a large extent bound to transport proteins.

T3
Triiodothyronine (3, 5, 3'-triiodothyronine) is, similarly to T4, present in the blood and for the most part bound to transport proteins. It is the thyroid hormone which, in its free form, is the most biologically active. Released in smaller quantities directly from the thyroid. The largest quantities of circulating T3 comes from the peripheral deiodination of T4.

rT3
Reverse triiodothyronine (3, 3', 5'-triiodothyronine). A metabolite of T4 which is biologically inactive.

Free T4
The fraction of thyroxine not protein-bound.

Free T3
The fraction of triiodothyronine not protein-bound.

List of Abbreviations and Definitions

Antibodies (Ab)
The abbreviation Ab is used in the text for antibodies.

TPOAb
Antibodies against thyroperoxidase. This is a sensitive marker for autoimmune thyroiditis.

TRAb
Antibodies against the TSH receptor. Stimulate or, in rare cases, block the TSH receptor.

TgAb
Antibodies against thyroglobulin.

Isotopes
The word isotope (from the Greek *isos* meaning the same and *topos* meaning place) is used to denote different forms of basic elements with the same atomic number, i.e. with the same position in the periodic table. Depending on the composition of the atomic nucleus (number of neutrons in relation to protons), a basic element can exist in different forms, or isotopes. Isotopes can be stable or unstable. Unstable isotopes decay spontaneously and emit radiation (radioactive radiation). Unstable isotopes are also called radionuclides (see definition below).

Common for the isotopes of a basic element is that they have the same number of protons and electrons, but different numbers of neutrons, which means that they have the same properties in chemical reactions.

Radionuclides
Radioactive unstable isotopes used for investigation and treatment.

Iodine (I)
The most common isotope of the basic element iodine is the stable isotope I-127. Radioactive isotopes include I-131, with a half-life of 8 days, and I-123 with a half-life of 13 h. The negatively charged ion, iodide (I$^-$), regardless of isotope number, is taken up by the thyroid from the blood through active transport via NIS, oxidized and bound to thyroglobulin in the follicle lumen.

By using radioactive iodine isotopes, it is possible to study both uptake of iodide by the gland and its hormone turnover. I-131 is most frequently used for diagnosis and treatment. The isotope I-123 is preferably used for diagnostic purposes in children and for diagnostic scans in thyroid cancer patients in order to avoid a stunning effect on subsequent 1-131 therapy. I-123 has a shorter half-life and in principle emits pure γ-radiation, which results in a lower impact to the thyroid gland. It is however, more expensive and more difficult to handle due to the shorter half-life.

Technetium (Tc)
Tc-99^m is a by-product of uranium fission and decays with emission of γ-radiation. It has a half-life of 6 h. Technetium has no stable isotopes. The pertechnetate ion, Tc-99^{m}O$_4^-$, is taken up by NIS in the thyroid in the same way as the iodide ion. In contrast

to I⁻, Tc-99mO₄⁻ does not undergo any further chemical reactions in the gland and is eliminated quickly. Investigations with a gamma camera after administration of Tc-99mO₄⁻ thus enables study of the uptake in the gland of iodide, but not of hormone synthesis.

> When Dmitri Mendeleev in about 1870 proposed grouping the basic elements with respect to their chemical properties, the periodic table, he was able to predict the existence of several basic elements which were discovered later. Among these was an element similar to manganese in group VIIa. This element, with atomic number 43, was the first to be synthesized artificially (in 1937), and was therefore called technetium (from the Greek technos, which means artificial).

Units and Terms Relating to Radiation

Radioactivity is ionizing radiation, generated during the decay of atoms. Ionizing radiation can be either electromagnetic radiation, such as gamma radiation, or particle radiation, such as alpha and beta radiation.

The power of a radioactive source is specified as the amount of activity, i.e. the number of radioactive transformations (decays) per second. Activity is measured in Becquerel.

Bq
Becquerel. Unit of amount of activity. 1 Bq = 1 decay/s.

MBq
Megabecquerel = 10^6 Bq.

Ci
Curie. Original designation of unit of activity. 1 mCi = 37 MBq.

When the radioactive radiation source accumulates in tissue, we define it as absorbed energy (absorbed dose), which is given in Gray. The term absorbed dose is used in connection with treatment using ionized radiation.

Gy
Gray. Unit of radiation dose absorbed by tissue (1 Gy = 1 J/kg tissue).

Rad
Original designation for unit for absorbed radiation dose. 1 Gy = 100 rad.

Radioiodine treatment
During radioiodine treatment, an amount of isotope I-131 activity (MBq) is administered with the purpose of attaining a desired absorbed dose (Gy) in the thyroid gland. The absorbed dose is dependent on the size of the gland, how much I-131 activity is administered, how much accumulates in the thyroid tissue and how long the isotope is retained (biological half-life).

Sievert (Sv)
In the radiation protection context, the unit Sievert is used to specify the equivalent or effective dose. The equivalent dose takes into account the type of radiation, i.e. alpha radiation, beta radiation or gamma radiation, while the effective dose also takes into account the different sensitivity of tissues to radiation.

1 Historical Background

The thyroid gland was described as early as the 16th century by Andreas Vesalius and probably even earlier by Leonardo da Vinci. It was named in 1656 by Thomas Wharton, who used the Latin designation *glandula thyreoidea*. The Latin form is derived from the Greek *thyr* (shield) and *eiodos* (appearance), referring to the shield-shaped cartilage in the larynx.

The hormone produced by the thyroid gland, thyroxine, is composed of tyrosyl residues (from the amino acid tyrosine). Tyrosine is an aromatic amino acid, the name of which is derived from the Greek *tyros*, meaning cheese. The name thyroxine is thus derived from tyrosine and not from thyroid.

1.1 Goitre and Iodine

People with an enlarged thyroid, goitre, have been portrayed in drawings, paintings and statues since the days of antiquity. It was only at the beginning of the 19th century, after Bernard Courtois discovered the basic element iodine, that a relationship between iodine, goitre and metabolic disorders was considered. During the 18th century, some physicians in Switzerland and France started to use iodine to treat goitre, but many regarded the treatment controversial. It was not until 1896 that Eugen Baumann demonstrated that the thyroid gland contained large amounts of iodine.

After resuming studies with iodine supplements to prevent goitre in 1910, iodized salt was introduced in some areas of Switzerland in 1922. An earlier study in the US led to the large-scale introduction of iodized table salt in Michigan in 1924.

Iodine supplementation studies were also initiated early in Sweden. The same year that iodized table salt was introduced in Michigan, a study began in Sandviken, Sweden that gave 1,000 school children iodine supplements, after which a significant drop in the incidence of goitre was noted. Similar results were obtained in a study in Falun, Sweden, that ran from 1927–1929. After extensive mapping of goitre prevalence in Sweden by Axel Höjer from 1928–31, the Royal Swedish National Board of Health decided in 1936 that iodized table salt (10 mg/kg) should be available to the general public. In 1966 it was decided to raise the iodine content in iodized table salt to 50 mg/kg.

1.2 Hypothyroidism

Theophrastus Paracelsus and Felix Platter described cretinism as early as the 17th century. However, it was not until the end of the 19th century that the connection was made between cretinism and myxoedema in adults and underactivity of the shield-shaped thyroid gland. Sir William Gull wrote the first classic description of myxoedema in 1873. The first successful treatment of hypothyroidism was performed in 1891 by

E. Nyström, G.E.B. Berg, S.K.G. Jansson, O. Törring, S.V. Valdemarsson (Eds.),
Thyroid Disease in Adults,
DOI: 10.1007/978-3-642-13262-9_1, © Springer-Verlag Berlin Heidelberg 2011

Chapter 1: Historical Background

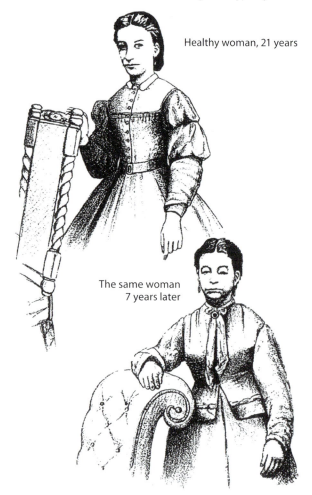

Fig. 1.1 A classic illustration of a woman suffering from hypothyroidism. **a** Healthy woman, 21 years. **b** The same woman 7 years later (from: Ord WM (1878) On myxoedema, a term proposed to be applied to an essential condition in the "cretinoid" affection occasionally observed in middle-aged women. *Medico-Chirurgical Trans* 57–61)

George Murray, who gave injections of sheep thyroid extracts to a woman with severe hypothyroidism. The same year, Murray published his results in the British Medical Journal in a paper entitled: "Notes on the Treatment of Myxoedema by Hypodermic Injection of an Extract of the Thyroid Gland of a Sheep." The following year, thyroid extract was administered orally to a patient for the first time.

As early as 1893, tablets with sheep thyroid extract were commercially available. In 1915 Edward Calvin Kendal successfully isolated crystalline thyroxine from a thyroid gland hydrolysate, and in 1926 the structure was determined and thyroxine was synthesized by Charles Harrington and George Barger. In 1952 Rosalind Pitt-Rivers and Jack Gross identified triiodothyronine. Two years later, synthetic thyroxine for human use was introduced.

1.3 Hyperthyroidism

Patients with thyroid overactivity were described as early as 1835 by the Irishman James Robert Graves who noted four patients with both goitre and heart palpitations. He presumed that the hypermetabolic symptoms were related to a heart condition. Interestingly, one of the patients also had exophthalmos.

In 1840, unaware of Graves' account, Carl Wilhelm Basedow described some patients with goitre, tachycardia and exophthalmos as the Merseburg triad (Merseburg is a small town near Halle in Germany). General, the patients' hypermetabolic symptoms were still not associated with goitre. It was not until the 19th century, after patients with severe thyroid enlargement underwent surgery, that convincing evidence for the significance of the thyroid gland for the symptoms was determined.

Around 1890, the name thyrotoxicosis arose because the symptoms were believed to be caused by an unnatural toxin from the intestine that the thyroid normally removed from the blood. When the thyroid, in spite of its endeavours, was unsuccessful in cleaning the blood sufficiently, the toxic symptoms and goitre arose. The name toxic goitre was therefore applied. Some people believed that the thyroid itself produced this toxin, because an operation resulted in improvement.

The introduction of three hyperthyroidism treatment modalities, surgery, antithyroid drugs and radioiodine, are presented here:

Surgery Before the end of the 19th century, surgery on the thyroid was associated with very high mortality. Causes of death were primarily uncontrolled bleeding during the operation and postoperative infections. It was only at the end of the 19th century, when Theodor Kocher improved the surgical techniques and reduced mortality figures to 0.5%, that surgical intervention on the thyroid became generally accepted. In 1909, Kocher received the Nobel Prize for his improved treatment of thyroid diseases.

Previously, the mortality rate for toxic goitre surgery was also high due to complications associated with the hypermetabolic state. When oral administration of an iodine solution was introduced to block the thyroid, toxic goitre operations could be performed relatively free of complications. For many years, surgery was the only form of treatment for hyperthyroidism.

Antithyroid drugs The effect of thioamides (methimazole, carbimazole and propylthiouracil) on hormone synthesis in the thyroid and their clinical use was discovered in the early 1940s by Edwin Bennett Astwood, Julia MacKenzie and C.G. MacKenzie.

Radioiodine Saul Hertz at Massachusetts General Hospital in the USA understood as early as 1936 that it should be possible to use radioactive iodine to examine the thyroid. Collaborating with Arthur Roberts and Robert Evans, physicists at the Massachusetts Institute of Technology, he produced I-128 for examination of the thyroid in rabbits. By 1939, it was possible to produce several iodine isotopes using a cyclotron.

I-131 was shown to have properties that made it suitable for therapeutic trials. In 1941, Hertz was the first person to administer I-131 for treatment of hyperthyroidism. During World War II, Hertz was called to the navy and his pioneering work was continued by Earle Chapman. Both men started treating patients with I-131 at the same clinic. Due to cooperation problems, however, they each submitted an article to the *Journal of the American Medical Association*. The editor decided to publish both reports in May 1946.

Introduction of Scintigraphy   At the beginning of the 1900s, Ernest Rutherford discovered that crystals with high density and transparency can absorb photons and by doing so produce light flashes called scintillations. The first scintillation detector used for the localization of radioactivity in biological systems was developed by Ben Cassen in 1947 in Los Angeles. In 1950, the first automated scanner was in use in the USA. In Gothenburg, Sweden, a scanner for thyroid examination was in use in 1955.

2 Anatomy and Physiology

2.1 The Embryologic Development and Anatomy of the Thyroid Gland

2.1.1 Embryology

The thyroid gland consists of two separate physiological endocrine systems. The first system, which comprises most of the thyroid, is responsible for the production of the thyroid hormones thyroxine (T4) and triiodothyronine (T3). The second endocrine cell system is responsible for production of the peptide hormone calcitonin. Knowledge of the embryonic development of the thyroid and its two physiological systems can facilitate the understanding of the final anatomical structure of the gland in adult humans.

The cells in the thyroid have two distinct embryological origins. The major part of the thyroid gland developed from epithelial cells originating in the endodermal cells of the primitive pharynx. Development starts with a diverticulum bulge in the median line from the embryonic floor of the pharynx. From here, the thyroid develops to become a bilobed encapsulated structure which descends down the median line eventually ending up at its final position anterior in the neck partly surrounding the trachea. During the descent, the embryonic thyroid lies adjacent to the structure which later becomes the aortic arch. The contact between the thyroid and the blood vessel is released, and the thyroid then moves cranially again before reaching its final position.

The thyroglossal duct, which is a small remnant of the primitive pathway down which the thyroid moved from the primitive pharynx, can still be seen in the median line. Sometimes, remains of thyroid tissue can be found along the thyroglossal duct. A thyroid remnant at the back of the tongue is called lingual thyroid.

The functional units of the thyroid for synthesis of T3 and T4 are the follicles. A follicle comprises one single layer of epithelial cells around a cavity, the follicle lumen, in which the colloid with thyroglobulin is stored (Fig. 2.1).

The neural ectoderm is the embryological origin of the parafollicular cells, or C cells, which are the second endocrine component of the thyroid. These C cells have migrated from the neural crest together with the ultimobrachial bodies from the fourth and fifth pharyngeal pouches. Together with the upper parathyroid glands, the C cells and ultimobrachial bodies migrate to their final position in the upper part of the thyroid gland, where the C cells reach their final position within the upper third of the thyroid lobes. The C cells comprise only 1–2% of the thyroid cell mass.

2.1.2 Anatomy

The thyroid gland in an adult weighs about 12–20 g, corresponding to a volume of 12–20 mL. It is slightly larger in men than in women. The upper limits were stated to be higher in older literature but, with the increased availability of iodine today, the average weight of the thyroid gland in the population has fallen slightly. The thyroid gland is shaped like a butterfly, with one right and one left lobe connected in the

Chapter 2: Anatomy and Physiology

middle by a bridge of tissue (isthmus). Occasionally, an outgrowth of glandular tissue stretches up in a cranial direction from the isthmus, the pyramidal lobe (Fig. 2.2). This lobe is comprised by glandular tissue which stretches up along the thyroglossus duct

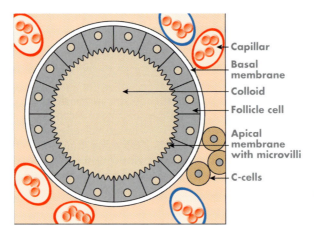

Fig. 2.1 Schematic representation of thyroid tissue

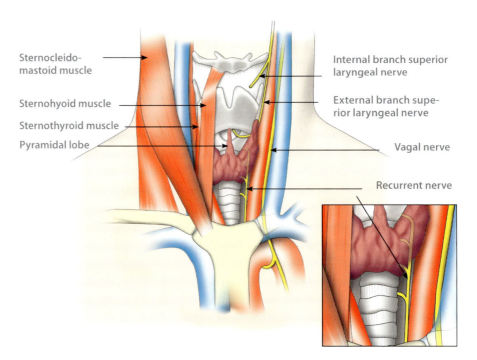

Fig. 2.2 Anatomy of the neck showing the thyroid gland, muscles and laryngeal nerves

2.1 The Embryologic Development and Anatomy of the Thyroid Gland

and, on occasion, may even reach up to the hyoid bone. Ventrally, the thyroid gland surrounds the upper section of the tracheal rings and larynx.

Each lobe rests medially in a bed between the tracheal wall and the oesophagus, and laterally between the carotid vessels, and is protected at the front by the straight neck muscles and the sternocleidomastoid muscle.

The normal thyroid gland is soft, has dark wine-red colour, and is covered by a thin capsule. It is loosely connected to its surroundings via connective tissue. The thyroid gland is normally attached at the ring cartilage and upper tracheal rings by a loose ligament (Berry's ligament).

2.1.3 Blood Supply

The arterial blood supply to the thyroid is provided primarily by two arteries, the inferior thyroid artery and the superior thyroid artery (Fig. 2.3a). The thyroid has a rich blood supply and the gland is one of the most well-vascularized tissues in the body. The superior thyroid artery passes in a caudal direction from the external carotid artery. The inferior thyroid artery passes from the thyrocervical trunk and stretches in a cranial direction dorsal to the carotid artery to later make a loop into the middle and caudal parts of the thyroid.

The veins draining the thyroid have a more varied structure than the arterial supply. The size of these thin-walled veins can vary greatly, and in pathologically enlarged glands, the vessels can be markedly dilated and widened. The thyroid capsule veins comprise an anastomizing network which covers the entire gland. Normally, there is one upper vein which passes alongside the superior thyroid artery. There is often a

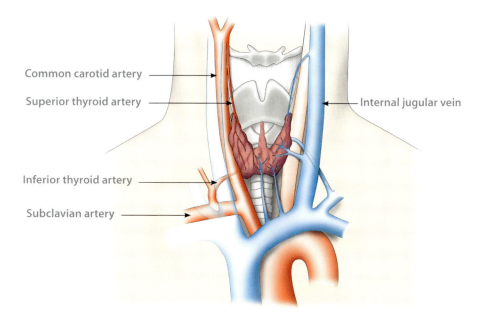

Fig. 2.3 a Vascular anatomy and the thyroid gland

prominent medial vein which drains directly into the internal jugular vein, and in addition, there are several caudal veins from the lower pole and isthmus which drain in a caudal direction to the inferior jugular vein or the brachiocephalic vein.

2.1.4 Lymph Drainage

The thyroid is supplied with a rich intraglandular and extraglandular network in which the lymph vessels anastomose freely. It is therefore not surprising that intraglandular spreading and multifocality of thyroid tumours is often observed.

The periglandular lymph network is primarily drained in two ways. The primary lymph drainage system (Fig. 2.3b, green area) comprises lymph nodes and lymph vessels in the central zone of the neck, between the carotid sheaths, which stretches down pre- and paratracheally. From here, the lymph drainage can communicate with the mediastinal lymph system. This central section of the lymph drainage system is normally considered to be the first zone into which the lymph drains from the thyroid.

The secondary lymph drainage system (Fig. 2.3b, pink area) is located in the lateral region and includes the lymph vessels and lymph nodes along the jugular vein and up towards the submandibular stations, and also tissue in the supraclavicular triangle. From here, communication can occur with the lymph node stations, which are located deeper and dorsally in and between the trachea and the oesophagus in towards the larynx.

Because of the anatomical structure of the lymph drainage system, metastases from tumours with a primary site in the thyroid are often seen in the lymph node stations in the central zone (pre- and paratracheal stations) and from there further laterally to lateral lymph node stations or down in the mediastinum. For tumours located in the cranial part of the thyroid lobes, lymph drainage can, however, go primarily directly to the lateral lymph node stations.

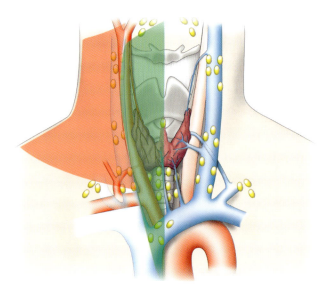

Fig. 2.3 b Lymphatic drainage of the thyroid gland

2.1.5 Nerves

The thyroid is located close to the path of the recurrent laryngeal nerve and the superior laryngeal nerve. It is important to be highly familiar with the anatomical pathways of these nerves in order to avoid damage at surgical intervention.

Patients can also be affected by sequalae from disease of the thyroid, most frequently cancer, which infiltrates or presses on the nerves resulting in impairment of function. The recurrent nerve passes from the vagal nerve and returns in a cranial direction in the groove between the oesophagus and the trachea up to the larynx. The nerve crosses the inferior thyroid artery close to the thyroid and then continues along the thyroid capsule up to where it enters the thyroid cartilage. In a small percentage, the nerve can exhibit a non-recurrent course on the right side, passing directly over from the vagus nerve to the entry point in the larynx, and can then be mistaken for a blood vessel. Damage to the recurrent nerve can result in paralysis of the vocal cord, and can affect the voice or breathing.

The superior laryngeal nerve is a thin nerve which runs in a caudal direction along the superior thyroid artery. This external branch of this nerve is a motor nerve which innervates the cricothyroid muscle. Damage to this nerve can result in voice changes in the form of reduced pitch, and a more monotonous voice which can cause great problems for people who require a good voice quality.

2.2 Iodine and the Thyroid

Iodine (from the Greek *iodes*, meaning violet) is a rare element in nature. Iodine was discovered in 1811 by Bernard Courtois and belongs to the chemical group of halogens, which can form salts. Iodine has 36 unstable isotopes of which I-131 is the most important in medicine. Like the other halogens, iodine is highly reactive and therefore does not occur in its free state in nature. However, a solid form of iodine exists, where the molecule consists of two iodine atoms (I_2) and appears as grey-black, violet, shiny crystals. Iodine is found in the largest quantities in the sea, bound organically in seaweed, for example, and as an iodide salt, sodium iodide (Na^+I^-). Otherwise, iodine is found in small amounts in nature as salts.

The thyroid is dependent on iodine to produce its life-essential iodine-containing hormones, thyroxine and triiodothyronine. Simple organisms which live in the sea with continuous access to iodine, synthesize hormones in open tubular structures, the so-called endostyle. In vertebrates, which can live in environments with fluctuating iodine availability, these structures have developed into follicles, which can store iodine and thyroxine bound to the thyroglobulin molecule. This allows continuous synthesis and release of the hormone, in spite of varying availability of iodine. The human thyroid normally contains between 3 and 20 mg of iodine, and sometimes even more. The size of the thyroid iodine pool has no association to thyroid function. However, the function of the thyroid can be affected if the supply is very low, or if there is a sudden increase in intake of iodide.

2.2.1 Transport of Iodine

Iodine in our food is reduced to iodide and taken up in the stomach and throughout the small intestine via the mucous membrane to the blood. It is then concentrated

Chapter 2: Anatomy and Physiology

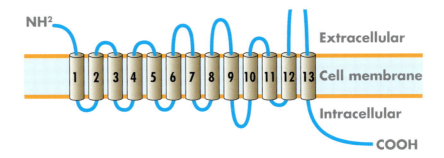

Fig. 2.4 The iodide pump NIS is situated in the basal membrane of the thyrocytes. NIS has 13 transmembrane transitions and forms the channel through which Na^+ and I^- are transported

in the thyroid against an electrochemical gradient over the basal membrane of the follicle cell via the so-called iodide pump. The process entails a significant increase in concentration (the concentration gradient for follicle cell:plasma is 20–40:1). The iodide pump has been characterized as a membrane protein designated NIS (Na^+/I^- symporter), a glycoprotein comprised of 618 amino acids. Thyroid stimulating hormone (TSH) regulates both the synthesis and the function of NIS. Intact NIS in the basal cell membrane (Fig. 2.4) is a prerequisite for accumulation of iodine in the thyroid. Iodide uptake via NIS is competitively inhibited by anions such as thiocyanate and perchlorate. A high intake of iodine indirectly blocks iodide uptake by down regulation of NIS.

NIS has also been found in other organs such as the mucous membrane of the stomach, choroid plexus, and in mammary gland tissue where NIS has an important function securing iodine supply to breast milk. In a nursing mother, the amount of iodine excreted in breast milk can reach 30% of the iodide intake.

Thiocyanate (SCN^-) is an anion that is a potent inhibitor of iodide transport via NIS. Thiocyanate accumulates in the blood and tissue of smokers and in people who consume large amounts of vegetables containing goitrogens, such as various sorts of cabbage, cassava, maize and sweet potatoes. If, in addition, iodine intake is low, an increased content of thiocyanate can be decisive for the iodine balance and hormone synthesis in the thyroid. In nursing mothers who smoke, the thiocyanate content of the tobacco smoke can cause an inhibition of iodide uptake in the mammary glands, and the nursing child can be at risk for iodine deficiency.

Iodide passes via passive diffusion from the basal membrane to the apical membrane of the thyrocytes. There, iodine enters and crosses the membrane to the extrafollicular lumen where thyroid hormone synthesis takes place. The mechanism for transport across the apical membrane has not been completely determined, but the membrane protein pendrin may play a role. In patients with pendrin deficiency, iodine is not organified (the so-called Pendred syndrome) and the capacity for hormone synthesis is affected.

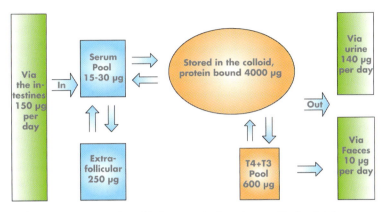

Fig. 2.5 Schematic representation of iodine metabolism at normal iodine intake

2.2.2 The Iodine Pool

At a recommended iodine intake of 150 μg/day, about 30% (45 μg) is taken up in the thyroid and the rest is excreted in urine. During catabolism of the thyroid hormone, about 25 μg is returned to the thyroid and 45 μg is excreted via urine and faeces. The total amount excreted via the urine will thus be about 140 μg/day, which provides an indirect measurement of the iodine balance. If there is insufficient iodine available, for example 70 μg/day, only about 35 μg are taken up in the thyroid in spite of a higher percentage uptake (50%) and the total excretion via the urine per day is reduced to 35–65 μg/day (Fig. 2.5).

During pregnancy, there is an increased demand for iodine at the same time as increased excretion via the kidneys. A low iodine intake therefore depletes the stores of iodine during pregnancy. The recommended daily intake of iodine for a pregnant woman is 200–250 μg/day. In recent years, we have come to understand that even mild iodine deficiency in the mother can affect the development of the foetal central nervous system.

2.3 TSH and TSH Receptors

TSH is a glycoprotein with an alfa subunit common to TSH, LH and FSH and a beta subunit specific to TSH.

The TSH receptor (TSH-R) belongs to the family of 7-transmembrane receptors, which also includes calcitonin, parathyroid hormone, glucagon, gastrin and the calcium sensing receptor among others. TSH-R (Fig. 2.6) is the mediator of the TSH effects on the follicle cell, but is also an important target for autoimmune processes, including stimulation via TRAb in Graves' disease. The number of TSH receptors per follicle cell is around 1,000. Binding of TSH to the TSH receptor triggers stimulation of the intracellular Gs protein and results in an increase in intracellular cyclic AMP. TSH can also stimulate phospholipase C, a component of another important intracellular signal system. In addition to activation by TSH, TSH-R is activated by high concentrations

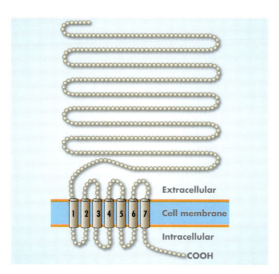

Fig. 2.6 The TSH receptor. Mutations can occur on both the extra and intracellular sections of the receptor and in the transmembrane part. Mutations can be activating, resulting in autonomous hormone secretion, formation of adenomas and hyperthyroidism. Mutations can also be inactivating, resulting in hypothyroidism

of hCG due to cross reactivity, for example, during the first trimester of pregnancy or in cases of molar pregnancy (hydatidiform mole). TRAb can not only stimulate but, less commonly, also block TSH-R and cause hypothyroidism. The precise molecular mechanism for this is not fully known.

2.4 Synthesis and Secretion of Thyroid Hormones

Normally, about 90 μg of T4 is produced per day exclusively in the thyroid. The daily production of T3 is about 30 μg, of which a small part comes directly from the thyroid and the rest from enzymatic 5'-deiodination of T4 to T3 in extrathyroidal tissues. The serum concentration of T4 is normally about 50 times higher than the concentration of T3 (reference range for T4: 70–150 nmol/L; for T3: 1.5–3.0 nmol/L; exact values depend on the analytical method used and population). Only about 0.1% of T4 and 0.3% of T3 occurs in a free form. The rest circulates bound to thyroxine binding globulin (TBG), transthyretin (prealbumin) and albumin. Altered concentration of the transport proteins, primarily TBG, affects the concentration of total T4 and T3, but not the concentration of the free hormone. Thus, high TBG concentrations result in high total levels of T4 and T3, but have only a negligible effect on free T4 and free T3.

The following factors are basic elements for synthesis of thyroid hormone (Fig. 2.7): iodide ions (I$^-$), thyroglobulin (Tg), thyroperoxidase (TPO) and hydrogen peroxide (H$_2$O$_2$). The structure and function of the follicle cell are critical in this process (Figs 2.7 and 2.8).

Synthesis of thyroid hormones takes place via the following steps: Tg and TPO are synthesized in the thyroid follicle cells. TPO is then bound to the apical cell membrane

2.4 Synthesis and Secretion of Thyroid Hormones

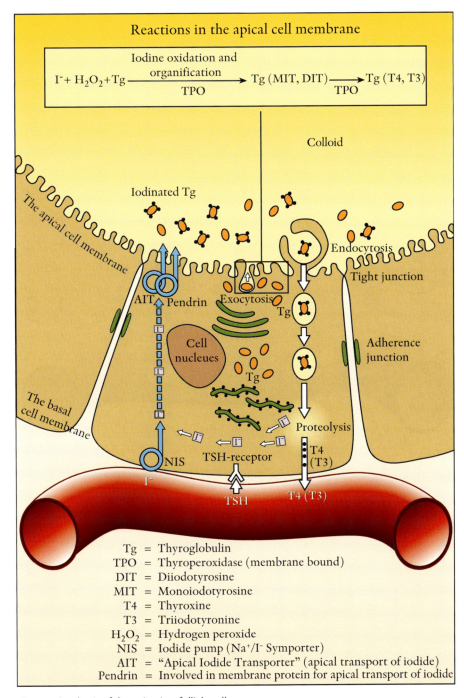

Fig. 2.7 Synthesis of thyroxine in a follicle cell

Chapter 2: Anatomy and Physiology

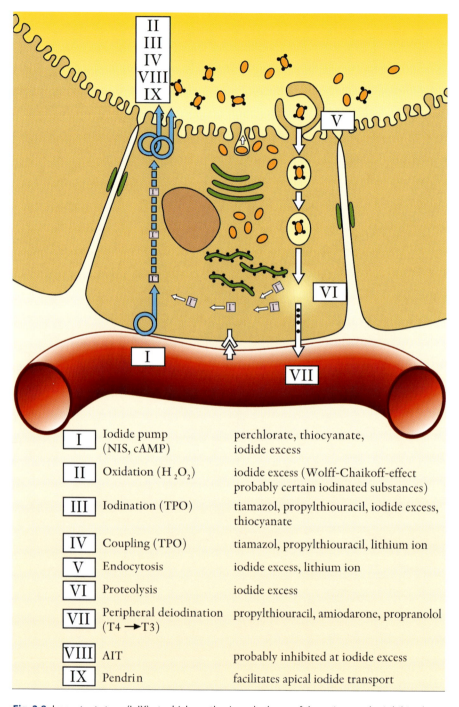

I	Iodide pump (NIS, cAMP)	perchlorate, thiocyanate, iodide excess
II	Oxidation (H_2O_2)	iodide excess (Wolff-Chaikoff-effect probably certain iodinated substances)
III	Iodination (TPO)	tiamazol, propylthiouracil, iodide excess, thiocyanate
IV	Coupling (TPO)	tiamazol, propylthiouracil, lithium ion
V	Endocytosis	iodide excess, lithium ion
VI	Proteolysis	iodide excess
VII	Peripheral deiodination (T4 → T3)	propylthiouracil, amiodarone, propranolol
VIII	AIT	probably inhibited at iodide excess
IX	Pendrin	facilitates apical iodide transport

Fig. 2.8 Important steps (I–IX) at which synthesis and release of thyroxine can be inhibited

while Tg is transported to the follicle lumen by exocytosis. Tg comprises an important component of the content of the follicle lumen, i.e. the colloid.

At the apical cell membrane, oxidation and organification of iodide occurs by iodination of tyrosyl residues in the large Tg molecule to monoiodotyrosine and diiodotyrosine. Iodination takes place extracellularly adjacent to the apical cell membrane in the colloid in the presence of TPO and H_2O_2. Next, iodothyronines are synthesized by coupling two diiodotyrosines in the Tg molecule to make T4, or monoiodotyrosine and diiodotyrosine to make T3. This reaction also takes place in the presence of TPO and H_2O_2.

2.4.1 Thyroglobulin

In addition to its role as the substrate for the synthesis of T4 and T3, thyroglobulin (Tg – molecular weight 660 kDa, Fig. 2.9) also functions as a storage molecule for these hormones and iodine. The thyroid gland usually has a store of hormone equivalent to the requirements for several weeks. The iodinated Tg molecule contains up to four T4 residues and 10–30 additional iodine atoms in the form of mono and diiodotyrosines. In the event of iodine deficiency, the molecule contains a higher proportion of T3.

T4 and T3 are released from Tg by endocytosis of the follicle contents and proteolytic release in the follicle cell of primarily T4, which diffuses through the follicle cell into the blood. Excess iodide from mono- and diiodotyrosines is retained in the follicle cell. Storage of thyroglobulin-bound iodine is proportional to availability. As previously mentioned, in euthyroid individuals the amount of iodine in the thyroid normally varies between about 3 and 20 mg. In hyperthyroidism due to Graves' disease, the amount of iodine in the thyroid is low, rarely above 3 mg.

If the integrity of the follicle is disturbed, for example through effects on the binding junctions (tight junctions and adherence junctions) as in cases of destructive thyroiditis, hidden antigen and iodinated and noniodinated thyroglobulin can leak into the blood, increasing the risk of autoimmunization through formation of TgAb in predisposed individuals. Furthermore, in thyroiditis the content of thyroid hormone in blood can increase due to this leakage. TPO, which is normally to be found in the apical cells, can also be exposed resulting in autoimmunisation. The NIS function is also dependent on follicle integrity and maintenance of basal and apical polarization of the thyrocytes.

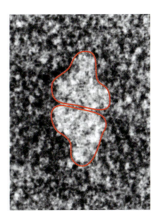

Fig. 2.9 Electron microscopic picture of a thyroglobulin molecule (Tg) magnified one million times. The molecule comprises two subunits (*red*) and constitutes the substrate for formation of thyroxine. Photo: Gertrud Berg

2.4.2 Regulation of Iodine Metabolism

Iodide uptake in the thyroid is primarily regulated by TSH. At moderately severe iodine deficiency, stimulation by TSH results in an increase in the number of NIS (iodide pumps) in the basal cell membrane. At long-term high iodine availability, the number of NIS drops. Thus, in nearly all cases, the individual adapts to a continuous high iodine intake via food because the thyroid is capable to cope with large differences in iodine availability. Accordingly, in the coastal regions of Japan, where the iodine intake may be extremely high, most people have normal thyroid gland function.

In addition to the Wolff-Chaikoff effect, exposure to high amounts of iodine results in an apical block of endocytosis as well as splitting of the thyroid hormone from Tg, the so-called Plummer effect. This results in a rapid inhibition of T4 and T3 release, an effect which can be utilized in clinical work in treatment with iodine in hyperthyroidism before surgery. The Plummer effect lasts about 7–10 days.

> For the thyroid, the term autoregulation mainly includes the regulation of iodine metabolism, which is independent of TSH and which occurs, for example, when the thyroid is subject to an overload of iodine. At intracellular exposure to high amounts of iodine (when the plasma concentration of iodine exceeds about 30 μg/dL) blocking of oxidation and organification of iodine occurs extracellularly at the apical border of the follicle cell, the so-called Wolff-Chaikoff effect (Fig. 2.8). It is believed that this blocking occurs via an organic iodine compound, an iodolipid, α-iodohexadecanal. The Wolff-Chaikoff effect has been interpreted as a protective effect against potentially toxic iodide levels. After a few days, oxidation and organification of iodide resumes when the intracellular iodine concentration has dropped independently of the plasma concentration of iodine. This adaptation is called "escape" from Wolff-Chaikoff. The mechanism is considered to be a down-regulation of the uptake of iodide across the basal membrane through a down-regulation of transcription of NIS. Inactivation of NIS can also occur through internalization of NIS which is thus moved from the cell membrane to the cytoplasm. The result is normalization of the intracellular iodide concentration and cessation of the Wolff-Chaikoff inhibition. Afterwards normal hormone synthesis can be resumed.

2.4.3 Selenium

Selenium was discovered by the Swedish professor in medicine and pharmacy Jacob Berzelius as early as 1817 and, like iodine, is a trace element occurring rarely in nature. There are geographical areas with severe selenium deficiency. It has been discovered that selenium deficiency in combination with iodine deficiency results in accentuated goitre development.

Selenium deficiency in pregnant women has been reported to cause relatively high T4 and low T3 levels. A low intake of selenium may therefore affect the foetal neurological development in early pregnancy.

The thyroid contains more selenium than any other organ (0.72 µg/g). Selenium is extremely important for thyroid function. It occurs in a large number of selenium proteins (about 30), of which glutathione peroxidase and thioredoxin reductase function as important antioxidants in connection with H_2O_2 production in the follicle lumen. The concentration of H_2O_2 increases in selenium deficiency which can result in destruction of thyroid cells, fibrosis in the thyroid, and thus hypothyroidism. Selenium is also incorporated in the deiodinase enzymes 1–3, of which the deiodinase type 2 and, to a certain extent, type 1 are responsible for the peripheral conversion of free T4 to T3.

2.5 Hypothalamus–Pituitary–Thyroid Axis

Thyroid activity is regulated by a series of external and internal factors, of which the pituitary thyroid stimulating hormone (thyrotropin, TSH) plays a central role (Fig. 2.10).

The synthesis and release of TSH from pituitary thyrotropic cells are regulated by the hypothalamus, are stimulated by thyroliberin (thyrotropin-releasing hormone, TRH), and are inhibited by dopamine. These substances are transported from the hypothalamus to the pituitary through the venous portal system in the pituitary stalk.

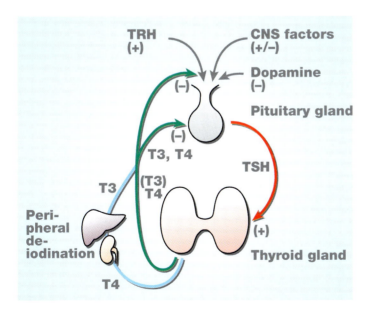

Fig. 2.10 Hypothalamus–pituitary–thyroid axis

T4 and T3 regulate the TSH release through negative feedback using various mechanisms, which directly affect the regulation of TRH, and the synthesis and release of TSH. The effect on TRH is exerted through effects on TRH release from the hypothalamus, and through inhibition of synthesis of TRH receptors in the pituitary thyrotropic cells.

The pituitary TSH-producing cells are inhibited by T4, which is taken up by the cell and deiodinated intracellularly to T3. Under normal conditions, the inhibitory effect is primarily exerted by the circulating T4. This is illustrated by the fact that in primary hypothyroidism, the TSH concentration increases early and is inversely related to the falling T4 concentration.

The T3 concentration is affected to a lesser degree (often not at all) in early stages of primary hypothyroidism. Normal T3 concentrations are maintained in such situations by an increased conversion of T4 to T3 instead of reverse T3 (rT3). Low T3 concentrations are therefore only seen in more pronounced hypothyroidism. Analogous to this, a slight increase in T4 can result in reduced TSH release in spite of normal T3.

2.6 Deiodinases

In healthy people, the thyroid produces mainly T4 (80–100 μg/day) and only a limited amount of T3 (25–32 μg/day). Most T3 is produced through deiodination of the outer ring of T4. In peripheral tissue, inactivation of T4 can also take place through deiodination of the inner ring, resulting in formation of rT3 (Fig. 2.11). Thus, deiodination of the outer ring of T4 results in activation, while deiodination of the inner ring results in formation of inactive metabolites. Three enzymes are responsible for the intracellular conversion of T4 to T3 and rT3, and their further inactivation and metabolism. These enzymes belong to a family of selenoproteins with one selenocysteine in the centre; type I (often abbreviated: D1), type II (D2) and type III (D3) (Fig. 2.12). See also Fig. 2.11

2.7 Mechanisms of Action of Thyroid Hormones

Thyroxine has an effect on the development, growth and function of all the cells in the body. T4 can be considered as a prohormone for T3, which exerts the main biological effects. T4 and T3 pass into the cell via specific transport proteins in the cell membrane. After passage across the cell membrane, T4 is converted to T3. T3 passes into the cell nucleus and is bound to intranuclear specific receptors which have a much higher affinity for T3 than for T4.

T3 primarily has two effects on the target cells, one genomic (protein synthesis, etc.), and one nongenomic (cell membrane and mitochondrial effects, Fig. 2.13). The nongenomic effects are highly transient and can be detected within a few minutes and last for a few hours. By this mechanism the activity of various transmembrane receptor complexes can be upregulated as well as important intracellular signal systems, such as cyclic adenosine monophosphate (cAMP) and phosphokinases (protein kinase A and C). In addition, T3 increases mitochondrial activity.

D2 is the most important deiodinase for T3 production. D2 is located in the central nervous system, the thyroid, the pituitary, the placenta, skeletal muscles and in brown adipose tissue, catalyzing outer ring 5´-deiodination of T4 to T3. D2 expression is thought to vary with thyroid function, thereby contributing to a relatively constant T3 concentration in spite of altering T4 availability. Thus D2 is upregulated in iodine deficiency and in hypothyroidism and downregulated in hyperthyroidism. D2 activity is also of particular importance in the brain and the pituitary, as it secures the availability of T3.

The main function of D3 is inner ring 5-deiodination of T4 to rT3 and of T3 to T2. D3 is located in most tissues especially the brain, the uterus, the placenta, the skin and the foetus. Decreased D3 activity in hypothyroidism and increased D3 activity in hyperthyroidism acts in concert with D2 to maintain adequate T3 concentrations. Furthermore, D3 seems to have an important role to protect certain tissues from excessive thyroid hormone levels during foetal life through deiodination of T4 to rT3 and of T3 to T2. A normal development of the pituitary thyroid axis is thereby secured. An appropriate joint regulation of T3 by D2 and D3 seems to be of importance also at the tissue level, e.g. the normal development of chochlear structures.

The role of D1 seems less distinct, being able to catalyze 5-deiodination as well as 5´-deiodination. D1 is primarily located in the liver, the kidneys, the pituitary and the thyroid and was previously supposed to be of main importance for T4 to T3 conversion. However, recent studies indicate the D2 is more efficient in this respect, having a 700-fold greater potency for this reaction compared to D1. Furthermore, D1 catalyzes deiodination of rT3 to T2 with a much higher efficiency than of T4 to T3. Thus, D1 seems more active in degradation of rT3 and other inactive iodthyronines, thereby acting as a scavenger enzyme, providing iodine for reutilisation, an effect of special importance in iodine deficiency.

As for regulatory mechanisms of deiodinase activities, TSH stimulation in hypotyreoidism and TRAb in Graves´ disease might increases D1 activity and thereby T3 synthesis. Increased D1 and/or D2 activities in thyroid nodules and in Graves´ could stimulate the conversion of T4 to T3 in the thyroid. The inhibitory effect of propylthiouracil is most pronounced for D1, while iopanoic acid impairs the function of D1, D2 and D3. Tissue injuries seems to affect deiodinase function. The final role of these enzymes for thyroid hormone regulation in the low T3 syndrome remains to be clarified.

Bioavailability of Thyroid Hormones Depends on Several Factors:

- Thyroid secretion of T4 and T3
- Extent of protein binding
- Activation of the prohormone T4 through deiodination of the outer ring to T3
- Inactivation of T4 and T3 through deiodination of the inner ring to rT3 and other metabolites

Chapter 2: Anatomy and Physiology

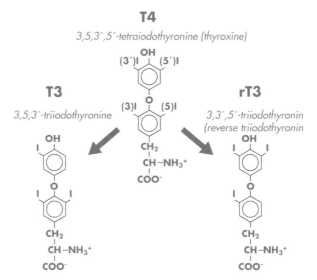

Fig. 2.11 Regulation of synthesis of thyroid hormones. Deiodination of thyroxine (T4) to its active metabolite triiodothyronine (T3) occurs by deiodination of the outer ring (deiodinase types I and II). Formation of the metabolically inactive form occurs by deiodination of the inner ring (deiodinase type III) giving formation of reverse T3 (rT3)

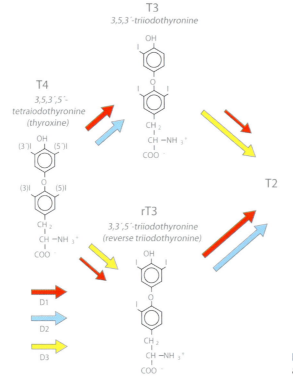

Fig. 2.12 Intracellular deiodinase activity regulates availability of T3.

2.7 Mechanisms of Action of Thyroid Hormones

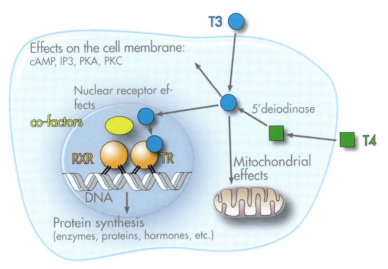

Fig. 2.13 The effects of thyroid hormones on the cell

The genomic effects of thyroid hormones are even more important, and it takes hours before the effect is seen. The result is a change in cell activity, protein expression, receptor and hormone production, which subsequently has consequences for thyroid hormone-dependent metabolic effects, brain and other body functions, over many days to weeks.

The genomic effects are exerted mostly through activation or inhibition of gene transcription of proteins and peptides which are regulated by thyroxine.

> The effect of T4 and T3 occurs through specific binding to intranuclear proteins, the thyroid hormone receptors (TRs). Binding affinity is about 40 times higher for T3 than for T4, which explains why T3 is the most bioactive.
> The TR belong to the same intranuclear receptor family as the receptors for glucocorticoids, testosterone, oestrogen and A and D vitamins. Two genes (α and β) code for 5 different TRs (α1, α2, β1, β2 and β3), of which α2 is inactive. The occurrence of the various isoforms of the receptors differ in different tissues, for example, the α receptors are strongly dominant in the heart and the β receptors in the liver. In addition, there are differences between the receptor's activating and inhibiting functions on thyroid hormone sensitive genes. An increase in serum T3 results in lower production of TRH and TSH. The different organs can therefore respond at different speeds to changes in the concentration of thyroxine.

T3 forms a dimer with its receptor (T3-TR), often with the retinol receptor complex (RXR). The dimer (usually T3-TR+RXR) binds to the area on DNA (thyroxine-response-element) that is specifically designed for its effects. Now, in interaction with a series of essential transcription factors (cofactors), transcription occurs at the gene for the proteins, peptides, etc., that are regulated by thyroid hormones. These proteins, enzymes, hormones (e.g. GH, TSH) and receptors (e.g. adrenergic receptors in the myocardium) may have a very long half-life in the body.

This explains why it normally takes several weeks (up to 6–8 weeks) from a change in T4 and T3 serum concentrations until the body is fully adapted to the biological effects of this change. This is important to keep in mind when thyroxine substitution is instituted in hypothyroidism, or when the dose is adjusted during thyroxine substitution therapy. Also, the often observed delay in improvement of thyrotoxic symptoms despite normalization of serum T4 and T3 when hypothyroidism is treated can be explained by the genomic T3 effect. The long half-life in serum for T4 (about 6 days) also contributes to this long adaptation time. In contrast, the half-life of T3 is considerably shorter (about 1 day).

2.8 Biochemical Indicators of the Peripheral Effects of Thyroid Hormones

The effect of an elevated concentration of thyroxine is reflected in the typical symptoms of thyrotoxicosis, and can generally be estimated by determination of the heart rate. It is, however, more difficult to objectively measure the effects of thyroxine on cell function or metabolic processes. Determination of the basal metabolic rate (BMR) using the measurement of oxygen consumption and carbon dioxide production was one method previously used and also comprised a diagnostic tool.

Present diagnostic methods for hypo- and hyperthyroidism are based on determination of the concentration of TSH and thyroid hormones, and not on variables that directly reflect the effect of thyroid hormones at cellular level.

Thyroxine concentration changes affect various organs:

Pituitary gland   Feedback regulation of TSH is a good example of the peripheral effect of thyroid hormones. Sensitive methods for TSH determination can indirectly diagnose high and low thyroid hormone concentrations.
Liver   Liver-synthesized plasma proteins, the concentration of which is affected by thyroid hormones, has been primarily studied in hyperthyroidism:
• TBG; lowered concentration
• Sex hormone binding globulin (SHBG); elevated concentration
There is, however, considerable overlap between values observed in normal individuals and those observed in hyperthyroidism, which reduces the value of these analyses as a diagnostic tool. Lowered SHBG is also observed in hyperandrogenism (in women), and in hyperinsulinism and obesity.

Lipids, lipoproteins   Falling concentrations of thyroxine result in successively greater effects on lipid metabolism. These effects are completely reversible with thyroxine substitution treatment.

Above all, in pronounced hypothyroidism that develops over a longer period, there is an increase in serum cholesterol, mainly in the form of an elevated LDL fraction. On the other hand, there is only a moderate increase in triglyceride levels. The mechanism of these lipoprotein disorders include a reduction in the intravascular metabolism of lipoproteins (reduced activity of lipoprotein lipase), and a slower elimination of cholesterol from HDL particles to the liver (reduced activity of hepatic lipase). Reduced function of LDL receptors with slower elimination of LDL particles is also observed.

In hyperthyroidism, the cholesterol concentration drops, in particular the LDL fraction due to increased metabolism and elimination. The effects on lipid metabolism are related to the levels of thyroid hormone, mostly T3.

Connective tissue   Thyroid hormones increase turnover, which leads to increased synthesis of collagen. During this synthesis, propeptides are split off from procollagens. These propeptides can originate from the amino-terminal or from the carboxy-terminal end of collagen, for example, in collagen type I (mostly in bone tissue) or collagen III (which is present in many organs).

Increased breakdown of collagen results in increased release of hydroxyproline and peptides, which constitute collagen cross links pyridinolines, deoxypyridinolines, sometimes designated pyridinium cross links, and telopeptides, which can be demonstrated in urine and in certain cases also in serum.

Skeleton   Bone tissue is maintained in a good shape throughout life by remodelling through local resorption followed by new bone formation. This process takes place in the osteon, the functional unit of the bone. After activation of the osteoclasts, bone resorption commences. After about 6 weeks, the osteon starts a new phase of about 4 months during which bone formation takes place by the osteoblasts forming new bone at the same place. The total cycle time for the osteon is around 150 days in a healthy person. At around 25–35 years of age, new bone formation is equivalent to bone resorption resulting in bone net balance.

Thyrotoxicosis results in increased cellular activity throughout the entire skeleton, thereby forming new osteons. In these and existing osteons, the osteoclast activity is augmented resulting in bone resorption. The increased cellular activity also results in a truncated cycle for each osteon (about 130 days). The osteoblasts that are responsible for bone formation will not fully replace the resorbed bone. Increased resorption also results in discontinuation of trabeculae which in certain areas are completely resorbed. This reduces the number of bearing and supporting pillars in the bridge construction of bone. The end result is therefore altered bone quality with reduced bone mass, altered microstructure and reduced strength. Many patients already have reduced or low bone density when they develop thyrotoxicosis and in these patients bone strength can lie below the fracture threshold. This may result in a fracture even when a fall is at the same level (low-energy fracture). These bone metabolic effects of high thyroid hormone concentrations are seen in particular in the vertebral bodies with their dominant trabecular tissue in which these processes are most pronounced. Increased bone remodelling also results in increased calcium release from the skeleton. Hypercalcemia occurs if the kidneys can not cope with the increased serum concentrations of calcium. Serum calcium normalizes when the patient becomes euthyroid.

> Treatment normalizes the thyroxine levels, as well as the activity of the osteon and bone remodelling. Therefore, bone density increases during the following 6 months to 1 year. A transient hypocalcemia and persistent increase in alkaline phosphatase can be observed, due to a transient increase in re-uptake of calcium into the bones which can persist several months.
> In hypothyroidism, the activity of the osteon is low (cycle time about 300–450 days) and bone density is usually normal or slightly increased.

2.9 Factors Affecting Thyroid Hormone Homeostasis

2.9.1 Circadian and Seasonal Variation

TSH secretion from the pituitary occurs in pulses at 1–2 h intervals and is lowest in the afternoon. TSH secretion increases in the evening and is highest at night from 22:00–02:00. A transient increase in free T3 follows upon the TSH surge. In central/pituitary hypothyroidism the circadian variation is reduced because the nightly surge in TSH disappears.

There might be a seasonal variation with a 10–15% increase in TSH above average values in the period from November to January and an equivalent drop from March to June for people living in the northern hemisphere. It also appears that T3 might display a similar seasonal variation with an increase of 3–5% from December to February and a drop of 3–5%, compared to the yearly average, during the warm season from June to August. In the southern hemisphere a similar seasonal variation should be expected.

2.9.2 Variation with Age

The prevalence of TPOAb positive individuals increases with age. The activity of the hypothalamus/pituitary axis declines slightly with increasing age. However, the circadian rhythm of TSH is maintained, and the pulsatility is mostly the same. The amplitude of the TSH variation is lower in older people and results in a certain reduction in TSH secretion at night with increasing age. Serum TSH, total and free T3 and BMR are reduced slightly in older people, while the rT3 concentration increases. Serum total and free T4 remains unchanged even with increasing age. However, taken together, these age-related minor changes in thyroxine and TSH secretion have no clinical significance, and mostly the same reference ranges are used as for young people.

2.9.3 Effects of Stress and the Environment

Fasting results in a reduction of TSH and T3. Chronic sleep deficiency lowers TSH. Living in a region with an outdoor temperature of −20 to −24°C results in a small reduction (4–7%) of T3, T4 and free T3, while free T4 is mostly unchanged. A TSH increase of 15–30% can be seen as compensation for increased peripheral T3 and T4 requirements. Altogether, these observations illustrate that the thyroid homeostasis participates actively and is well suited to adapt to and compensate for different types of environmental physical stress.

The Thyroid – Anatomy and Physiology

- Follicular cells (T4 and T3 production) and C cells (calcitonin production)
- Normally the gland weighs 12–20 g
- Highly vasculated through two main arteries (common carotid artery and subclavian artery)
- In close contact with nerves (recurrent laryngeal nerve, superior laryngeal nerve)
- Recommended daily intake of iodine (adults) is 150 µg daily, and 200–250 µg during pregnancy and lactation
- Iodide uptake is regulated via the iodide pump (NIS)
- TSH stimulates iodide uptake, hormone synthesis and gland growth by activating the TSH receptor
- T4, and smaller amounts of T3, are released from the follicle cells by TSH stimulation
- T4 is peripherally converted to T3 via deiodination
- TPO is a follicular enzyme important for T4 and T3 synthesis
- Presence of antibodies against TPO (TPOAb) indicates autoimmune thyroid disease
- T3, T4 are stored in the follicle lumen bound to thyroglobulin
- Thiamazol and propylthiouracil inhibit the synthesis of T4 and T3
- Hypothalamus/pituitary/thyroid: feedback regulation of thyroid hormone secretion via TSH
- T3 exerts its effect through nuclear receptors
- T3 has effects on all cells of the body and therefore affects all organ functions

2.10 Effects of General Illness and Pharmaceuticals (NTI)

The hypothalamus-pituitary-thyroid axis can be affected in various ways by common acute and chronic diseases as well as trauma and major surgical intervention. This often causes difficulty in interpreting the results of biochemical analyses of TSH and thyroid hormones. The consequences of such changes are called nonthyroidal illness (NTI) or euthyroid sick syndrome.

As mentioned above, in healthy individuals the prohormone thyroxine (T4) is metabolized to the active hormone triiodothyronine (T3) through outer ring 5'-deiodination. In NTI, this conversion is reduced and inner ring 5'-deiodination takes over, in which thyroxine is converted to the inactive metabolite reverse T3. This results in a decreased production of T3, which therefore drops (low T3 syndrome). In more serious acute and chronic diseases, secretion of TSH at hypothalamic level is also inhibited via effects of various cytokines.

Certain medicines can also affect the hypothalamus-pituitary-thyroid axis. For example dopamine and dopamine agonists, as well as glucocorticoids, inhibit TSH secretion at the hypothalamic level. Furthermore, propranolol, glucocorticoids, amiodarone and propylthiouracil affect the peripheral conversion of thyroxine to triiodothyronine. The picture is further complicated by the fact that some analytical methods can be affected by substances that are released in NTI, including free fatty acids. This applies primarily to methods for analysis of the free hormone fraction of T4 and T3.

In less severe forms of NTI, the main observation is a reduction of free T3, while TSH and T4 are not noticeably affected. A similar drop in T3 can be seen when fasting. In more pronounced NTI, an initial rise in T4 is observed related to the reduction of T4–T3 conversion, while at the same time T3 drops and the concentration of biologically inactive reverse T3 increases (Fig. 2.14). Analysis of this hormone is, however, rarely carried out routinely.

As the disease progresses, a drop in TSH is observed and, as a consequence, T4 levels are reduced. It has been demonstrated that falling T4 is related to the severity of the disease and to an unfavourable prognosis. Some weeks after the acute phase, there is generally a rebound increase in TSH secretion when the thyroid homeostasis reasserts itself. In this phase, TSH can increase temporarily, sometimes to about 10–12 mIU/L, for a few weeks after the acute phase.

Because of the changed TSH regulation and T4/T3 metabolism, evaluating thyroid samples is always difficult in NTI. Furthermore, methodological problems can occur due to analytical interference. During progression of NTI, test results may indicate hyperthyroidism, central hypothyroidism or primary hypothyroidism. A good piece of advice is to always wait, if possible, with thyroid biochemical tests until these patients have recovered from their nonthyroid-related illness. If a test of thyroid function is

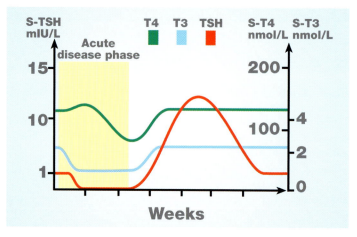

Fig. 2.14 Schematic representation of the changes which can be seen in serum concentrations of TSH and thyroid hormones in serious illness. In less serious conditions, only a reduction in T3 is observed; TSH and T4 remain unchanged

nevertheless carried out on a sick patient, hyperthyroidism can be excluded with great certainty if the TSH concentration is not suppressed. Similarly, normal concentrations of T4 would suggest that hypothyroidism is not present.

It is not settled whether the reduction in thyroid hormone concentrations observed in NTI means that there really is a deficit of thyroxine at the tissue level. Attempts to administer triiodothyronine (thyroxine is unsuitable because conversion to triiodothyronine is reduced) to very sick patients in an attempt to alter the progression of the underlying disease have not given clear results. Similarly, attempts to treat patients with T3 after major surgical intervention have not given unequivocal positive results.

> **The Thyroid and Common Illness, NTI**
>
> *During* common illness, the serum concentration of
> - T3 falls (most pronounced and most common)
> - TSH falls initially
> - T4 increases temporarily or remains normal in most cases
> - In cases with difficult and protracted common illness T4 falls successively
> - In extremely protracted common illness (intensive care cases) a pronounced drop in T3, T4 and TSH is often observed
> - Methodological problems can occur.
> - *After* a common illness, the serum concentration of TSH rises temporarily for a period (weeks).

3 Biochemical Investigations

This chapter starts with a description of the analyses used in the diagnosis of thyroid diseases. Subsequently, analytical strategies for various diseases will be discussed. Diagnostic information and indications for the respective analyses are given in Table 3.2 at the end of this chapter.

3.1 TSH

Normally, there is a negative feedback relationship between TSH secretion by the pituitary and hormone secretion by the thyroid. For various causes of hyperthyroidism and, for example, in the case of excessive thyroxine supply, the concentration of TSH drops (Fig. 3.1). In hypothyroidism, when the thyroid produces low amounts of thyroxine, TSH increases. Raised or lowered TSH concentrations can also be a consequence of adaptive changes in nonthyroid illness (see Chap. 2).

During a slight increase in release of thyroid hormones, a marked decrease of TSH is observed, and in more pronounced hyperthyroidism, TSH can not be detected. In this book, we have chosen to denote a TSH value below the lower reference range limit as suppressed. When TSH is so low that it can not be determined by the method used, the description can be further defined as not detectable (Fig. 3.2).

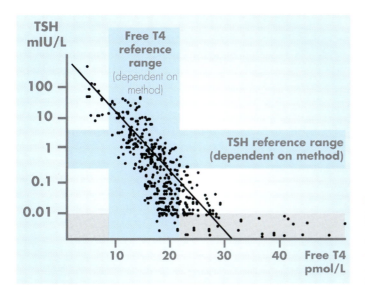

Fig. 3.1 Relationship between log TSH/free T4 in serum (from: Spencer CA et al. (1990) J Clin Endocrinol Metab 70:453–460)

E. Nyström, G.E.B. Berg, S.K.G. Jansson, O. Törring, S.V. Valdemarsson (Eds.),
Thyroid Disease in Adults,
DOI: 10.1007/978-3-642-13262-9_3, © Springer-Verlag Berlin Heidelberg 2011

Chapter 3: Biochemical Investigations

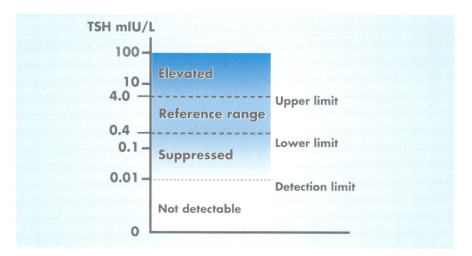

Fig. 3.2 Terminology for the evaluation of various TSH concentrations. The reference range limits are dependent on both the selected reference population and the analytical method used. The detection limit is dependent on the analytical method

The "set-point" for the relationship between TSH and free T4 is gentically determined. Figure 3.1 shows that a small change in free T4 has a very large impact on TSH. Doubling the concentration of free T4 results in a pronounced reduction in the concentration of TSH. Determination of TSH is therefore a sensitive method that is used to indirectly demonstrate changes in the concentration of thyroxine.

TSH can not be used alone to evaluate the degree of thyrotoxicosis. This is better reflected by determination of the thyroid hormone concentration, which in practice means free T4. A graphical representation of the relationship between TSH and free T4 can be of great value in diagnosing various types of thyroid dysfunction (Fig. 3.3).

With falling T4 concentrations, the pituitary secretion of TSH increases. In mild hypothyroidism, decreasing T4 secretion from the thyroid can be compensated for by increased peripheral conversion of T4 to T3, which will maintain the normal hormone effect at the cellular level. The major part of the T3 pool in the TSH producing cells originates from intracellular deiodination of T4 to T3. This means that decreasing availability of T4 results in increased TSH secretion, even if the circulating level of biologically active T3 remains mostly normal during the early stages of hypothyroidism as well as subclinical or mild hypothyroidism.

3.1 TSH

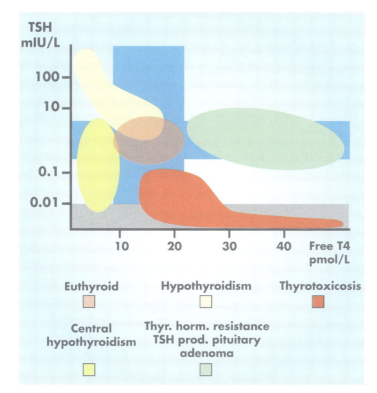

Fig. 3.3 Schematic representation of the relationship between TSH and free T4 in euthyroid individuals and in diseases of the thyroid

The high analytical specificity attained by the modern TSH methods (based on monoclonal antibodies) can cause problems. Circulating TSH is heterogeneous. Different TSH methods can therefore determine various immunoreactive parts of the TSH populations in patient samples, which results in different reference ranges for healthy people, depending on the TSH method used. In addition, the immunological methods can be affected by interference. The most significant interference for TSH determination is caused by heterophilic antibodies. Animal antibodies, such as human antimouse antibodies (HAMA), in patient samples can create the bridge that is normally formed by the analyte (TSH) in the analytic reaction, thereby giving a false increase in the TSH value. Heterophilic antibodies occur in low concentrations in about 50% of the population, but the effect of these are eliminated in routine diagnostics by addition of immunoglobulins from nonimmunized animals or humans. In cases where it is difficult to interpret the results (unexpectedly high/low TSH values) the laboratory should be consulted.

3.2 TRH-Stimulated TSH Secretion

This test, also known as the TRH stimulation test or simply the TRH test, was once commonly used to diagnose hyperthyroidism. Since sensitive methods have become available for the determination of TSH, this stimulation test is rarely used for that purpose.

In the TRH test, thyroliberin (thyrotropin-releasing hormone) is administered and TSH determined over a period of 30 min, or longer. In euthyroidism, an increase of TSH is seen after about 20 min, while in thyrotoxicosis the TSH concentration remains low. The test can be of value if, for example, analytical interference is suspected (inappropriate TSH in a patient with high thyroxine concentrations). The latter is only seen in pituitary hyperthyroidism (TSH-producing tumour) and in thyroid hormone resistance, an extremely rare condition. In pituitary hyperthyroidism, TRH-stimulation is not expected to result in an increase in TSH. In thyroid hormone resistance, on the other hand, increasing TSH can be demonstrated using this test (see Chap. 34).

A TRH stimulation test can also be valuable when diagnosing central/secondary hypothyroidism, in which a low glycosylated TSH with low biological activity and long half-life but unchanged immunological detectability can be secreted. This explains why TSH concentrations can occasionally be observed within or even above the reference range in central hypothyroidism. It also explains why in the extended TRH test (3 h) an increase in TSH can be observed that is pronounced and persistent (hours) due to the long half-life of this TSH variant.

3.3 Thyroid Hormones

In hyperthyroidism, secretion of T4 increases in most patients. There is often an even more pronounced increase of T3 if the patient is otherwise healthy. An isolated increase of T3 can be seen at mild hyperactivity, for example, in autonomous nodules and in individuals with hyperthyroidism and iodine deficiency.

> **Thyroid Hormones and Plasma Protein Binding**
>
> Both T4 and T3 are bound more than 99% to plasma proteins:
> - Thyroxine binding globulin (TBG): binds both T4 and T3
> - Prealbumin (transthyretin): binds T4
> - Albumin: binds T4 and T3

Therefore, the concentrations of circulating T4 and T3 do not depend only on the balance between secretion and elimination of the hormones, but also on the concentration of binding proteins and the presence of disease, medicines or other substances that affect protein binding.

Factors that change the binding protein concentrations change the total hormone concentrations without affecting the free (active) hormone concentrations, provided that the hormone secretion or metabolism is not affected by the disease or medicines.

> The concentration of the dominating binding protein, TBG, is affected by oestrogens. High concentrations of TBG are seen in pregnancy and during treatment with oestrogen-containing contraceptive drugs. For this reason, higher concentrations of total T4 and total T3 are observed in these situations.
>
> Low TBG concentrations can be seen, for example, in nephrotic disease or liver cirrhosis, but can also have a genetic cause. This condition results in low concentrations of total T4 and total T3, and can affect measurement of the free hormone concentrations to varying extents, depending on the analytical method used (see below).
>
> An effect on the binding protein's affinity for thyroid hormones is exerted primarily by some anticonvulsive medicines. During chronic treatment with anti-epileptic medicines, low total T4 and total T3 concentrations are seen. With some methods, subnormal concentrations of free T4 may be found. Opposite effects can be seen after the intake of high doses of salicylic acid and in certain patients receiving heparin, even low molecular weight heparin. In the latter case, fatty acids are released, which compete with T4 for binding to albumin.

3.4 Free Thyroid Hormones

In order to avoid problems in interpreting analytical results arising from changes in binding proteins, most clinical chemistry laboratories now analyse the free fraction of T4 or T3 (free T4, free T3). Because the free fraction comprises one component in an equilibrium relationship with the bound fraction, each measurement results in alteration of the equilibrium, and methodological problems have been common. With current routine methodology, it appears adequate to regard the results as an estimate of the free hormone concentrations. However, these methods are robust and well-suited for clinical use. The determination of free T4 can thus be considered as one of the basic analyses in clinical work.

Today, because analyses of free T4 and free T3 occur to a far greater extent in routine clinical work than total hormone analyses, we have chosen to primarily focus on these analyses in the chapters directly concerning diagnostic work-up. Many laboratories continue, however, to use total hormone analysis in routine clinical work.

3.5 Analytical Problems

It is important to be familiar with the limitations of the methods used for analyzing the free fraction of thyroid hormones. In cases of deviating values, it is often wise to consult the laboratory physician or supplement with analyses of total hormone, T4 or T3, and if necessary also conduct analyses at a different laboratory using other analytical methods.

As indicated above, sometimes analytical interference by heterophilic antibodies can occur when measuring free thyroid hormones. This is however relatively uncommon (probably <1% of all analyses). Importantly, the measurement method for the determination of total thyroid hormones may not be affected.

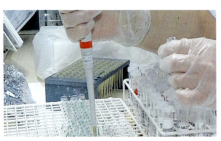

The determination of free hormone can also be affected by substances that affect binding to serum proteins (primarily to albumin and TBG), for example, certain medicines and free fatty acids (FFA). The latter is relevant after heparin administration (see above), which results in the release of endothelial-bound lipoprotein lipase. The presence of this enzyme in the blood sample in vitro results in the release of FFA from triglycerides which, with some methods, results in raised free hormone values, and with other methods, lowered values (depending on the FFA concentration). In severe NTI, it is believed that circulating inhibitors of thyroid hormone binding protein are present. The biochemical nature of these inhibitors is disputed.

Congenital TBG deficiency is a condition which strongly affects modern methods for determination of the free hormone fractions. In these fairly uncommon cases incorrect values of thyroid hormones are observed.

> **Analytical Problems When Evaluating Thyroid Function:**
>
> (1) TSH
> - Heterophilic antibodies (incorrectly elevated values)
>
> (2) T4 and T3
> - High concentration of binders, due for example to oestrogen effects (e.g. results in higher T4 and T3)
> - Changed affinity for binders (e.g. through effects of antiepileptic medicines, results in lower T4 and T3)
> - Thyronine antibodies may give incorrect values
> - Dysalbuminemic hyperthyroxinemia (high T4 due to increased albumin binding of T4)
> - Low concentration of binders (nephrosis, congenital low TBG, results in low T4 and T3)

> **(Continued) Analytical Problems When Evaluating Thyroid Function:**
>
> (3) Free T4 and free T3
> - Thyronine antibodies may give incorrect values (elevated free T4 and free T3 with many methods)
> - Heparin administration gives incorrectly high values
> - Congenital TBG deficit

Determination of free T3 has, together with TSH, the highest diagnostic sensitivity for hyperthyroidism, provided that the free T3 measurement is not affected by other factors such as analytical interference, NTI or certain medicines. Total T4 has the lowest diagnostic sensitivity. Measurement of free T3 has been associated with technical problems which vary between the methods. For routine diagnostic work-up many laboratories prefer determination of free T4 together with TSH, which today is seldom affected by analytical interference.

3.6 Reference Ranges (Normal Values) for Thyroid-Associated Hormone Analyses

When determining the reference range of one variable, the analysis is performed on a relatively large number of healthy individuals (at least 200). For some variables, the range must be specified for different ages and/or sex. There are no clinically significant differences in thyroid hormone levels at various ages or between the sexes.

The reference range may be affected by pregnancy. Primarily, falling hormone levels are observed when determining free T4 with most routine analytical methods used. Only a few laboratories, however, provide reference ranges for free T4 for the three trimesters of pregnancy.

When selecting the population for determining the reference range for thyroid-associated hormone, individuals with thyroid disease must be excluded. Therefore, individuals comprising the study population must be confirmed to be free of thyroid disease (including goitre), free of thyroid antibodies, and without an iodine deficiency. This has been shown to be of particular significance with respect to the TSH reference range. Using the normal methods, the reference range with an unscreened population normally lies in the range of 0.3–4.2 mIU/L. If individuals with TPOAb are excluded, a reference range of about 0.3–3.5 mIU/L (or lower) is obtained. It is therefore important to know how the laboratory recruits its reference population. An obvious requisite is that the reference range for thyroid-associated hormones is always determined on a healthy population without TPOAb.

The reference ranges for TSH and thyroid hormones illustrate that thyroid-associated ranges are unusually wide when compared with other ranges. For example, the range spans an order of magnitude for TSH (0.4–4.0 mIU/L). It should be noted that reference ranges for individuals, i.e. the variation in repeated analyses of TSH and thyroid hormones in an individual, is genetically determined, and is significantly nar-

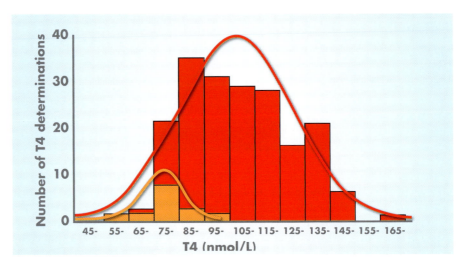

Fig. 3.4 Distribution of T4 concentrations in 16 healthy individuals (*red*) compared to the distribution for one of these individuals (*yellow*). Each individual was sampled once per month over 1 year (modified after: Andersen S et al. (2002) J Clin Endocrinol Metab 87:1068–1072)

rower than the reference range for the entire population (Fig. 3.4). In practice this means that an individual can demonstrate hypothyroid symptoms when he or she has low/normal free T4, while another person with the same value is euthyroid. The situation with respect to TSH is the same. An individual therefore has a fairly narrow range of TSH values and can exhibit symptoms when the values rise or fall and deviate over a longer time from this individual range by more than 0.75–1.0 mIU/L for TSH.

3.7 Antibodies Against Thyroperoxidase (TPOAb)

Measurement of antibodies against the membrane enzyme thyroid peroxidase (see Fig. 2.7) is currently the most sensitive and most commonly used biochemical method (diagnostic sensitivity ≥95%) for diagnosing autoimmune (lymphocytic) thyroid disease. TPOAb are often also present in patients with Graves' disease. Individuals with TPOAb are common in the euthyroid population among women (in Sweden 15–20%). The prevalence of TPOAb-positive individuals is higher in areas with high iodine intake and increases with increasing age.

During pregnancy, decreasing concentrations of TPOAb are observed. After giving birth, TPOAb normally returns or rises and predicts the possible development of postpartum thyroiditis. A high TPOAb value in the later stages of pregnancy indicates that the woman is at high risk for postpartum thyroiditis (see Chap. 31).

Thyroid antibodies were previously detected using immunofluorescence on tissue sections (cytoplasmic antibodies), and later with agglutination techniques using membrane fractions from a thyroid homogenate as an antigen source (antimicrosomal antibodies). These methods are seldom used today.

3.8 Antibodies Against the TSH Receptor (TRAb)

Antibodies against the TSH receptor can bind to receptors on the basal membrane of the follicle cells. of the follicle cells. This binding can induce a TSH-like activation. This receptor activation is the mechanism behind Graves' disease which is thus a consequence of an autoimmune disorder. Determination of TRAb is used to clarify the etiology of hyperthyroidism/thyrotoxicosis and establish whether Graves' disease is present or if there is another cause for the elevated hormone levels.

Methods for determination of TRAb are based on the measurement of binding to receptor preparations. It is important to note that routine TRAb methods do not differentiate between stimulating and inhibiting TRAb.

Using modern methods, TRAb are demonstrated in 95–99% of all patients with Graves' disease (Table 3.1). Patients with hyperthyroidism due to other causes, such as toxic nodular goitre, lack detectable TRAb. In these patients, antibodies can sometimes be detected after treatment with radioiodine. After radioiodine treatment, an increase in TRAb is nearly always observed in patients with Graves' disease.

Table 3.1 Antibodies in autoimmune thyroid disease

	Graves'	Hashimoto/ autoimmune thyroiditis
TRAb	About 95–99%	–
TPOAb	About 60%	95%

TRAb are of clinical importance not only in patients with Graves' disease. Some types of TRAb lack the ability to activate the receptor; in these cases they may inhibit thyroid function through preventing TSH binding, in which case they behave as blocking antibodies. TRAb-dependent hypothyroidism is rare, but one should be aware of this possibility. Some patients with TRAb can present with a fluctuating picture of hyperactivity and hypoactivity, which can possibly be ascribed to variations in the relation between stimulating and inhibiting TRAb. TRAb can pass from the placenta to the foetus. This is associated with a risk of the foetus being affected by thyroid dysfunction during the foetal stage or after birth. (See also Chap. 31).

3.9 Thyroglobulin (Tg)

Thyroglobulin is a protein that can only be formed by differentiated thyroid follicle cells. Only small amounts of thyroglobulin leak from the healthy thyroid gland into the blood. In hypothyroidism and thyroxine administration, Tg concentrations in blood can fall. During excessive exogenous intake of thyroxine, the Tg concentration can fall to values around the lower limit of the reference range or even lower. High concentrations of Tg can, on the other hand, be observed in hyperthyroidism, thyroiditis, multinodular goitre and in differentiated follicular and papillary cancer.

With modern methods, the lower detection limit is around 0.5 µg/L. Antibodies occur in 25–30% of patients, and these antibodies can affect the analysis. Falsely high Tg values are obtained for measurements using competitive methods (classical radioimmunoassay) and falsely low levels with immunometric methods (IRMA, ELISA). The interaction of Tg antibodies with the latter method is illustrated by a low recovery test (measurement of Tg concentration after adding in vitro a certain amount of thyroglobulin to the sample to be analyzed). A recovery of <70% is achieved in the presence of interfering Tg antibodies. A sensitive IRMA method with a functional sensitivity of 1.0 µg/L is currently recommended.

Determination of Tg is performed only for special indications, mostly when following up with patients with differentiated thyroid cancer who have undergone total thyroidectomy. Tg is thereby used as a marker for remaining tumour tissue or recurrence (see Chap. 30).

3.10 Antibodies Against Thyroglobulin (TgAb)

The presence of antibodies that react with intact Tg indicates an autoimmune thyroid disease; the diagnostic sensitivity is, however, less than the determination of TPOAb. Autoimmunization against iodothyronine in the Tg molecule can also occur and give rise to iodothyronine antibodies. These can cause interference when determining thyroid hormones. Determination of TgAb is valuable after treatment for thyroid cancer, as a complement to the analysis of Tg.

3.11 Thyroxine-Binding Globulin (TBG) and Transthyretin (Prealbumin)

Measurement of these proteins may be indicated when an unexplainable deviation of total T4 values and/or a discrepancy between free and total T4 is observed. TBG analysis is also indicated for unexplainable discrepancies between measured free and total T3. For the same reasons, protein analyses can be indicated when concentrations of T4 (T3) are elevated in the presence of normal TSH. Oestrogen stimulates synthesis of TBG. Low TBG concentrations can have genetic origins or depend on increased losses (nephrosis) or reduced synthesis (cirrhosis of the liver).

3.12 Calcitonin

Calcitonin is formed in the C cells of the thyroid and has a pharmacological effect on calcium regulation. Its significance in normal physiological concentrations is not clarified. Because medullary thyroid cancer arises in the C cells, calcitonin is a valuable marker for this form of cancer. Patients with this tumour disease usually have elevated serum calcitonin levels. Persistently high values after surgery indicate remaining tumour tissue or metastases.

Calcitonin is either determined in a basal test or after provocation with pentagastrin or calcium infusion, which can release calcitonin even from small tumours. These methods were previously used at diagnosis of individuals with a family history for this disease. With the arrival of genetic analytical methods, the above mentioned tests have become less important for early identification of carriers of the hereditary mutation.

3.13 Iodine in Urine

The measurement of iodine in urine is an indirect method for measuring iodine intake. The measurement is made on a 24-h urine collection. It is also possible to estimate the average iodine intake in a population by analysing random samples of urine from a large number of people (about 200–1,000) and then calculating the median value of iodine concentration. The most common analytical method is based on the Sandell–Kolthoff reaction in which iodide catalyses the reduction of cerium ammonium sulphate, causing a colour change. Measurement of iodine in urine has been suggested for use before radioiodine treatment in thyroid cancer in order to exclude iodine overload.

3.14 Genetic Diagnostics

In patients with medullary thyroid cancer, the gene which causes multiple endocrine neoplasia type 2, the RET gene, is analysed. This gene carries the code for a tyrosine kinase receptor located on the cell surface. Point mutations in the genetic sequence results in changes in the extra or intracellular part of the receptor. This leads to a constitutional activation of the receptor even without ligand binding and continual growth stimulation of the cells in which the receptor is expressed.

In patients with thyroid hormone resistance, it is now possible to demonstrate and characterize the mutation in the nuclear beta 1 receptor, which causes lowered binding of T3 to the T3 binding domain in the receptor.

3.15 Analytical Strategy

> **Investigations available for the diagnosis of common thyroid diseases:**
>
> - TSH
> - Thyroid hormones
> - TPOAb
> - TRAb

TSH is the basic analysis when thyroid dysfunction (hypo- or hyperthyroidism) is suspected. It has been suggested that analysis of TSH should be used as the only first-hand analysis at primary care level investigation. However, this strategy will not detect individuals with thyroid dysfunction due to disease at the hypothalamic-pituitary level. A strategy that combines analysis of TSH with TPOAb has also been proposed. This provides the possibility of directly determining the significance of elevated TSH levels. In our opinion, the combination TSH and free T4 is optimal for initial thyroid diagnosis at primary care level.

3.15.1 Hypothyroidism

TSH is the preferred analysis, both for the diagnosis of primary hypothyroidism and when performing a thyroxine substitution follow-up. Concomitant determination of free T4 will supplement the information on the severity of the hypothyroidism. In hypothyroidism, the T3 concentration is often initially maintained, but falls at more pronounced thyroid hormone deficit.

If TSH is slightly raised, TPOAb should be analysed. If TPOAb are present, the patient has autoimmune thyroid disease. Repeated TSH determinations are recommended, particularly after 3-4 weeks, if an elevated level is found after a general illness (NTI). If an adult with no history of thyroid disease is found to have typical hypothyroidism with pronounced TSH rise, TPOAb does not need to be analysed. The cause is almost always autoimmune thyroid disease.

The analysis of TPOAb is useful in determining the cause of slightly elevated TSH values, partly to confirm an autoimmune origin and partly to predict the risk of developing hypothyroidism, with a need for thyroxine substitution.

3.15.2 Thyrotoxicosis

TSH and free T4 are preferred analyses in diagnosis of thyrotoxic conditions. A suppressed/nondetectable TSH must always be investigated, even if the total and free hormone levels lie within the reference range. TSH is the most sensitive analysis for determining the presence of thyroid dysfunction, while free T4 provides information on the severity of the disorder.

If the laboratory tests indicate thyrotoxicosis, determination of T3 provides valuable supplementary information. Determination of free or total T3 may also be more sensitive than free T4 at diagnosis of modest hyperactive conditions due to toxic nodular goitre and toxic adenoma.

TRAb verifies that the cause of hyperthyroidism is Graves' disease.

Chapter 3: Biochemical Investigations

Table 3.2 Overview of biochemical investigations

Serum component		Diagnostic information[1]
Indicators for autoimmune thyroid disease		
TPOAb (Antibodies against thyroperoxidase)		Provides information on presence of autoimmune thyroid disease[2] and the risk of developing thyroid dysfunction
TRAb (Antibodies against TSH receptors)		Presence of immunoglobulins which bind to TSH receptors and which stimulate or rarely inhibit follicle cell activity
TgAb (Antibodies against thyroglobulin)	1	Provides information on presence of autoimmune thyroid disease[3]
	2	Affects the results when measuring Tg through (**a**) effect on Tg concentration in vivo and (**b**) effect on analysis in vitro[4]
	3	Increasing concentrations of TgAb in a patient who has undergone total thyroidectomy for differentiated cancer indicate metastases
Indicators of thyroid dysfunction		
TSH (Thyrotropin)	1	Provides information on thyroxine availability in the tissues (primarily pituitary and CNS) assuming normal function of the hypothalamus and pituitary. The TSH concentration is inversely related to the T4 concentration
	2	Manifest high concentrations are diagnostic for primary hypothyroidism, while low, normal or slightly elevated TSH concentrations can be found in hypothalamic hypothyroidism[5]
TSH hormone secretion (thyroliberin stimulated)	1	Provides information on TSH secretion after administration of thyroliberin (TRH)
	2	Is there feedback inhibition of TSH secretion?

1. Highly schematised.
2. In this case, analysis of TPOAb have greater sensitivity than TgAb with current methods.
3. Autoimmune/non-autoimmune etiology? Silent thyroiditis?
4. The methods routinely used today to determine Tg cannot be used if antibodies for Tg are present. Therefore a known amount of thyroglobulin is regularly added, after which recovery can be determined and the presence of interference assessed. If TgAb are present, Tg is often determined using older RIA methods. RIA.

3.15 Analytical Strategy

Indication for testing[1]

1. Unclear TSH increase
2. Goitre of unknown etiology[3]
3. Investigation of suspected polyglandular autoimmune disease (pernicious anaemia, Addison's disease, vitiligo, diabetes mellitus type 1, etc.)
4. Family history for autoimmune thyroid disease
5. Treatment with medicines that affect the immune system (risk for development of thyroid dysfunction) and with medicines that affect thyroid function (e.g. lithium salt)
6. Differential diagnosis of thyrotoxicosis of unknown etiology

1. Differential diagnosis of thyrotoxicosis[3]
2. Investigation of thyroid-associated ophthalmopathy
3. Unclear thyroid dysfunction with varying clinical picture
4. Follow-up of pregnant women who have/have had autoimmune hyperthyroidism

1. Supplement to analysis of Tg
2. Follow-up of differentiated thyroid cancer

1. Preferred analyses at suspicion of primary hypothyroidism and thyrotoxicosis
2. Follow-up of thyroxine treatment
3. Supplement to analysis of free T4 at suspicion of secondary hypothyroidism[5]
4. Supplement to analysis of free T4 and free T3 at suspicion of thyroid hormone resistance

1. Suspect interference at determination of TSH in some tests (incorrectly normal values at thyrotoxicosis? Incorrectly high values in euthyroid patients?)
2. Secondary hyperthyroidism (acute psychiatric illness, selective pituitary thyroxine resistance, TSH-producing tumour)
3. Thyroid hormone resistance
4. Central hypothyroidism

5. In hypothalamic hypothyroidism with TRH deficit, TSH can be immunochemically reactive but biologically inactive. At TRH test, a protracted response is observed because the low-glycosylated TSH has an extended half-life.

Chapter 3: Biochemical Investigations

Serum component		Diagnostic information
Indicators of thyroid dysfunction, cont.		
T4 (free, total)	1 2	Reflects the actual hormone secretion from the thyroid [6] Provides information on thyroxine availability in tissues during thyroxine treatment [6]
T3 (free, total)	1 2 3	Reflects thyroid hormone secretion at thyrotoxicosis [6] Elevated concentrations during thyroxine treatment indicates autonomous activity in the thyroid with hyperactivity [7] Reflects the conversion of T4 to T3 [6]
rT3		Reflects the conversion of T4 to rT3 or conversion of rT3 to T2
TBG (Thyroxine binding globulin)		Dominating carrier protein for T4 and T3
Transthyretin (prealbumin)		High affinity binder for T4
Tg (Thyroglobulin)		Reflects leakage from normal or neoplastic thyroid tissue with the capacity to synthesize Tg
Investigation of suspected analytical interference at thyroid investigation		
Heterophilic antibodies (including HAMA)		Can lead to incorrect values measured at analysis of TSH and/or thyroid hormones
Antibodies against iodothyronine (e.g. T4, T3)		Provides information on the risk for incorrect results at analysis of free or total T4 and/or T3 (method dependent)
Albumin-associated thyroid hormone binders		Provides information on incorrect results at analysis of hormones
Hormones from thyroid C cells		
Calcitonin	1 2	Provides information on the quantity of C cells in the thyroid, elevated at medullary thyroid cancer Presence of calcitonin producing tumours external to the thyroid, for example in the pancreas

6. If total T4 (T3) is analysed, but not free hormones, interpreting problems may arise if abnormal protein binding of thyroid hormones occurs (to TBG, transthyretin, anti-iodothyronine antibodies, albumin-associated thyroid hormone b
7. In uncomplicated cases of thyrotoxicosis, the diagnostic sensitivity for free T3>T3 = free T4>T4; at concomitant NTI ("Non Thyroidal Illness", see Chapter 3), the diagnostic sensitivity for free T3 is lower.

3.15 Analytical Strategy

Indication for testing

1. Supplement to analysis of TSH at suspicion of primary hypothyroidism
2. Suspicion of hyperthyroidism (alternative to T3)
3. In the initial stages at follow-up after treatment for thyrotoxicosis (because TSH can be suppressed during the first period after treatment)
4. Fine adjustment of thyroxine treatment and check-up of compliance with thyroxine treatment.
5. Suspicion of secondary hypothyroidism[6]

1. Investigation of thyrotoxicosis[7]
2. Suspicion of autonomy during thyroxine treatment
3. Differential diagnosis of low TSH concentration[8]
4. Assessment of severity of primary hypothyroidism

Low conc. of free T3 of unclear origin

1. Discrepancy between total and free T4 and/or T3 findings at incorrectly interpreted high T4 conc (e.g. if at the same time TSH conc is normal)
2. Determination using both immunochemical and binding methods can be indicated at suspicion of presence of variation in the TBG (primarily with low affinity, for example, investigation of unexplainably low total T4 and discrepant results for T4 with different methods, and also unexplainably low TSH concentrations)

1. Discrepancy between total and free T4
2. Unexplainably high total T4

1. Diagnosis and follow-up after thyroidectomy for thyroid differentiated cancer
2. Metastases from adenocarcinoma with unknown primary tumour
3. Diagnosis of thyrotoxicosis of unknown etiology
   (thyrotoxicosis factitia has low Tg concentration)

If deviating results at analysis of TSH, free or total T4 and/or T3
(in relation to other analyses or clinical pictures)

If divergent results from analysis of free or total
T4 and/or T3 (in relation to other analyses or clinical pictures)

1. Investigation of unexplainably high T4 (or T3, rT3)
2. Family history for dominant inheritance high T4

1. Diagnosis and follow-up of medullary thyroid cancer
   (basal, after administration of pentagastrin and/or calcium)
2. Diagnosis and follow-up of multiple endocrine neoplasm type 2
3. Diagnosis and follow-up of neuroendocrine tumours

---

8. High concentration at hyperthyroidism (or within the reference range upper section). For T3, low concentrations are present in "Non Thyroidal Illness"; for free T3, normal or low concentrations are observed at NTI depending on the method used. Normal or low concentration at secondary hypothyroidism.

4 Other Investigations

4.1 Investigations Using Radionuclides

Investigations using radionuclides are based on the ability of the thyroid gland to actively take up iodide ions and similar, negatively charged ions via the iodide pump (NIS). They also utilize the fact that iodine isotopes bind to the thyroglobulin molecule during hormone synthesis and are subsequently stored in the colloid.

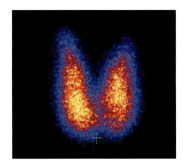

Fig. 4.1 Scintigraphic image of the normal thyroid gland

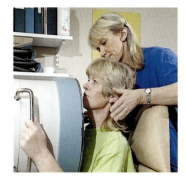

Fig. 4.2 The patient positioned in front of a gamma camera

Table 4.1 Radioactive isotopes used at investigation of the thyroid

Nuclide	Main radiation	Range	Half-life of decay	Application
I-131	γ radiation	Long	8 days	Visualization
				Uptake test
	β radiation	0.5 mm	8 days	Therapy
I-123	γ radiation	Long	13 h	Visualisation
Tc-99m	γ radiation	Long	6 h	Visualisation

E. Nyström, G.E.B. Berg, S.K.G. Jansson, O. Tørring, S.V. Valdemarsson (Eds.),
Thyroid Disease in Adults,
DOI: 10.1007/978-3-642-13262-9_4, © Springer-Verlag Berlin Heidelberg 2011

Chapter 4: Other Investigations

Isotopes of iodine or technetium are used in the investigations (Table 4.1). Isotopes which emit γ radiation are used for diagnostic purposes. These have a long range and will reach outside the body. β emitters are used for treatment. These have a short range and are absorbed by the tissue.

4.1.1 Gamma Camera Investigations (Scintigraphy)

Investigations of the thyroid using nuclear medicine technology require equipment that can detect gamma radiation. Scintillation techniques make use of crystals that absorb photons and simultaneously release flashes of light. These light flashes can be registered and counted by a scintillation detector as an iodine uptake test, but can also be used to display images using a gamma camera over the thyroid gland or, using earlier technology, a rectilinear scanner.

Most centres now utilize technetium for scintigraphy. The patient receives an intravenous injection of about 150 MBq (Tc-99^m) pertechnetate (radiation dose about 2 mSv), followed by investigation of the thyroid gland about 15 min later (Figs. 4.1, 4.2).

The investigation with technetium is based on the uptake via NIS. Thyroid scintigraphy using Tc-99^m thus provides information on function (isotope uptake) and morphology (isotope distribution), but not on the extent of hormone synthesis.

Questions that can be answered using gamma camera investigations include:
- Is the entire gland functional (Graves' disease) or only in certain areas (one or more "hot" nodules)?
- Is thyrotoxicosis a consequence of hyperthyroidism (high uptake of isotope) or thyroiditis (low/no uptake)? Considering that thyroiditis can be a temporary process and because uptake increases in the recovery phase, investigations to answer this question should be done early in the disease progression.
- Can inactive areas be detected?
- Is a palpable lump in the neck caused by isotope absorbing thyroid tissue (hot autonomous nodule) or nonisotope absorbing thyroid/tumour tissue ("cold" nodule)?
- Is residual thyroid tissue present after thyroidectomy in thyroid cancer or are there metastases with avid uptake of isotope?
- Where is the active thyroid gland tissue located? At the site of the normal gland or outside of this site, for example, a lingual thyroid?

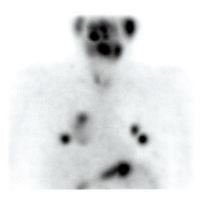

Fig. 4.3 Patient with thyroid cancer and iodine uptake in lung metastases. Image taken with a gamma camera after radioiodine treatment with I-131

4.1 Investigations Using Radionuclides

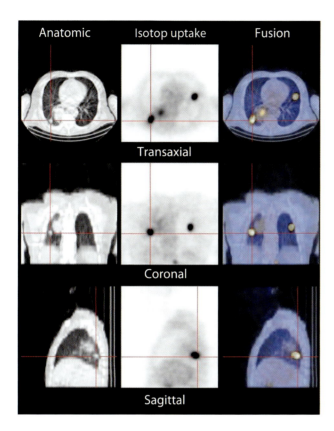

Fig. 4.4 Investigation performed using SPECT to anatomically locate the iodine absorbing changes (same patient as in Fig. 4.3). *From left to right* X-ray-CT image, gamma camera image, and fusion image of CT + gamma. *From top to bottom:* transaxial view, coronal view, sagittal view

At present, single photon emission computed tomography (SPECT) is a method that can be used in nuclear medicine investigations for improved localization of anatomical changes (Fig. 4.4). This study can be combined with X-ray CT to acquire information on the localization of the lesion.

4.1.2 Radioiodine Uptake Investigation (Radioiodine Uptake Test)

Measurement of I-131 uptake (Fig. 4.6a) is a simple method to determine how much of an administered quantity of iodine isotope has been retained by the gland. By measuring at several points of time, information can also be obtained on how long the iodine isotope remains in the thyroid.

The patient receives an oral test dose of sodium iodide (I-131, about 0.5 MBq) as an aqueous solution with neutral taste. Measurement of uptake (scintillation technology) by the thyroid is normally performed after 24 h (and thus called the 24 h I-131 uptake test).

Repeated measurements after 4–7 days allows for the calculation of the effective half-life, which is a function of the half-life of decay of the radioactive isotope (8 days) and the biological half-life (metabolism of the iodide taken up). The biological half-life is normally around 60 days, but can be considerably shorter (20 days) in cases

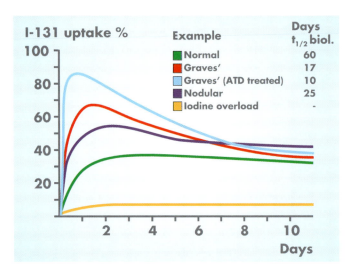

Fig. 4.5 Uptake of radioiodine in the thyroid and approximate half-life of I-131 in various clinical conditions. Treatment discontinued 1 week before measurement of uptake (ATD = antithyroid drug)

of hyperthyroidism, such as Graves' disease. Figure 4.5 presents graphs of uptake in various clinical conditions.

Radioiodine uptake investigations are most commonly performed for dose calculations before radioiodine therapy in hyperthyroidism. Thyroid scintigraphy and radioiodine uptake investigations are performed at the same time, and the patient is investigated using two different radioactive substances, Tc-99^m and I-131, on the same occasion. The patient then returns for measurements on one or more occasions.

Absence of (I-131) iodide or pertechnetate uptake (Sect. 4.1.1, Fig. 4.7d) in a patient with thyrotoxicosis indicates that the thyrotoxic condition may not be the result of increased hormone production in the thyroid gland as in hyperthyroidism. The most common cause of this is subacute or silent thyroiditis during the destructive phase. The condition can also be caused by a high intake of iodine or thyroxine.

4.1.3 Uptake of Radioiodine by the Thyroid in Various Clinical Conditions

As a consequence of differences in iodine availability between geographical regions and between individuals within a region, there is a large interindividual variation in normal uptake of (I-131) iodide. The possibility of distinguishing between low, normal and high uptake is therefore comparatively poor, and is the reason why iodine uptake investigations as a quantitative method for function assessment are not as useful as biochemical analyses of TSH, T4 and T3.

One important indication is uptake measurement for radioiodine therapy dose calculation. The method can also quickly provide information on whether the thyrotoxicosis is the result of hyperthyroidism (such as Graves' disease), in which a high uptake is seen after 24 h (Table 4.2), or of destructive thyroiditis in which uptake in the destructive phase is 0–6%.

4.1 Investigations Using Radionuclides

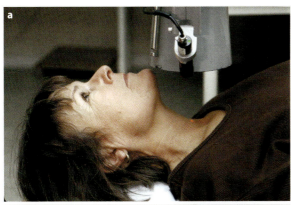

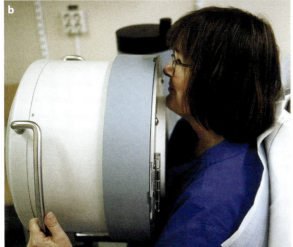

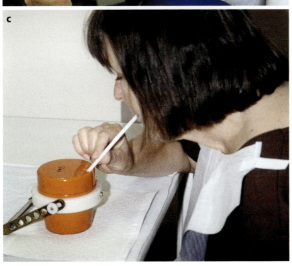

Fig. 4.6 a–c **a** Measurement of I-131 uptake using a scintillation counter.
b Investigation with gamma camera after intravenous administration of Tc-99^m.
c Therapy with I-131 where the solution is sipped using a straw from a lead beaker

Chapter 4: Other Investigations

Table 4.2 24 h I-131 uptake in the thyroid gland

Individuals in areas without iodine deficit	9–30%*
Patient with diffuse autoimmune hyperthyroidism (Graves' disease)	40–80%
Patient with destructive thyroiditis	0–6%
Iodine overload	0–6%
Autonomous nodule, nodular goitre	varies, about 10–60%

*Please note that the above values are approximate, and depend on the iodine status of the individual.

4.1.4 Perchlorate Test

The perchlorate test is rarely used except in cases of suspected Pendred's syndrome, in which there is defective iodide transport apically from the follicle cell to the follicle lumen. The test involves administration of a test activity of I-131 perorally to the patient. Uptake by the thyroid gland is measured after a given length of time. Next, the patient is given a solution of perchlorate. In individuals with a normal thyroid, the retention of I-131 is nearly always unchanged, because the iodine is incorporated into the thyroglobulin molecule. Patients with defective apical iodine transport exhibit a basal leakage of iodide and therefore have a lower amount of residual iodide in the gland. Thus, the I-131 uptake measurement gives a significantly lower value after perchlorate administration.

4.1.5 Important Features of Radionuclide Investigations

- *Iodine overload* Disturbed function of iodine uptake can persist for about 3 months after administration of large amounts of iodine. During this time, radionuclide investigations of the thyroid will give misleading results. Important groups of iodine-containing preparations are: contrast media (e.g. for CT, angiography, urography), health food preparations (algae products), and medical preparations (amiodarone, iodine-containing wound dressings)
- *Antithyroid drugs* Treatment with antithyroid drugs, which are primarily inhibitors of iodine organification, should be stopped for about a week before any investigations to avoid unnecessary inhibition of isotope uptake in the thyroid
- *Pregnant women must not be investigated* The isotopes cross the placenta, and after the 10th week of pregnancy iodine isotopes will also be taken up by the foetal thyroid gland

4.1 Investigations Using Radionuclides

- *Breastfeeding* Breastfeeding women must not be given radioiodine (I-131). Scintigraphy with Tc-99^m can be performed, but requires a 24-h interruption of breastfeeding
- *Iodine allergy* Patients with iodine allergy often react to the administration of iodine compounds, e.g. iodine-containing contrast media. On the other hand, there is no known hypersensitivity to iodine in the form of iodide. Therefore I-131 uptake tests and radioiodine treatment can be performed in patients with iodine allergy
- *Patients being treated for, or who have been treated for, hyperthyroidism* If persistent autonomous activity is suspected (suppressed TSH), this can be clarified by measuring uptake even during ongoing thyroxine treatment. If the uptake is high, this is a sign of residual autonomy in the gland
- *Hypothyroidism* In patients with hypothyroidism (with or without thyroxine treatment), isotope investigations are not indicated (low uptake of isotope)

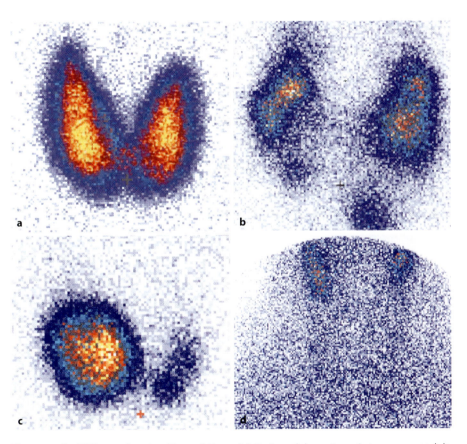

Fig. 4.7 a–d a Diffuse toxic goitre (Graves´ disease). **b** Toxic nodular goitre. c Autonomous nodule (hot adenoma). **d** Inhibited uptake, e.g. at iodine overload or destructive thyroiditis (note uptake in the salivary glands)

Chapter 4: Other Investigations

4.2 Positron Emission Tomography (PET)

Positron emission tomography (PET) has been proven to give valuable diagnostic information in patients with thyroid cancer in which there are biochemical indications of metastases, but where the tumours do not take up iodine. Here, it is not possible to demonstrate metastases using iodine scintigraphy.

PET can be used to show areas with increased tissue metabolism. A positron is a positively charged particle, which is annihilated when it meets a negatively charged electron in tissue. During the reaction, annihilation energy is generated as gamma radiation and is emitted in two opposite directions. The event can be recorded by coincidence imaging using a ring of gamma camera detectors around the patient.

Usually, 18 fluoro-deoxyglucose (18-FDG) is used for PET investigations (Fig. 4.8). 18-FDG is a radioactive sugar molecule with a half-life of about 110 min. 18-FDG is produced in a cyclotron shortly before the investigation. The substance accumulates in higher concentrations in cancerous tissue than in normal tissues because of the high metabolism of the tumour cells. It must be pointed out that other conditions with increased glucose metabolism, such as an inflammatory process, can also result in increased uptake of 18-FDG, and this must be taken into consideration. PET imaging can be combined with CT.

4.3 X-ray, CT, and MR

An X-ray examination can provide information on whether an enlarged thyroid gland, or goitre, compresses or causes side displacement or deviation of the trachea. These observations are often detected as incidental findings. X-ray investigation of the neck with an oral contrast medium can provide an idea of the extent of the mechanical effects of a goitre on the oesophagus and trachea (dislocation, compression).

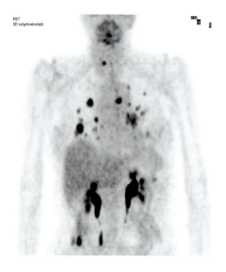

Fig. 4.8 PET investigation with 18-FDG of a patient with noniodine-accumulating lung metastases from thyroid cancer. Frontal image showing 18-FDG uptake in lung metastases. Note the normal uptake of 18-FDG by the kidneys

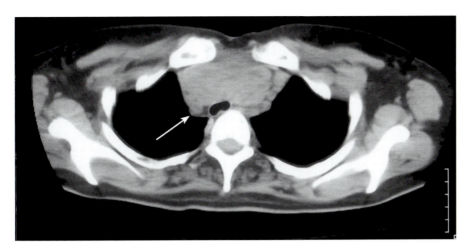

Fig. 4.9 Computer tomography image showing an intrathoracic goitre extending down into the upper mediastinum. The trachea is compressed and deviated from the median line (*arrow*)

Computer tomography (CT, Fig. 4.9) or magnetic resonance tomography (MR) is generally preferred to map intrathoracic goitre and malignant processes. Using these techniques, it is possible to evaluate the impression on the oesophagus, trachea and blood vessels, and also to determine intrathoracic extension. Note, however, that the iodine-containing contrast used for CT can cause long-term interference with uptake, thus making subsequent nuclear investigations or radioiodine treatment impossible until many months later. Furthermore, there is also a risk that the administered iodine will induce hyperactivity in a nodular goitre or latent Graves' disease.

4.4 Ultrasound

Ultrasound investigation of the thyroid and neck (Figs. 4.10, 4.11) enables the determination of
- The shape, size and location of the thyroid gland
- The presence of abnormal areas in the thyroid, e.g. solid or cystic areas
- The presence of pathological lymph nodes in the neck e.g. in patients operated for thyroid cancer
- Homogenous (diffuse) or irregular gland structure (e.g. nodular goitre and autoimmune thyroiditis)
- Blood flow at investigation of certain forms of thyroiditis or focal lesions
- Structures in connection with fine-needle biopsy

Ultrasound investigations have been increasingly used for morphological investigation and can be a valuable aid to guide cytological investigations of difficult-to-palpate lumps in the thyroid. It is important to remember that ultrasound, in contrast to

Chapter 4: Other Investigations

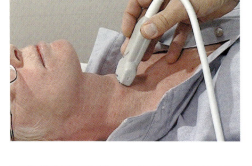

Fig. 4.10 Ultrasound investigation of the thyroid

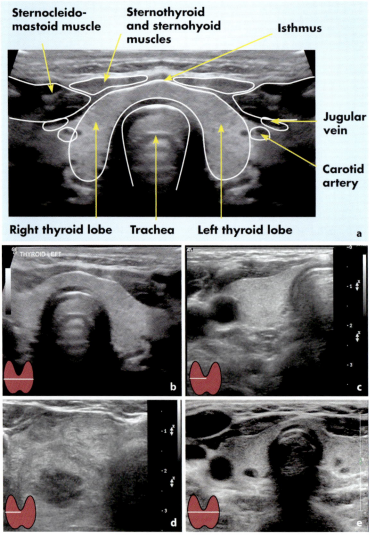

4.4 Ultrasound

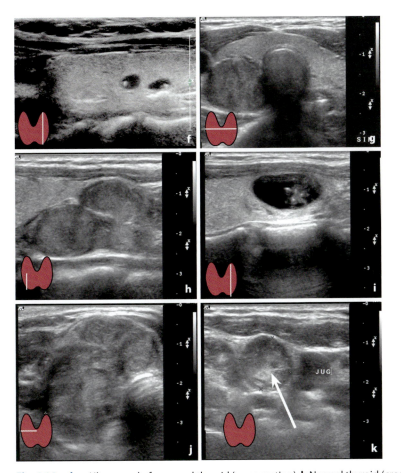

Fig. 4.11 a–k a Ultrasound of a normal thyroid (cross section). **b** Normal thyroid (cross section) in which both the right and left lobes are of normal size without focal parenchymal changes. **c** Right thyroid lobe (cross section) without pathological focal changes. The tracheal wall can be seen on the right of the image and the carotid artery on the left laterally to the lobe. **d** Right thyroid lobe (cross section) with nodular colloid goitre. The right lobe is enlarged due to the nodular changes. A low-attenuating colloid nodule can be seen in the middle. **e** Right and left lobes (cross section). A small cyst with a small calcification can be seen in the right lobe. Two small, similar cysts can be seen in the left lobe (benign). **f** Left lobe (longitudinal section) containing two small cysts each with a small calcification (same patient as in Fig. 4.11e). **g** A rounded, nonhomogenous low attenuating border structure can be seen dorsally in the right thyroid lobe (cross section). Histopathological diagnosis: papillary thyroid cancer. **h** Two pathologically enlarged, rounded lymph nodes can be seen in the lower thyroid pole (longitudinal section). Histopathological investigation reveals metastases of papillary thyroid cancer (same patient as in Fig. 4.11g). **i** A 1.5 × 1 × 1.7 cm cyst containing irregular tissue can be seen centrally in the left lobe (longitudinal section). Histopathological diagnosis: cystic papillary thyroid cancer. **j** A lobular nodule about 4 cm in diameter with a surrounding thin border of thyroid tissue can be seen in the right lobe (cross section). Histopathological diagnosis: Hürthle cell cancer. **k** A pathological lymph node which partly compresses the vein can be seen laterally to the jugular vein (cross section). Histopathological diagnosis: metastases (same patient as in Fig. 4.11j)

isotope investigations, does not provide any information on the functional status of a lump, i.e. whether it is cold or hot.

If the colour-flow Doppler technique is available, it is possible to show differences in the thyroid between Graves' disease with high vascular flow and Hashimoto thyroiditis with low flow in the chronic phase (might be high in the acute phase). The method can also be useful at diagnosing amiodarone-induced thyroid dysfunction type 1 (iodine-induced thyrotoxicosis with high blood flow) or type 2 (thyroiditis with low blood flow). Ultrasound findings that may indicate malignancy in a lump are hypoechogenicity, microcalcification and irregular borders. None, however, have 100% specificity or sensitivity.

4.5 Fine-Needle Biopsy

Fine-needle biopsy is routinely performed today for cytological diagnosis with fine-needle aspiration cytology (FNAC, Fig. 4.12) of abnormalities in the thyroid. The main indications are: diagnosis/exclusion of malignancy when palpating a lump; uncertainty with regard to findings at palpation; or a wish to investigate a cold area in a scintigraphy image. In these cases, fine-needle biopsy should be performed after thyroid scintigraphy, partly to better target the biopsy and partly to avoid postbiopsy bleeding, which could introduce artifacts in the scintigraphic image.

Thyroiditis (chronic, subacute) can be advantageously demonstrated by cytological investigation (without prior scintigraphy).

The diagnostic accuracy of cytological investigations of changes in the thyroid is very high. However, it should be emphasized that the quality of the investigation does depend on the training and competence of the person executing the technique. The value of the fine-needle biopsy for thyroid changes is fully dependent on the quality of the aspirated cells. It is an advantage to perform ultrasound-guided fine-needle biopsies when investigating difficult-to-palpate, small or deep-lying tissue changes.

4.5.1 Sampling Technique

The instrument has a pistol handle (Fig. 4.13) which is easy to manoeuvre with one hand. The puncture needle normally has a diameter of only 0.6 mm. In most cases,

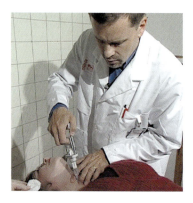

Fig. 4.12 Fine-needle biopsy of the thyroid

local anaesthetic is not required, but a topical anaesthetic can be used, primarily on children. When the investigator is sure the needle tip is positioned within the target area, the pistol handle is used to slightly reduce the pressure in the syringe, which results in the cells being aspirated into the needle tip.

The needle is then moved carefully backwards and forwards at different angles from the puncture point in order to collect an adequate number of cells. It is important to release the reduced pressure when the needle is withdrawn to ensure that the cell sample remains in the needle tip. The needle is disconnected from the syringe which is filled with air, and the needle contents are then ejected onto a microscope slide using the air-filled syringe. The fine-needle aspirate on the microscope slide is immediately smeared out to achieve a thin layer of cells for investigation. The smear is air-dried and stained (e.g. May-Grünwald-Giemsa).

It is recommended that several fine-needle biopsies of changes in the thyroid are taken in order to obtain a representative material. Both sides of the thyroid should be routinely biopsied even if only one-sided changes are present in order to provide a reference material for the investigator.

4.5.2 Cytological Findings

Normally, varying amounts of blood cells and thyrocytes are observed in a smear. The fine-needle aspirate in *hyperthyroidism* is rich in cells with scanty colloid and follicle structures are often observed. The picture can therefore be similar to that seen in follicular neoplasm, but the aspirate is identical in the entire gland, and a distinct palpable lump is often absent. There is a closer binding of follicular cells, and at the edge of the cytoplasm of the cell, there are often small fine vacuolar vesicles and a reddish material (fire flares). Furthermore, there is large variation in the diameter of the nuclei, but none are excessively enlarged or have pronounced changes. The cell picture is thus active, but the extent of the activity can not be determined cytologically. Signs of inflammation are often scarce.

In *benign colloid goitre* there is plentiful colloid in the background, and formations of follicle cells and macrophages, as well as some inflammatory cells, as an expression of regressive changes.

Typical findings of lymphocyte accumulation occur in *autoimmune thyroiditis* and *Hashimoto's disease*. In *subacute thyroiditis (de Quervain)* findings of granular epitheloid cells and polynuclear giant cells support the diagnosis.

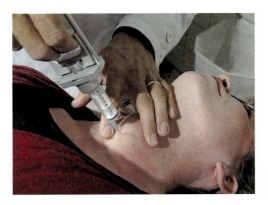

Fig. 4.13 Fine-needle aspiration biopsy using an instrument with a pistol handle

In *tumours (benign or malignant),* the fine-needle aspirate is commonly cell-rich. There is often a background material that is scant in colloid and clusters of cells that keep together in formations which may look like papillae or follicle structures. The cells can vary with different nuclear sizes. In malignant tumours, the cells can exhibit typical changes in the cytoplasm or cell nuclei. In *follicular tumours*, it is not possible to distinguish between malignant and benign changes in a cytological investigation using fine-needle biopsy. Tumours are discussed further in Chaps. 29 and 30.

4.5.3 Complications

Complications after fine-needle biopsy of the thyroid are very few. Some patients may get a hematoma, which can cause some local discomfort in the neck, but very rarely threatens the airways. Anti-coagulation treatment is not a contraindication, but testing for PK/INR before biopsy is recommended. The investigator should, however, be informed that the patient is undergoing such treatment. Infections and abscesses after fine-needle biopsy of the thyroid have been reported, but are extremely rare.

4.5.4 Histological and Cytological Diagnostics

Figures 4.14–4.17 present histological and cytological images (from fine-needle biopsy) of the normal thyroid, diffuse toxic goitre (Graves' disease), subacute thyroiditis, lymphocytic thyroiditis, follicular neoplasm, papillary thyroid cancer, Hürthle cell adenoma and Hürthle cell cancer.

4.5 Fine-Needle Biopsy

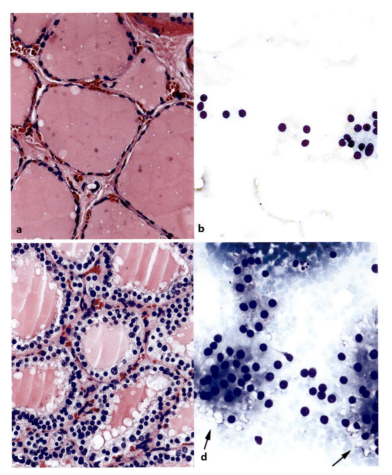

Fig. 4.14 a–d **a** Histological image of a normal thyroid fixed in formalin, embedded in paraffin and stained with hematoxylineosin. The epithelial cells are flat and the nuclei small and dark. The follicles are rich in colloid. **b** Cytological biopsy of a normal thyroid. The preparation is air-dried and stained using May-Grünwald-Giemsa. Epithelial cells are scanty and the cells small. The nuclei are small, dark and equal-sized. **c** Image of toxic diffuse goitre (Graves' disease). The epithelium is cubic and the follicles colloid content is relatively scarce (compare with Fig. 4.14a). The edge of the colloid, is rich in vacuoles. Note that the nuclei are large, relatively bright and vary somewhat in size. **d** Cytological picture of toxic diffuse goitre. Epithelial cells are plentiful and the cells lie in follicle-like formations. The cells are relatively large with light nuclei which vary greatly in size. Distinct vacuoles can be seen around the cell connections (*arrow*, compare with Fig. 4.14a)

Chapter 4: Other Investigations

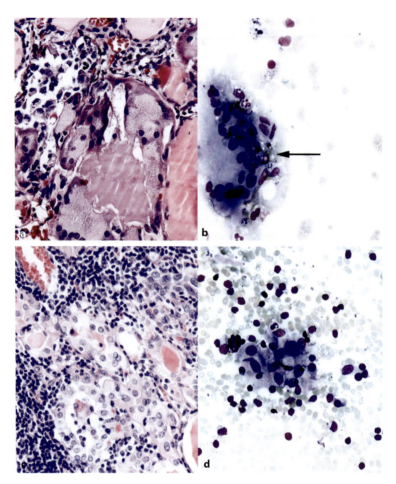

Fig. 4.15 a–d a Image of subacute (granulomatous) thyroiditis. Centrally in the image, giant cells can be seen which are phagocytosing the colloid. Furthermore, there are inflammatory cells, primarily lymphocytes and plasma cells. b Cytological biopsy reveals a few multinucleated giant cells (*arrow*) and lightly reactive changed epithelial cells but few inflammatory cells. c Image of lymphocytic thyroiditis of type Hashimoto. The image is dominated by an inflammatory cell infiltrate and destruction of the follicles can be seen. Large areas of the tissue have been replaced by lymphocytes, plasma cells and macrophages, and in the remaining area of follicular epithelium, a distinct oxyphile metaplasia can be observed, i.e. the cells are large with densely red-stained cytoplasm and relatively large cell nuclei. d Cytologically, a group of oxyphilic changed epithelium with a dense cytoplasm and large nuclei which vary in size is observed. Numerous inflammatory cells, primarily lymphocytes, can be seen in the background

4.5 Fine-Needle Biopsy

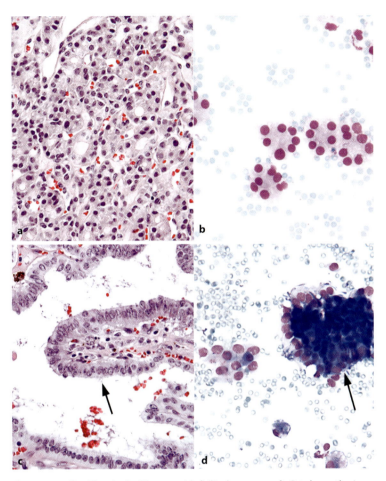

Fig. 4.16 a–d **a** Histological image with follicular tumour. **b** Cytology: the image reveals distinct follicular formations. **c**, **d** Papillary thyroid cancer. The *arrows* demonstrate papillary formations at both histology **c** and cytology **d**

Chapter 4: Other Investigations

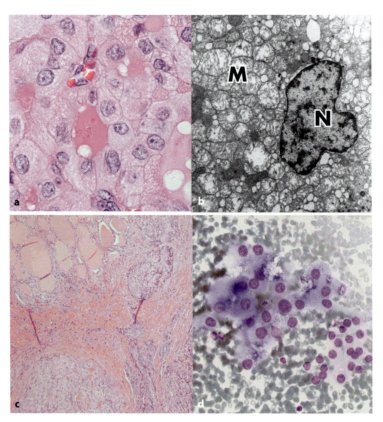

Fig. 4.17 a–d **a** Histology image of Hürthle cell adenoma. Note pronounced eosinophilia due to mitochondrial enrichment. **b** Electromicroscopy of Hürthle cell adenoma. The entire cytoplasm is filled with mitochondria (*M*). Cell nucleus: *N*. **c**, **d** Oxyphile cells in Hürthle cell cancer, histology **c** and cytology **d**

Non-biochemical Thyroid Investigations

- Radionuclide investigations of the thyroid are based on isotope uptake via the iodide pump (NIS)
- The isotopes used are I-131, Tc-99^m and I-123
- Thyroid scintigraphy with a gamma camera is performed after intravenous administration of Tc-99^m
- Thyroid scintigraphy is used in the diagnosis of thyrotoxicosis. Provides information on size, enlargement and activity
- I-131 uptake tests provide information on how much of an administered activity of I-131 is taken up by the thyroid gland
- Large amounts of iodine, e.g. iodine contrast media, can inhibit uptake
- Pregnant and breastfeeding patients must not be investigated with radionuclides
- PET is a nuclear medicine method which demonstrates increased tissue metabolism and is valuable for detecting non-iodine-accumulating metastases in thyroid cancer
- CT and MR can be used for mapping, for example in intra-thoracic goitre
- Ultrasound can be used to assess the size and shape of the thyroid gland and to distinguish between solid and cystic areas. It is excellent for guided fine-needle biopsy. Useful for detection of pathological lymph nodes
- The main indication for fine-needle biopsy is investigation of a lump in the thyroid to demonstrate/exclude malignancy
- Fine-needle biopsy is valuable for diagnosis of lymphocytic and subacute thyroiditis

5 Clinical Investigation of the Thyroid

5.1 Medical History

The medical history taken at the first consultation should comprise information about thyroid disease in the family, smoking habits, iodine intake (including for X-ray investigations), external radiation and consumption of herbal medicines (e.g. algae preparations).

The assessment should also include general toxic symptoms and eye symptoms, which indicate thyroid-associated ophthalmopathy. Descriptions of these symptoms are found in their respective dedicated chapters. For female patients, information should also be obtained about their menstrual cycle, use of contraceptive pills, pregnancy plans, pregnancy, giving birth or having an abortion within the last year.

5.2 Physical Examination

An important part in the investigation of patients with thyroid disease is palpation of the thyroid gland. The purpose of this examination is to determine whether the patient has a goitre and, if so, what type. The examination starts by observing the patient's neck when swallowing (Fig. 5.1).

In many cases, the investigator can determine whether there is diffuse enlargement or irregularities in the thyroid by studying the contour and shadows on the neck. In most people, the thyroid lies easily accessible for palpation (Fig. 5.2). The neck should be palpated with the patient's head held in a normal position with the head bent backwards and the patient swallowing.

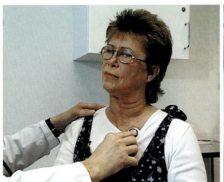 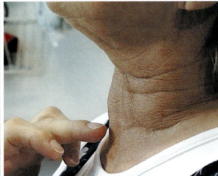

Fig. 5.1 a, b Physical examination of the patient and inspection of the thyroid region

E. Nyström, G.E.B. Berg, S.K.G. Jansson, O. Tørring, S.V. Valdemarsson (Eds.),
Thyroid Disease in Adults,
DOI: 10.1007/978-3-642-13262-9_5, © Springer-Verlag Berlin Heidelberg 2011

Chapter 5: Clinical Investigation of the Thyroid

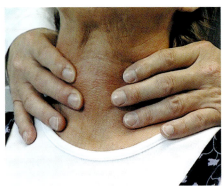

Fig. 5.2 Palpation of the thyroid

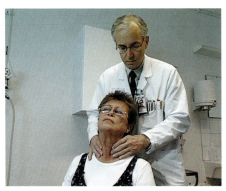

Fig. 5.3 The patient positioned with her back towards the examiner

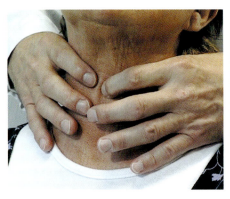

Fig. 5.4 The tip of the thyroid cartilage is localised

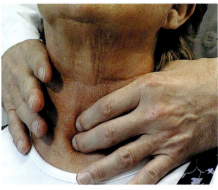

Fig. 5.5 The isthmus is felt on the front of the trachea usually over or just below the cricoid cartilage

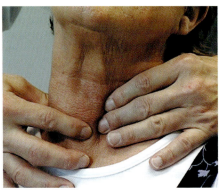

Fig. 5.6 Each side lobe is examined separately

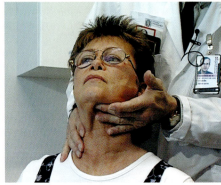

Fig. 5.7 Assessment of any enlarged regional lymph node on the front of the neck

5.2 Physical Examination

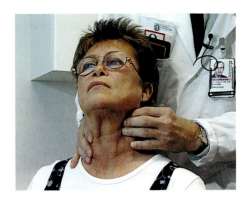

Fig. 5.8 Assessment of any enlarged regional lymph node in the lateral side of the neck

The patient should sit on a chair with their back towards the examiner (Fig. 5.3). It is important that the patient's back is straight, and the neck muscles relaxed. Palpation is normally performed using the index and middle finger pads of both hands.

First, the isthmus is localized by gently moving the fingers along the front of the trachea (Fig. 5.4). The best way to start palpation is by localizing the tip of the thyroid cartilage and then, just below, the cricoid cartilage. The isthmus normally lies connected to or immediately below the cricoid cartilage.

Normally the isthmus is felt only as a soft cushion on the front of the trachea (Fig. 5.5). The side lobes are frequently not palpable; this is a normal finding if goitre is not present.

To palpate the side lobes, stabilize the trachea in a side position by using gentle counter pressure with the fingers of one hand (Fig. 5.6). This prevents the trachea and thyroid from being pushed away. Each side lobe is examined separately.

It is often an advantage to ask the patient to swallow during palpation. Allowing the patient to take a few sips of water enables the examiner to feel the thyroid during swallowing, during which it will first move upwards, and then downwards. In children and patients whose thyroid is difficult to palpate, the thyroid can be palpated while the patient is lying on her/his back with a pillow under their neck, which helps the patient to relax the muscles in their neck.

During palpation, the size and consistency of the thyroid is noted. The surface of the gland should also be examined with respect to whether it is smooth, grainy, irregular or knobbly. In a diffusely enlarged thyroid, the isthmus and side lobes can be felt as a soft to firm expansion. Sometimes, the pyramid lobe, which is the remnant of the thyroglossus duct, can also be felt as an extension from the isthmus along the front of the thyroid cartilage. An experienced examiner can thereby make at least an approximation of the thyroid volume.

If the thyroid is asymmetrically enlarged, it should be decided whether any lumps are solitary or multiple, and whether they are localized in one or both of the lobes. When assessing a lump and its position, the examiner should assess the size and consistency of the lump, and whether it adheres to skin, muscle or the tracheal wall.

The clinical examination should also include assessment of any enlarged regional lymph nodes on the front and lateral sides as well as the proximal posterior triangle of the neck (Figs. 5.7, 5.8). It should be pointed out that, in principle, if a lump is found in the thyroid further investigations using fine-needle biopsy, ultrasound or scintigraphy must always be considered in order to exclude a malignant process.

In Graves' disease, the thyroid gland can have a highly increased blood flow, which can be heard using a stethoscope. A pulse-synchronized flow bruit can be heard over the thyroid or down the front of the precordium. Sometimes this bruit can be misinterpreted as originating in the heart.

Iodine and the Thyroid Gland in Health and Sickness

6

Access to an adequate amount of iodine is important if an individual is to fully maintain production of thyroid hormones. In areas with low availability of iodine in food (Fig. 6.1), a deficiency of iodine can result in TSH stimulation of the thyroid and development of goitre. This enables an adult to initially compensate for low iodine supply and maintain adequate hormone production. Iodine deficiency during childhood and adolescence can thereby result in irregular growth of the thyroid and formation of multinodular goitre.

However, iodine deficiency has its most serious effects on the foetus and the developing child. This may result in cretinism, which is a developmental disorder due to inadequate supply of thyroid hormone during foetal development. The foetus is supplied with thyroxine from the mother during the first half of pregnancy. From about the 16th week of pregnancy, the foetus synthesizes thyroid hormone itself, but is subsequently dependent on a supply of iodine from the mother. If the mother can not supply a sufficient amount of thyroxine or supply the foetus with iodide, normal development of the foetal central nervous system (CNS) is hindered. The development of the central nervous system is most sensitive to lack of iodine during the first trimester.

However, later during foetal development and during the early postnatal period, thyroxine and an adequate supply of iodine continue to be important for normal development of the CNS. The various consequences of thyroxine deficiency are thus dependent on when the deficiency occurs during foetal development (Fig. 31.5).

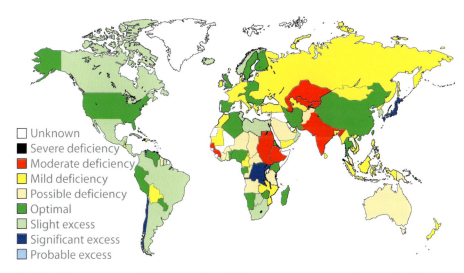

Fig. 6.1 Global iodine availability (natural availability and iodine consumed as food additives)

E. Nyström, G.E.B. Berg, S.K.G. Jansson, O. Törring, S.V. Valdemarsson (Eds.),
Thyroid Disease in Adults,
DOI: 10.1007/978-3-642-13262-9_6, © Springer-Verlag Berlin Heidelberg 2011

Even a slight iodine deficit in the mother and later in the newborn child have been shown to result in a lower IQ of the child and impaired cognitive and motor functions. The collective name for conditions due to iodine deficiency is iodine deficiency disorders (IDD). In addition to iodine deficiency, simultaneous selenium deficiency may also contribute.

6.1 Global Aspects of Iodine Intake

In many regions of the world, the natural availability of iodine is extremely low. In 1999, the World Health Organization (WHO) estimated that 740 million people, i.e. about 13% of the global population, have goitre due to iodine deficiency. Goitre and cretinism occur, for example, in the Himalayas and the Andes. These are areas once covered by glaciers, the melt waters of which have leached iodine from the soil. Iodine deficiency is also a major health problem in isolated regions of Asia and Africa. Before iodine supplementation programs were initiated, iodine deficiency caused goitre in Scandinavia and many Central European countries. Mild iodine deficiency still occurs in several European countries.

Iodine deficiency can be prevented by iodination of basic commodities such as salt and flour. In areas with extreme iodine deficiency, depot injections or capsules of iodinated oil can be given at 6–18 month intervals.

Studies with prophylactic iodine supplements to schoolchildren started in Utah as early as 1916, and the first public iodination program was introduced in Michigan in 1924. Now, there is an ongoing global iodination program in a collaboration between the International Council for Control of Iodine Deficiency Disorders (ICCIDD), UNICEF and WHO, with the goal of eradicating iodine deficiency throughout the world. The iodination program also includes monitoring goitres and measuring the concentration of iodine in the urine in the population as quality assurance of the program (Tables 6.1, 6.2).

From the Swedish perspective, as early as in the 18th century, Carl von Linné described cases of goitre in Sweden. The prevalence of goitre has probably varied over the years, depending on the availability of iodine-rich fish.

Table 6.1 Iodine intake and urinary iodine compared to iodine status

Iodine intake µg/day	Iodine in urine µg/L	Iodine status
< 30	< 20	Severe deficiency
30–70	20–49	Moderate deficiency
75–100	50–99	Mild deficiency
150–300	100–199	Optimal intake
300–500	200–299	Slight excess
> 500	> 300	Significant excess

6.2 Thyroid Dysfunction Caused by Excessive Iodine Intake

Table 6.2 Recommended daily iodine intake (WHO)

90 μg	Preschool children < 6 years old
120 μg	School children 6–12 years old
150 μg	Adults
200–250 μg	Pregnant women
200–250 μg	Breastfeeding women

The regions with the highest prevalence of goitre in Sweden have been Dalarna, Värmland, Västernorrland and Gästrikland. In 1920, Axel Höjer, a well-known general director of the Royal Swedish National Board of Health, estimated that 300,000 people in Sweden had goitre, and the total number of cretins was estimated to be as high as 1,000. The Swedish population was at this time close to six million.

In 1924, a pilot project for iodine supplements for school children in Sandviken was successfully implemented. This resulted in the introduction of a public iodination program in Sweden in 1936 through table salt iodination at a level of 10 mg/kg (the Royal Swedish National Board of Health circular 30/1936). In 1960, the dose was increased to 50 mg/kg. Sweden's salt iodination program continues, but noniodized salt is also available.

6.2 Thyroid Dysfunction Caused by Excessive Iodine Intake

High iodine intake can both block and stimulate thyroid hormone production. If a person with a normal thyroid gland consumes, or is in some way exposed to large amounts of iodine, a transient inhibition of thyroid hormone production can be expected. This is known as the Wolff-Chaikoff effect and is counteracted gradually through autoregulation of NIS in the thyroid so that production of the hormone is normalized (see Sect. 2.4.2).

In certain thyroid diseases, e.g. autoimmune thyroiditis, or in the immature thyroid tissue of a foetus, this "escape" mechanism is not always effectuated (see Chap. 2) at long-term exposure to excessive iodine concentrations. This results in a persistent inhibition of follicle cell hormone synthesis and secretion, with the associated risk for development of hypothyroidism.

When a population with a relative iodine deficiency and increased occurrence of nodular goitre increases their iodine intake, this frequently results in the development of autonomous or toxic nodular goitre, i.e. hyperthyroidism. These experiences are well-documented in several regions of the world, including Central America, Tasmania,

Swedish mountain areas, and also in recent years in Denmark, after introduction of the iodination program.

Large quantities of iodine can also trigger or exacerbate latent Graves' hyperthyroidism. This is seen in particular in patients with small iodine reserves.

In patients with nontoxic multinodular goitre, or an autonomous nodule, a high load of iodine via medical preparations can lead to increased hormone synthesis – hyperthyroidism. Normally, thyrotoxicosis is not seen until several weeks after the time of iodine exposure and it is then common that the iodine uptake of the gland remains low. This can also be observed after extended treatment with amiodarone.

The integrity of the thyroid follicles can also be damaged at exposure to large amounts of iodine, resulting in transient leakage of thyroid hormone which appears clinically as thyrotoxicosis. Because the NIS has been made nonfunctional, diagnosis using radionuclides or treatment with radioactive iodine can not be applied in these cases.

Increased iodine intake in a population has different effects depending on the initial status of the population with regard to iodine intake. The incidence of iodine-induced hypothyroidism is higher in countries with high iodine intake, which provides individuals with a large iodine reserve (e.g. USA). A higher prevalence of latent autoimmune thyroiditis is also observed. The opposite is seen in areas with low availability of iodine (e.g. Central Europe), where iodine-induced hyperthyroidism is more common.

6.3 Iodine in Foodstuffs and Medical Preparations

Iodine consumed in food is mainly found in fish and shellfish, eggs and dairy products, and iodized table salt (Table 6.3). Some seaweeds, such as those used in Japanese cooking, contain very large quantities of iodine (about 200,000 µg/meal).

Some substances with very high iodine content and of clinical significance include:
- *X-ray contrast media*   Water-soluble iodine containing contrast media are only retained in the body for a short time, but substantial iodine quantities can be deposited. A study with 200 mL of a water-soluble iodine contrast medium containing 300 mg iodine/mL can give up to 7 mg free iodine. Furthermore, the iodine contrast can undergo deiodination in the body which contributes further to iodide in the blood. An intravenous urography investigation can therefore give rise to iodine-induced thyrotoxicosis, and prevent iodine/technetium uptake in the thyroid follicle for several months. Contrast media used for gallbladder investigation are fat-soluble and therefore remains in the body for even longer.
- *Amiodarone*   An antiarrhythmic agent that contains 37% by weight iodine (amiodarone chloride) and has a half-life of about 100 days. The normal daily dose is 200 mg, which is equivalent to 74 mg iodine (see Chap. 33)
- *Iodine containing preparations*   Preparations for dressing wounds may contain 10–60 mg iodine/compress
- *Algae products* These may contain large amounts of iodine

Table 6.3 Examples of iodine content in food (µg/100 g consumable part)

Lobster	700	Milk	8
Mussels	180	Coffee	7
Salt water fish	40	Cheese	25
Eggs	21	Pineapple	10
Beef	4	Bananas	7
Chicken	0.5	Dried peas	45
Wheat flour	2	Potatoes	1
Tea	30	Rice	1

- *Potassium iodide tablets* Commonly these are 65 mg KI tablets and contain 50 mg iodine. Used to block iodine uptake in diagnostic procedures and as protection against radioactive iodine isotopes in the event of nuclear power plant accidents
- *Iodine solutions for oral use* Iodine–potassium iodide solution; A 5% solution (iodine 5; potassium iodide 10, aq. dest. 85) contains about 2.2 mg iodine per drop (see Chaps. 17 and 24)

6.4 Iodine Blocking

6.4.1 Nuclear Accidents

Iodine administration is recommended in the event of nuclear power plant accidents in order to reduce the uptake of radioactive iodine isotopes in the thyroid (Table 6.4). The mechanism is primarily based on diluting the radioactive iodine with stable iodine. Iodide in the form of potassium iodide (KI) tablets containing about 50 mg iodine is recommended. If treatment is given at the same time as exposure to radioactive iodine, the radioactive uptake can be reduced by about 90%. The protective effect declines rapidly.

Administration of KI will also immediately inhibit the organification of iodine and inhibit the release of hormones from the colloid (Plummer effect). This effect is, however, short-lived. The effect of KI administration therefore decreases quickly and, after a couple of days, radioactive uptake is only reduced by 50%. If administration of excess iodine is continued, downregulation of NIS persists with subsequent continued lower total iodine uptake.

Undesired effects of treatment with KI tablets can constitute a considerable problem. It is important to give KI prophylactically to women, children and adolescents in order to prevent radiation-induced cancer in the thyroid. However, children and the foetus may acquire persistent hypothyroidism through a noneffectuated immature escape. In adults, the advantage of a potassium iodide prophylaxis may be less than the risk of

Table 6.4 Recommended single doses of stable iodine as prophylaxis in the event of a nuclear power plant accident (WHO)

Age	mg KI	mg iodine
Newborn ≤1 month	16	12.5
Children 1 month–3 years	32	25
Children 3–12 years	65	50
Children and adults 12–40 years	130	100

developing an iodine-induced thyroid dysfunction in individuals with a pre-existing thyroid disorder, mostly multinodular goitre.

6.4.2 Radionuclide Investigations and Treatments

Certain nuclear medicine investigations and treatments for organs other than the thyroid make use of a radionuclide bound to a carrier molecule. If the free isotope is taken up by the thyroid, it can be appropriate to block this uptake using iodine prophylaxis. Normally, when the isotopes I-123 or Tc-99^m are used, no iodine prophylaxis is given because these involve gamma radiation with insignificant radiation to the tissue. For diagnostics using the I-131 isotope, iodine prophylaxis can be recommended for people younger than 40. At therapy with I-131 (e.g. I-131 MIBG in neuroblastoma), iodine prophylaxis is always given in advance. The prophylaxis is started at least 4 h before therapy and is given for a couple of days (Table 6.4).

Iodine and the Thyroid Gland

- Iodine deficiency continues to be a global public health problem
- Iodine deficiency can result in TSH stimulation of the thyroid gland and development of goitre
- Iodine is important for normal foetal development, in particular development of the CNS during pregnancy
- Iodine and/or selenium deficiency during pregnancy and in the newborn child can cause a persistent reduction in IQ
- Recommended iodine intake is 150 µg/day in adults
- During pregnancy and lactation the recommended intake is 200–250 µg/day
- High iodine intake can trigger hyperthyroidism in patients with nodular goitre
- High iodine intake can unmask/trigger or exacerbate latent Graves' hyperthyroidism
- An increase in iodine intake will increase the prevalence of autoimmune thyroid disease in the population
- High iodine intake can trigger hypothyroidism in autoimmune thyroiditis
- Administration of peroral KI is used to block the thyroid gland iodine uptake (NIS) to avoid accumulation of radioactivity in the thyroid in the event of a nuclear power plant accident and in certain nuclear medicine investigations/therapies

7 Autoimmunity and the Thyroid Gland

Immunological mechanisms are critical for the occurrence and progression of autoimmune thyroiditis (AIT) and diffuse toxic goitre (Graves' disease), with or without thyroid-associated ophthalmopathy (TAO) (see Chaps. 9 and 18).

As in other autoimmune diseases, the pathophysiological background of the development of autoimmune thyroid disease has not been entirely clarified. It's likely that some individuals have a predisposition which, in conjunction with triggering factors, starts the process. In addition to genetic factors, predisposing factors can include reduced immunological tolerance, which could have arisen during maturation of the immune competent cells in the thymus.

It is thought that autoimmune reactions against the thyroid can develop in various directions. In AIT, the immunological process is dominated be a lymphocyte mediated cell-damaging processes, leading to destruction of follicular cells; in Graves' disease the immunological process is dominated by synthesis and release of antibodies that stimulate the TSH receptor.

7.1 Immunological Background

7.1.1 Antigen-Presenting Cells

Macrophages and dendrite cells are antigen-presenting cells (APCs) that deal with foreign material in the body tissues. The remains of the particles taken up are transported to the surface of the cell to be exposed to immune competent cells, primarily T-lymphocytes, using major histocompatability complex (MHC) molecules (Figs. 7.1 and 7.2).

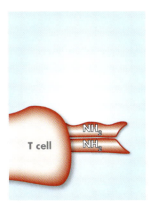

Fig. 7.1 Immune competent T-lymphocyte with specific receptors (NH2) for antigens

E. Nyström, G.E.B. Berg, S.K.G. Jansson, O. Tørring, S.V. Valdemarsson (Eds.),
Thyroid Disease in Adults,
DOI: 10.1007/978-3-642-13262-9_7, © Springer-Verlag Berlin Heidelberg 2011

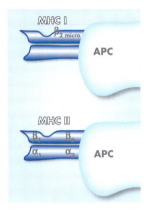

Fig. 7.2 Major histocompatability complexes (MHC I and MHC II) on antigen-presenting cells (APCs)

7.1.2 MHC Molecules
MHC molecules or human leucocyte antigen (HLA) are specific molecules on the surface of the antigen-presenting cells. MHC molecules are proteins whose structures are specific to the individual and are genetically determined. There are two types of MHCs (Fig. 7.2).

MHC I is present in almost all cells with a cell nucleus and binds residues of foreign materials after a relatively extensive degradation in the cell. MHC II is found primarily on APCs and binds to the foreign material being dealt with.

MHCs play a critical role in the exposure of foreign material to immunocompetent cells. The immune system reacts strongly when cells with foreign MHC molecules enter the body, for example, after transplantation.

7.1.3 T and B Lymphocytes
T and B lymphocytes develop from lymphoid stem cells. T cells mature in the thymus and, normally, only T cells that do not react against the body's own material are released into the circulation. T lymphocytes can be divided into two main subgroups, cytotoxic T lymphocytes and helper T lymphocytes. (Natural killer cells comprise another group of lymphocytes.)

Helper T cells can, in turn, differentiate into two distinct subgroups:
- T helper cells type 1, which induce cell-mediated immune reactions through stimulation to development of cytotoxic T lymphocytes; and
- T helper cells type 2, which induce development of B cells to antibody producing plasma cells and, thus, a humoral immunoreaction.

Helper T lymphocytes interact with APCs. T cells have specific external receptors, which can interact with the MHCs, the foreign material transported by the APC to the surface, and the MHC molecule (Fig. 7.1).

7.1.4 Interaction Between T Cells and APC (Simplified Model)
In addition to specific receptors for antigens, T cells have several other external structures that control their interaction with APCs. These external structures are often called cluster determinants (CDs) with a number code (Fig. 7.3).

7.1 Immunological Background

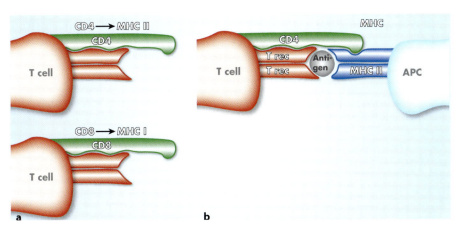

Fig. 7.3 a,b T cells have external membrane bound structures called cluster determinants (CDs), which control their interaction with APCs. CD 4 fits MHC II and CD 8 fits MHC I

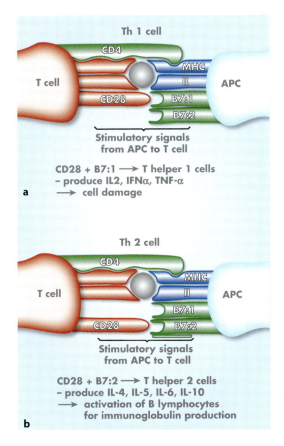

Fig. 7.4 a, b Interaction between T-cells and APCs, which occurs either through B7:1 or B7:2

CD4 is present on the exterior of T helper cells, and specifically fits the MHC II complex. Cells with CD4 are therefore directed to APCs with MHC II.

CD8 is present on cytotoxic T lymphocytes and directs the lymphocytes to APCs with MHC I (Fig. 7.3).

After the T helper cell has bound to the correct APC via the CD4 and MHC the interaction between them must be further regulated. Once again, specific molecules enter the appropriate cells, and regulate the continued interaction between the T helper cell and the APC. One such molecule on T cells is CD28 (Fig. 7.4).

The APC containing MHC II also has molecules on the exterior that can interact with CD28 on the T helper lymphocytes. The molecules on the APCs are called B7 with subgroups B7:1 (Fig. 7.4b) and B7:2 (Fig. 7.4b). Interaction between CD28 and B7:1 results in differentiation of the T helper lymphocyte to a T helper cell type 1 (which mediates cell-mediated immunoreactions), while interaction between CD28 and B7:2 results in differentiation of the T helper lymphocyte to a T helper cell type 2, which mediates humoral immunoreaction (Fig. 7.4).

7.1.5 Cytolytic T Lymphocyte-Associated Antigen 4 (CTLA-4)

After the T helper lymphocyte binds to MHC II on the APC, a specific molecule on the surface of the T cell, cytolytic T lymphocyte-associated antigen 4 (CTLA-4), can be upregulated. CTLA-4 can compete with CD28 for binding to the B7 complex on the APC. CTLA-4 is thought to have a blocking effect and is thus able to inhibit the immunological reaction (Fig. 7.5).

CTLA-4 has received particular attention in the pathophysiology of autoimmune thyroid disease, especially for Graves' disease, because genetic polymorphism of this protein has been demonstrated in some of these patients. A dysfunctional CTLA-4 would thus impair the normal inhibitory effect of this molecule (anergy) on the immune process.

In addition, studies have suggested also other genes outside the HLA-region to be possibly associated to autoimmune thyroiditis and to Graves' disease.

7.1.6 Fas/Fas-L and the Destruction of Cells

Fas is a complex of molecules present on the outer surface of certain cells. Fas-L ligates with Fas. Interaction between Fas-L and Fas results in the activation of a cascade of intracellular reactions with release of caspase among other compounds (Fig. 7.6). This process results in apoptosis (organized cell death).

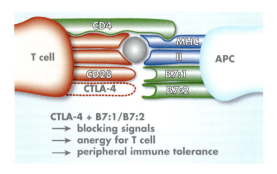

Fig. 7.5 A specific molecule on the T-cell, CTLA-4, can inhibit the immunological reaction

7.2 Autoimmunity

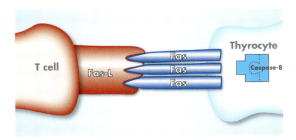

Fig. 7.6 Fas is a complex of molecules present on the outer surface of certain cells. Interaction between Fas-L and Fas results in activation of a cascade of intracellular reactions

Thyrocytes can express Fas. Induction of Fas-L on follicle cells has been discussed as a possible explanation of why the follicle cell is not damaged by lymphocytes.

7.2 Autoimmunity

For unknown reasons, antigen structures in the thyroid are thought to be exposed to APCs in the thyroid. These cells appear to be able to move to regional lymph nodes where exposed antigen will be presented to lymphocytes.

If an immunological tolerance is absent, i.e. lymphocytes are present that can react with the exposed intrinsic antigen, specific T lymphocytes are activated. Genetic polymorphism for CTLA-4 has been mentioned as a possible factor important in allowing the immunological process to proceed.

Cytokines from activated T lymphocytes are thought to subsequently stimulate cells in the thyroid to act as APCs with MHC II. This development could contribute to maintaining and reinforcing the autoimmune process, thereby enabling it to continue even within the thyroid.

7.2.1 Hashimoto or Graves' Disease?

Whether the autoimmune process results in autoimmune thyroiditis or Graves' disease may depend on how the process proceeds after it has been initiated. Basically, the autoimmune reaction can develop in two different directions (Fig. 7.7).

Figure 7.8 outlines a simplified picture of the paths of the immunological process with regard to the thyroid. Depending on genetic and environmental factors, the antigen is exposed in the thyroid. The immunological response involves lymphocyte activation and movement of lymphocytes into the thyroid. It is believed that a specific mechanism then determines the differentiation of the T lymphocytes to either Th1 or Th2 cells.

Induction of T helper type 1 cells involves activation of cytotoxic T cells with cell destruction as a consequence, i.e. development of tissue damage as in autoimmune thyroiditis, Hashimoto's disease or variants of this disorder.

Induction of T helper type 2 cells involves an antibody mediated immune reaction. If these antibodies target the TSH receptor, diffuse toxic goitre (Graves' disease) arises if the effect is stimulation of the receptor (but in rare cases results in hypothyroidism or atrophic thyroiditis if the antibody has a blocking effect on the TSH receptor). It has been suggested that the follicle cell in the thyroid may also develop Fas-L. If this is the case, it may also prevent the cells from being destroyed during the immunological process.

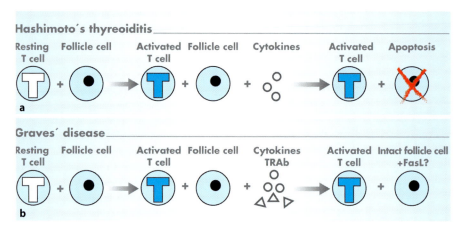

Fig. 7.7 a, b a Activated T cells damage follicle cells **b** Follicle cells avoid apoptosis but are affected by TRAb

7.2.2 Antithyroid Drugs and the Immunological Process

During treatment of Graves' disease with antithyroid drugs, the concentrations of TRAb, TPOAb and TgAb often declines. Infiltration of lymphocytes in the thyroid drops. The relationships between the various lymphocyte populations are re-established. The mechanism of this effect has not been determined. Antithyroid drugs are not considered, however, to have any pronounced immunosuppressive effect. Neither is it proven that the effect is a consequence of the drop in thyroid hormone concentrations during treatment.

One hypothesis is that under the influence of the antithyroid drugs, there is less exposure of follicle cell antigens.

7.3 Predisposing Factors

Factors that initiate and continue the autoimmune process are still unclear. Genetic, endogenous and exogenous factors are considered to be important in the occurrence of autoimmune thyroid disease.

7.3.1 Genetic Predisposition

The importance of genetic factors is supported by the increased prevalence of autoantibodies in relatives of affected patients, and because several members of one family can be affected by autoimmune thyroid disease. In some way, certain changes in the MHC/HLA system are thought to be associated with these diseases. Twin studies have, however, demonstrated a higher occurrence of the disease in siblings than can be explained by the HLA system alone.

Apart from the HLA system, the gene for CTLA-4 (see above) has also been linked to autoimmune thyroid disease, primarily Graves' disease, but also autoimmune

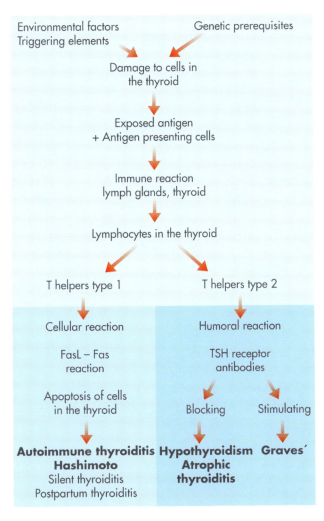

Fig. 7.8 A simplified picture of the paths of the immunological process with regard to the thyroid

thyroiditis and other autoimmune disorders. It is speculated that the polymorphism found for CTLA-4 in Graves' disease lowers the molecule's blocking action so that the attack by the T cells on the APCs proceeds. A significant alteration in the gene for the TSH receptor protein has not yet been demonstrated.

Patients with Turner's syndrome have a slightly higher prevalence of antithyroid antibodies and autoimmune thyroid disease. This could indicate that the X chromosome may be important in the occurrence of autoimmune thyroid disease. The relationship is, however, not clear. An increased presence of thyroid antibodies has also been observed in Down's syndrome.

7.3.2 Other Endogenous Causes

It is possible that oestrogens are of importance in autoimmune thyroid disease because the condition is more prevalent in women and is often seen when oestrogen concentrations vary. Thus, an increased incidence of hypothyroidism is observed in women during and after menopause. Remission of Graves' disease during pregnancy, relapse after pregnancy and postpartum thyroiditis are other examples. The cause of the increased incidence of autoimmune thyroid disease in women and, more specifically, the effect of changes in oestrogen levels has still not been determined.

7.4 Exogenous Factors

7.4.1 Iodine

A high intake of iodine can affect the progression of both Graves' disease and autoimmune thyroiditis. Defective autoregulation of follicle cell iodine management probably plays the most important role for disease progression, but iodine itself may also affect the immunological processes.

Thus, the prevalence of autoimmune thyroiditis is higher in populations with a high intake of iodine than in populations with a low intake. Other data indicate that iodine supplementation in populations with low iodine intake can increase the incidence of thyroiditis.

Several different mechanisms have been proposed. Changed configuration of thyroglobulin could possibly create new antigen epitopes. Another possibility is that TPO-dependent oxidation of supplementary iodide releases oxidative molecules (free acid radicals), which can damage membranes thus exposing antigens. Finally, it has been pointed out that iodine can have direct effects on APCs.

7.4.2 Smoking

Smoking is thought to affect the immunological process so that the risk of developing autoimmune thyroiditis (TPOAb) will decrease, while the risk of getting Graves' disease will increase. Smokers have also been reported to run a higher risk of relapse after treatment with thyrostatic drugs for Graves' disease, especially in men. Furthermore, smoking will increase the risk of ophthalmopathy and will also limit the benefit of medical treatment. This also applies to I-131 treatment. The mechanism has not been completely elucidated. It has been speculated that tissue hypoxia can induce synthesis of glucosamino-glycans, which in turn results in local oedema in the orbit. Another hypothesis is that the thiocyanate in the smoke may have a mild toxic effect.

7.4.3 Stress

Stress and major negative life events have been reported to occur more frequently among people who have Graves' disease. Pathophysiologically, it has been speculated whether an increased activity of the pituitary-adrenal axis can affect the immune system. It must be noted that the cases reported have been subject to extreme disturbances and/or stress.

7.4.4 Infections/Cytokines

It has previously been suggested that Yersinia enterocolitica and coxsackie-B infections could induce autoimmune thyroid disease. Even if this theory is supported by certain findings, the relationship between these infections and occurrence of the disease in the thyroid has not been convincingly confirmed. Neither does it appear that a cross reaction between an antigen associated with one infectious agent and the thyroid plays a role.

Congenital rubella is considered to be associated with an increased incidence of autoimmune hypothyroidism.

An increased prevalence of TPO antibodies is seen in hepatitis C. When treated with interferon, these patients can develop thyroid autoimmunity. Hypothyroidism is most common, but hyperthyroidism can also occur. Pathophysiologically, both thyroiditis and Graves' disease may be observed.

In patients with multiple sclerosis, treatment with monoclonal antibodies against T cells has been found to increase the risk of acquiring Graves' disease. In this patient group treatment with β interferon may be a triggering factor.

7.5 Autoimmune Polyglandular Syndrome

If two autoimmune diseases are found in a patient, the condition is named polyglandular autoimmune syndrome (PAS). Also nonendocrine organs may be damaged by similar autoimmune mechanisms: stomach (atrophic gastritis with lack of cobalamines), intestine (coeliaci), skin (vitliligo, alopecia) and the ovaries (premature menopause).

There are two variants of PAS of which PAS type 1 is less common. The patient is affected early in age and the clinical picture dominated by mucocutane candidadiasis, hypoparathyroidism and primary adrenal insufficiency (Addison's disease), while diabetes-type and thyroid autoimmune disease are less common.

PAS 2 is more common at 1–2 cases/10,000/year. It may be seen early in life, but individuals affected are most often diagnosed at an age of 20–40 years. Autoimmune thyroid disease is dominating and seen in 70–75% of individuals affected. Diabetes type 1 is seen in 50–60%, Addison's disease in 40%, and hypoparathyroidism rarely.

7.6 Immunological Markers in Clinical Work

Antibodies against microsomal thyroid antigen, thyroglobulin and long-acting thyroid stimulating (LATS) factors were previously used as indicators of autoimmunity in Hashimoto's and Graves' disease.

7.6.1 TPO Antibodies

Presence of antibodies against thyroperoxidase, TPOAb, are considered to be the most sensitive marker for autoimmune thyroiditis. TPOAb are detected in about 95% of affected people. TPOAb are also found in about 60% of all patients with Graves' disease. The pathophysiological role of TPOAb have not been clarified but most probably TPOAb does not have a direct causal effect on the immunological process. Thus, newborn babies are not affected by hypothyroidism if TPOAb passes from the mother to child.

TPOAb are often present for a long time in affected patients, but the concentration can slowly drop in hypothyroid patients receiving thyroxine substitution. Women who have TPOAb run an increased risk of spontaneous abortion even if their TSH levels are normal.

An increased occurrence of antibodies against thyroglobulin, TgAb, are also seen in autoimmune thyroiditis. These antibodies are considered to be less specific for autoimmune thyroid disease.

7.6.2 TSH Receptor Antibodies

The TSH receptor is the target for stimulating antibodies, TRAb, in Graves' disease. TRAb can be demonstrated in nearly all patients with this disease. Blocking antibodies directed against the TSH receptor may also occur and cause hypothyroidism. In some patients, switching between blocking and stimulating TRAb can explain why the patient may first be affected with hypothyroidism and later by hyperthyroidism due to Graves' disease, or vice versa.

Thus in contrast to TPOAb, TRAb have a causal effect with resultant hyper- or hypothyroidism depending on their stimulating or blocking properties.

If a woman is affected by Graves' disease during pregnancy and has elevated TRAb levels, or if she has persistent elevated TRAb concentrations after previous treatment for Graves' disease (surgery or I-131), there is a risk that the TRAb will pass from the placenta to the foetus. The foetal thyroid can then be stimulated (or blocked) by transferred antibodies with resultant foetal/neonatal hyperthyroidism (or hypothyroidism if the antibodies are blocking). Routinely used methods for determining TRAb will not distinguish between stimulating or blocking antibodies.

A decrease in the concentration of TRAb may indicate decreasing immunological activity of the disease and determination of TRAb can thus be used as an indicator of remission (and withdrawal of antithyroid drugs). This applies in many cases, but not all.

7.6.3 Clinical Applications

Graves' disease In Graves' disease, antibodies are produced that react with the TSH receptors. This causes stimulation of the follicle cells with resultant hyperthyroidism. Antibodies against TSH receptors (TRAb) can be demonstrated by routine analyses. This can be used to determine the cause of a patient's hyperthyroidism.

Autoimmune thyroiditis In autoimmune thyroiditis, the immunological reaction causes damage to the follicle cells with resultant hypothyroidism. There is no known causal antibody. Demonstration of antibodies against thyroperoxidase (TPOAb) are a marker for this process. Depending on the progression of the immunological process, autoimmune thyroiditis can present clinically as Hashimoto's disease, atrophy of the thyroid, silent thyroiditis, postpartum thyroiditis and focal thyroiditis.

Thyroid-associated ophthalmopathy (TAO) In spite of intensive research, it has not been possible to demonstrate that any single antibody is the cause of TAO. The occurrence of TSH receptors in the orbital tissues does support the hypothesis of concomitant immunological reactivity against the thyroid and the orbital tissue. TAO can be seen in autoimmune thyroiditis, but this is relatively rare. Thyroid-associated ophthalmopathy is discussed in Chap. 19.

Thyroid acropachy and pretibial myxoedema These are other unusual extrathyroidal manifestations, which also probably have an immunological background, and which are in practice only seen in patients who also have TAO.

7.7 Treatment Strategy

7.7.1 Autoimmune Thyroiditis

A specific treatment of the immunological process behind autoimmune thyroiditis is of limited value because TPOAb are not thought to have a direct effect. The occurrence of TPOAb in autoimmune thyroiditis is therefore not given any special attention except for diagnostic use. So far, treatment targets the subsequent thyroid dysfunction that may affect these patients.

7.7.2 Graves' Disease

The choice of treatment in Graves' disease has important effects on the concentration of TRAb (Fig. 18.5). In patients whose disease is well-controlled with thyrostatic drugs, a drop in TRAb is often observed. Radioiodine treatment is followed by a clear and long-term (months or years) increase in these antibodies.

In some patients, onset or progression of TAO is observed after treatment with radioiodine (Fig. 7.9). Development or exacerbation of TAO is seen in particular in patients with highly active disease, i.e. high T3 levels at disease onset. The risk of deterioration of TAO is also thought to apply to a patient who, in spite of treatment with antithyroid drugs and thyroxine, have a disease which is not under control and therefore fluctuating thyroid hormone levels. The relationship between the increase in TRAb and development of thyroid-associated ophthalmopathy is, however, unclear.

After surgical intervention with subtotal thyroidectomy, TRAb levels often drops. Individual progression varies somewhat more than the gradual reduction in TRAb seen in well-controlled patients on medical therapy. The possibility to reduce the risk of thyroid-associated ophthalmopathy after total thyroidectomy in Graves' disease has not been clearly determined.

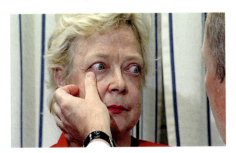

Fig. 7.9 This figure illustrates clinical investigation of moderate TAO

7.7.3 Pregnancy

During pregnancy, the concentration of both TPOAb and TRAb will decrease, often to increase again after delivery. This explains why autoimmune diseases in the thyroid often abate in intensity during pregnancy (both thyroiditis and Graves' disease) only to be reactivated some months after giving birth with postpartum thyroiditis or onset/exacerbation of the Graves' type of hyperthyroidism. High concentrations of TPOAb in the mother in the later stage of pregnancy entails an increased risk of postpartum thyroiditis (see Chap. 31).

Autoimmunity and the Thyroid Gland

- Immunological reactions are considered to cause autoimmune thyroiditis and Graves' disease with or without TAO
- Neither the triggering factors nor the exact immunological mechanisms have been mapped in detail
- Development of thyroid disease is caused by both cytotoxic and antibody-mediated effects
- TPOAb are seen typically in autoimmune thyroiditis and is believed to reflect the autoimmune process, but not to have a direct causal effect on the reaction. On the other hand, high concentrations of TPOAb in an euthyroid patient, indicates an increased risk of later development of hypothyroidism
- TRAb have a causal function in the occurrence of hyperthyroidism in Graves' disease. In unusual cases, TRAb can exhibit blocking properties and cause atrophy of the thyroid and hypothyroidism
- In Graves' disease, the immunological reaction is dominated by the formation of antibodies which stimulates the TSH receptors and thus cause hyperthyroidism
- The mechanism of the inflammatory reaction in TAO has not been clarified

8 Growth Regulation of the Thyroid Gland

Homeostasis of thyroid gland tissue is controlled by many factors (Table 8.1). Thyroid stimulating hormone (TSH) from the pituitary is the most well-known factor that has a direct and indirect effect on the function and growth of the thyrocytes. Other examples of growth stimulating factors are epidermal growth factor (EGF), transforming growth factor α (TGF-α), insulin like growth factor (IGF), fibroblast growth factor (FGF), hepatocyte growth factor (HGF), platelet-derived growth factor (PDGF) and the growth inhibiting transforming growth factor β (TGF-β). In addition there are factors that regulate cell death (apoptosis) in the thyroid gland. Furthermore, the availability of iodine has a significant effect on homeostasis. All of these factors can affect thyroid tissue volume and its ability to meet the requirements of the body.

Locally, growth can be affected by disturbances within the various growth regulating mechanisms. Genetic events and/or specific mutations can result in development of neoplasms in the thyroid.

Growth regulation in the thyroid is a complicated and intricate network of mechanisms of which much is known, but many gaps still remain in understanding this complex interaction.

Table 8.1 Growth regulating factors

Factor	Signal system	Effect
TSH	Cyclic AMP	Stimulates function and probably growth
EGF	Tyrosine kinases	Stimulates
TGF-α	Tyrosine kinases	Stimulates
IGF-I	Tyrosine kinases	Stimulates
FGF	Tyrosine kinases	Stimulates
HGF	Tyrosine kinases	Stimulates
PDGF	Tyrosine kinases	Stimulates
TGF-β	Tyrosine kinases	Inhibits

E. Nyström, G.E.B. Berg, S.K.G. Jansson, O. Törring, S.V. Valdemarsson (Eds.),
Thyroid Disease in Adults,
DOI: 10.1007/978-3-642-13262-9_8, © Springer-Verlag Berlin Heidelberg 2011

8.1 TSH

Traditionally, TSH has been considered to be the primary stimulating factor for thyroid function. Thyrocytes are stimulated by the binding of TSH to a specific receptor on the surface of the thyrocyte (TSH-R). Activation of TSH-R results in an increased cellular content of cyclic AMP, which acts as a second messenger for the effects of TSH. However, it has also been demonstrated that TSH, via activation of TSH-R, will give an increased phosphatidyl inositol turnover, which also activates intracellular signal systems.

TSH-R is a G-protein coupled receptor with seven membrane transitions (Fig. 2.6). For a long time, TSH has been considered a trophic pituitary hormone which regulates both function and growth in the thyroid. It has been established that TSH activates the function of the thyrocytes. On the other hand, the extent to which TSH has growth promoting effects in the human thyroid is more controversial. It appears that there are synergy effects between TSH and EGF, for example, on thyroid cell proliferation in in vitro studies. Furthermore, both activating and inactivating mutations have been demonstrated in TSH-R. Activating mutations have been demonstrated in patients with autonomous thyroid adenoma.

8.2 Hyperplasia and Goitre

The development of hyperplastic, lumpy areas with increasing age is normal. Here, the gland contains nodular areas in which the tissue becomes soft and often gelatinous. A cross-section of a nodular enlarged thyroid gland can be granulated and, histologically, hyperplasia is observed. There is often a large variation in the size of the follicles with areas with increased cell density. Such hyperplastic follicles exhibit a heterogeneous picture of functional characteristics and growth potential.

There appears to be a large variation between individual thyrocytes in the same follicle. The thyrocytes, which have an ability for faster growth, are kept together in a segment of the follicle cell wall, and give rise to a locally increased growth potential that is inherited from the individual cell to surrounding cells in the follicle wall.

A variety of mechanisms have been suggested to explain the occurrence of nodular formations in a multinodular goitre:
- Cells with rapid growth are kept together and constitute growth centres in the follicles.
- A somatic mutation can be expressed in different generations of thyrocytes, which can result in local or regional growth in the gland.
- The presence of connective tissue zones, necrosis and haemorrhage in growing thyroid glands can lead to an altered structure of the gland.

Further growth stimulation, such as increased TSH release during iodine deficiency and presence of immunoglobulins or other growth stimulating factors, will induce hyperplasia and growth of tissue resulting in the development of goitre. Theories have been proposed that certain thyrocytes develop a reduced sensitivity for TSH. The opposite, increased sensitivity for TSH or other growth factors, can arise through mutations that change the growth rate. Increased growth can also arise through defect apoptosis.

8.3 Neoplasms and Tumours

Cell replication is controlled by genes and if these genes are subjected to mutation, this can result in uncontrolled cell division. These mutated genes are called oncogenes. Tumour suppressor genes are genes that normally function as brakes on uncontrolled growth. Activation of oncogenes and/or loss of tumour suppressor genes result in tumour development.

Most neoplasms in the thyroid, both the highly common benign and the less common malignant tumours, normally have a monoclonal origin, which indicates a single underlying genetic event as the initial cause. A number of different genetic changes have been demonstrated in human thyroid gland tumours (Fig. 8.1).

Chapter 8: Growth Regulation of the Thyroid Gland

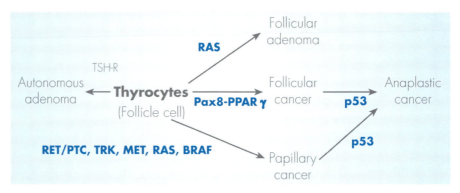

Fig. 8.1 Schematic representation of different genes associated with tumour development in case of genetic mutation events

A single mutation may act as the triggering pathophysiological mechanism. Subsequent mutations and other genetic events can be additive, which results in a changed growth pattern in the tumour. The information stored in the genetic code can affect the production of proteins necessary for cellular function.

Growth factors often exert their effect via membrane bound receptors which, at activation, results in an intracellular signal to the cell nucleus and normally stimulated growth. Oncogenes can cause a change in the external receptor protein, which in turn results in an altered signal to the cell nucleus. A common family of such external receptors are tyrosine kinase receptors, which can be altered through mutations in the RET gene, the TRK gene or the MET gene, for example. Other oncogenes include the family of RAS genes or point mutations in the BRAF gene. A hybrid gene formed from two genes has been demonstrated in follicular thyroid carcinoma, the fusion gene (PAX 8-PPAR g 1).

The purpose of the p53 gene, popularly called the guardian of the genome, is to regulate apoptosis. A mutation affecting the p53 gene can result in defect apoptosis and tumour growth, which has been demonstrated in poorly differentiated and anaplastic tumours.

Growth Factors

- Several different growth factors control the growth of the thyroid
- The exact interaction between, and significance of, the various growth regulating factors in the thyroid are not fully understood
- In addition to promoting growth, TSH also regulates thyroid hormone production
- Certain follicle cells in the thyroid are thought to have higher growth rates than others in the formation of goitre
- Activation of oncogenes and/or inhibition of tumour suppressor genes results in tumour development

9 Thyroiditis and Pathogenesis

9.1 Thyroiditis

Thyroiditis is a collective name for several inflammatory conditions in the thyroid. In most cases, thyroiditis is caused by autoimmune mechanisms as discussed in Chap. 7. Subacute thyroiditis, which is thought to be triggered by a viral infection, is dealt with in Chap. 26. Bacterial infections of the thyroid are rare. Other causes of inflammatory reaction in the thyroid include treatment with I-131, which is sometimes associated with an inflammatory-like reaction, and external trauma to the thyroid. In some instances, medicines can cause thyroiditis.

When managing patients with thyroiditis, it is essential to clarify if the cause is autoimmune, since these patients are at risk of developing permanent hypothyroidism.

A common consequence of several forms of thyroiditis is an inflammatory reaction effect on the integrity of the follicle structure. The follicle epithelial cells connection points, the tight junctions, can be damaged so that thyroglobulin and stored hormone leaks out into the blood. The increase in serum thyroid hormone levels may give symptoms of thyrotoxicosis. When the inflammatory reaction abates, the hormone leakage drops. This could be the result of a phase with a diminished hormone production, partly due to damage of the follicle and partly due to persistent inhibition of TSH secretion after the toxic phase.

The clinical progression, as well as the length and intensity of the various phases, differs with various forms of thyroiditis (Fig. 9.1). As mentioned previously, the phase with hypothyroidism may persist, primarily in autoimmune thyroiditis, while in other types of thyroiditis the thyroid generally resumes hormone production.

Many forms of thyroiditis have been classified using terms that focus more on the process of the disease than the underlying etiology, such as *destruction thyroiditis* or *biphasic thyroiditis*.

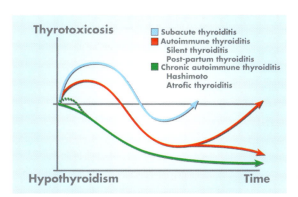

Fig. 9.1 Schematic representation of progression with time for various types of thyroiditis

E. Nyström, G.E.B. Berg, S.K.G. Jansson, O. Törring, S.V. Valdemarsson (Eds.),
Thyroid Disease in Adults,
DOI: 10.1007/978-3-642-13262-9_9, © Springer-Verlag Berlin Heidelberg 2011

9.2 Autoimmune Thyroiditis

The term autoimmune thyroiditis covers the following forms with a common etiology (see also Table 9.1, 9.2):
- Chronic autoimmune thyroiditis – Hashimoto's disease (with goitre)
- Atrophic thyroiditis (without goitre)
- Silent thyroiditis (painless thyroiditis)
- Postpartum thyroiditis
- Juvenile thyroiditis
- Focal thyroiditis

In addition, local areas of autoimmune inflammatory reactions are found in the thyroid in Graves' disease, the other dominating autoimmune form of thyroid disease in which antibodies against the TSH receptor cause hyperthyroidism (see Chap. 18).

The diagnosis of autoimmune thyroiditis is founded on clinical examination and the presence of antibodies against thyroperoxidase (TPOAb). Cytologic investigations will show an inflammatory reaction with enrichment of lymphocytes (lymphocytic thyroiditis is therefore another name for autoimmune thyroiditis).

TPOAb should primarily be determined when autoimmune thyroiditis is suspected. Most analytical methods for TPOAb demonstrates antibodies in around 95% of patients with autoimmune thyroiditis. Analysis of antibodies against thyroglobulin, TgAb, have lower sensitivity (see Chaps. 3 and 7) and is now rarely used in the diagnosis of autoimmune thyroid disease.

TPOAb can be demonstrated in a relatively high proportion of the population. In iodine-replete nations like Sweden, the prevalence in the female population is between 15 and 20%. The presence of TPOAb or lymphocyte infiltration in the thyroid does not necessarily entail a risk of clinical disease in the form of hypothyroidism. Nonetheless, TPOAb should be considered a risk factor for the development of hypothyroidism.

It should be pointed out that TPOAb can be demonstrated in around 60% of patients with Graves' disease; in these patients this finding most probably reflects a general expression of the autoimmune process against the thyroid.

The predisposition for autoimmune thyroid disease can be expressed in different ways within a family – some members develop autoimmune thyroiditis while others develop Graves' disease. As with several other diseases of the thyroid, there is a female predominance (see Chap. 27).

9.2.1 Hashimoto's Disease

Hashimoto's disease, chronic autoimmune thyroiditis with goitre, was described in 1912 in four patients (struma lymphomatosa). The enlarged thyroid gland is characterized by a pronounced lymphocyte infiltration, which generally affects the whole gland or sometimes one lobe more than the other. The lymphocyte infiltration is occasionally very dense, and forms reaction centres in about half of the cases (Fig. 9.2). Typically, atrophy of the follicle epithelium and development of fibrosis in the thyroid are observed. Uniform enlargement of the thyroid, diffuse goitre, is characteristic, as is development of hypothyroidism.

Sometimes at an early stage of the disease, a brief toxic phase is observed in the patient known as Hashitoxicosis. This is most probably caused by a leakage of stored

Table 9.1 Autoimmune mechanisms for thyroiditis (inflammation in the thyroid gland)

Type	Cause	Clinical development	Diagnostic tests (except for TSH, T4 and T3)	Therapy
Hashimoto	Infiltration of lymphocytes, inflammatory permanent effects	Hypothyroidism Goitre Chronic	TPOAb Cytology	Thyroxine
Atrophic	Inflammation resulting in apoptosis	Hypothyroidism Atrophic gland Chronic	TPOAb Blocking TRAb (rare)	Thyroxine
Silent (painless)	Transient inflammatory effects	Biphasic progression* with or without remission	TPOAb Cytology Scintigraphy/ measurement of uptake	Must be followed! Risk of permanent hypothyroidism Thyroxine as required
Postpartum	Transient inflammatory effects within 12 months after giving birth	Biphasic progression* with or without remission	TPOAb Cytology	Must be followed! Risk of permanent hypothyroidism Thyroxine as required
Focal	Limited area with lymphocyte infiltration	Thyroid dysfunction or goitre does not need to be present	TPOAb Cytology and histopathology	Must be followed! Thyroxine as required
Medicine-induced Interferon Amiodarone Iodine	Demasking of latent autoimmune thyroid disease	Varying progression	TPOAb, TRAb Scintigraphy/ measurement of I-131 uptake	Individualized

*Biphasic progression: initially a toxic phase followed by a hypothyroid phase

Chapter 9: Thyroiditis and Pathogenesis

Table 9.2 Other triggering factors for thyroiditis

Type	Cause	Clinical development	Diagnostic tests (except for TSH, T4 and T3)	Therapy
Subacute: De Quervain Granulomatous (painful)	Thought to be associated with virus. Intense inflammatory reaction – often transient	Goitre Local tender Pain on swallowing Fever Biphasic progression* with remission in 95%	SR/CRP, LPK Cytology Scintigraphy/ measurement of uptake	Beta blockers NSAID Glucorticoids if severe symptoms If hypothyroid: Thyroxine (in 5% permanent)
Acute bacterial	Gram positive most common	Fever/general signs of infection Local inflammation/ abscess Normally euthyroidism	SR/CRP, LPK Fine-needle biopsy for cytology and culture	Antibiotics or drainage
Radiation-induced after treatment with radioiodine	Cell damage Autoimmune reaction	Biphasic progression* with or without remission	Scintigraphy/ measurement of uptake TRAb, if necessary	Beta blockers Must be followed! Risk of permanent hypothyroidism Thyroxine as required
Radiation-induced after external radiation upon the neck	Cell damage and/ or autoimmune reaction	Slow development of hypothyroidism over several years	Medical history radiation treatment TPOAb, if necessary	Thyroxine
Iodine-induced	Cell damage and/or autoimmune reaction (See above under medicines)	Biphasic progression* with or without remission	Medical history iodine exposure TPOAb, TRAb Scintigraphy/ measurement of uptake	Iodine withdrawal Must be followed! Risk of hyper/ hypothyroidism
Amiodarone	Cell damage	Varying progression	TPOAb, TRAb Scintigraphy/ measurement of I-131 uptake Ultrasound Doppler	Individualized
Trauma	Cell damage due to external violence against the gland	Biphasic progression* with remission	Medical history course of events	Beta blockers, if necessary
Riedel's thyroiditis	Unclear	Hypothyroidism Hard goitre Extrathyroidal fibrotisation	Biopsy for histological diagnosis	Thyroxine Glucocorticoids Tamoxifen

*Biphasic progression: initially a toxic phase followed by a hypothyroid phase

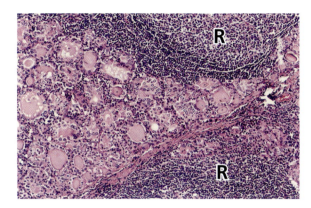

Fig. 9.2 Hashimoto's thyroiditis. The cross-section reveals parts of the reaction centres (R) and diffuse interfollicular lymphocyte infiltration in between

thyroxine from the follicles, as discussed at the beginning of this chapter. In certain cases, receptor-stimulating antibodies can occur.

As in other autoimmune processes, it is unclear what triggers the immunological process in Hashimoto's disease. Typically, TPOAb are detected but also antibodies against other antigens, such as the thyroglobulin molecule.

Symptoms are mostly dominated by an enlarged thyroid gland, with loss of hormone production. Hypothyroidism will sooner or later affect many of these patients. The thyroid is normally more or less diffusely enlarged with a firm consistency. However, there are some cases which present with a more pronounced inflammation and fibrotic changes which make the thyroid irregularly enlarged and uneven, and sometimes with firm/hard areas in the gland.

Diagnosis and treatment are discussed in Chap. 25.

9.2.2 Atrophic Autoimmune Thyroiditis

This manifestation of autoimmune thyroiditis, chronic autoimmune thyroiditis without goitre, is also known as idiopathic hypothyroidism or atrophic Hashimoto thyroiditis, and was previously referred to as primary myxoedema.

The association with Hashimoto's disease indicates that atrophic autoimmune thyroiditis could be considered as a final stage of Hashimoto's thyroiditis, where changes in the thyroid structure had not been noticed earlier. In this type of thyroiditis, there is an early onset of apoptosis and fibrotisation.

It is not clear why the autoimmune process in the thyroid in certain cases presents with goitre and gradual loss of follicle function and in other cases with atrophy. Probably, the interaction between various types of cytokines, lymphocytes and thyroid cells is of importance.

It is not unusual that TSH receptor antibodies are detected in patients with atrophic autoimmune thyroiditis. In these patients, the histological picture is also characterized by fibrosis and lymphocyte infiltration, as is found in Hashimoto's disease.

9.2.3 Silent Thyroiditis and Postpartum Thyroiditis

Silent thyroiditis is a more acute form of autoimmune thyroiditis, with a probably identical variant, postpartum thyroiditis, occurring in the months after giving birth.

Chapter 9: Thyroiditis and Pathogenesis

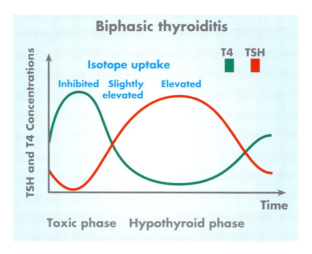

Fig. 9.3 Schematic representation of progression with time for thyroiditis

Clinically, both conditions are characterized by an initial toxic phase due to a leakage of thyroid hormones followed by a hypothyroid phase (see Sect. 9.1 and Fig. 9.3). Silent thyroiditis is also described in the literature as painless thyroiditis.

During the initial toxic phase, the patient can experience mild symptoms which spontaneously remit only to be followed by a phase with hypothyroidism. If the patient is first diagnosed in the later part of the disease progression, with signs of hypothyroidism, information on earlier transient toxic symptoms can be the guide to the correct diagnosis.

In contrast to autoimmune thyroiditis with goitre (Hashimoto's disease) or autoimmune atrophic thyroiditis, the inflammatory process in silent thyroiditis will often recede for unknown reasons. Thus, up to 50–70% of these patients regain normal thyroid function and are euthyroid with no need for thyroxine substitution. Because of the autoimmune etiology, these patients do, however, run the risk of later developing permanent hypothyroidism.

In these forms of thyroiditis, the thyroid is often slightly enlarged with a slightly increased consistency at palpation. Serum inflammatory indicators are normal or only slightly elevated.

TPOAb are demonstrated in most cases and indicate the autoimmune etiology. During the toxic phase, determination of TRAb will discriminate between silent/postpartum thyroiditis and Graves' disease. The progression of the disease (a short toxic phase in silent/postpartum thyroiditis) will also support a correct diagnosis. Further diagnostic aspects and treatment are discussed in Chap. 25.

High levels of TPOAb during later stages of pregnancy indicate a risk of increased autoimmune disease activity after delivery, postpartum thyroiditis, which is discussed in more detail in Chap. 31.

9.2.4 Juvenile Thyroiditis

A diffuse thyroid enlargement is occasionally seen in adolescents. In geographic regions without iodine deficiency the most common cause is lymphocytic infiltration, Hashimoto's disease. It is important in these cases to conduct basal biochemical tests with determination of thyroid function and TPOAb, particularly if thyroid disease is present in other members of the family (see Chap. 32).

9.2.5 Focal Thyroiditis

Lymphocyte infiltration can be limited to certain local areas in the thyroid, which is known as focal thyroiditis. The prevalence in the female population is around 15–20%.

Areas with focal infiltration of lymphocytes are often found upon microscopic examination of the thyroid gland and also after Graves' disease surgery.

Occasionally, a pronounced accumulation of lymphocytes in the thyroid is observed during histological examination of tissue from the thyroid after surgery for other reasons, such as multinodular goitre. This should alert the physician/surgeon that the patient may also have autoimmune thyroid disease with an increased risk of developing hypothyroidism (see also Chap. 25).

9.2.6 Steroid-Sensitive Encephalopathy Associated with Autoimmune Thyroiditis

This condition has previously been called Hashimoto's encephalopathy, but in recent years, the term steroid-sensitive encephalopathy associated with autoimmune thyroiditis has been proposed. The association with thyroid disease is suggested by the presence of TPOAb. However, the patient does not necessarily present with clinical hypothyroidism or increased TSH. It is not established if this really is an expression of Hashimoto's disease or a condition with a completely different etiology.

Two forms of this uncommon condition have been described: one with acute neurological symptoms such as seizures and stroke-like signs similar to that in vasculitis, and one with a more chronic onset of disturbances with effects on mental condition, confusion and even coma. The symptoms most commonly reported are tremor, temporary aphasia, myoclonia, effects on gait, cramps and sleep disturbance. Signs of inflammation are present in cerebrospinal fluid in about 25%. High cerebrospinal fluid concentration and abnormal electroencephalographic findings are seen in 78% and 98%, respectively. The condition is reported to respond to treatment with glucocorticosteroids.

This encephalopathy must be distinguished from the severe mental disturbance, myxoedema madness, which can be seen in severe hypothyroidism.

9.3 Other Triggering Factors for Thyroiditis

9.3.1 Subacute Thyroiditis (de Quervain's Disease)

Subacute thyroiditis, sometimes known as giant-cell thyroiditis or granulomatous thyroiditis is, with regard to the thyroid dysfunction, similar in its clinical appearance to silent autoimmune thyroiditis. The clinical picture is, however, much more aggressive with a painful thyroid gland and a pronounced inflammatory reaction with fever and elevated inflammatory parameters such as C-reactive protein or erythrocyte sedimentation rate. The condition differs pathophysiologically from autoimmune silent/postpartum thyroiditis and is probably associated with a viral infection. Subacute thyroiditis is discussed in Chap. 26.

9.3.2 Iatrogenic Thyroiditis

Some medicines affect the function of the thyroid by inducing an inflammatory process with an increase in TPOAb or through a tissue reaction that is reminiscent of various forms of autoimmune thyroiditis or subacute thyroiditis. This applies, for example, to amiodarone (see Chap. 33).

During treatment with interferon, for instance for hepatitis C, an exacerbation of hypothyroidism or hyperthyroidism may be observed. An inflammatory reaction similar to that in autoimmune thyroiditis is seen and also occasionally hyperthyroidism similar to that in Graves' disease with increased uptake of isotope in the thyroid.

9.3.3 Radiation-Induced Thyroiditis

Radiation-induced thyroiditis can occur 4–12 weeks after radioiodine treatment. The condition should be distinguished from the acute radiation reaction in the thyroid which appears within a week as a result of the direct radiation effects of the treatment.

The process is often long lasting, sometimes several weeks, with leakage of hormone from the thyroid and thus mild thyrotoxic symptoms in the patient. In most cases, the condition eventually progresses relatively quickly to permanent hypothyroidism. Local symptoms from the thyroid are often scarce. During the phase with hormone leakage and toxic symptoms, I-131 uptake tests will give low values and scintigraphy show low uptake. During this period, the patients may require symptomatic treatment with beta blockers.

External radiation treatment can also have an effect on the healthy thyroid tissue. Up to 40% of patients who receive external radiation treatment for tumours in the region of the neck, develop hypothyroidism after about 2 years. Patients with autoimmune thyroiditis may presumably have an increased risk of decreased thyroid function after external radiation treatment in the thyroid region (see Chap. 25).

9.3.4 Trauma-Induced Thyroiditis

Direct trauma to the thyroid can, in certain cases, trigger an inflammatory reaction in the thyroid. This can occur, for example, in traffic accidents when a seat belt is tightened and pressed against the thyroid (seat belt thyroiditis).

After surgery for primary hyperparathyroidism, a transient thyrotoxicosis has been observed in some patients. However, a definitive relationship to the surgical trauma has not been demonstrated. Patients with autonomous areas in the thyroid, multinodular goitre, are thought to have a higher risk of being affected. This reaction spontaneously regresses after a few weeks.

9.3.5 Riedel Thyroiditis

In 1896, a chronic sclerosing form of thyroiditis was described. This is an extremely rare disease, mostly affecting middle-aged people. It is slightly more common among men than women. The disease is dominated by extensive fibrosis in the thyroid and adjacent structures.

The progression of the disease can vary with continuous or intermittent course. Either the entire thyroid or parts of it are affected by fibrosis. In spite of this, the follicles can remain intact, which is the reason why hypothyroidism does not occur in more than 30–50% of the cases.

The symptoms are dominated by a local, progressive fibrosis. The thyroid can acquire a very firm consistency. The inflammation can attack surrounding tissue, such as the oesophagus, trachea, the parathyroids and blood vessels. This will cause problems such as tautness, pain, swallowing and breathing problems as well as other symptoms. Clinically, the condition can be difficult to distinguish from a malignant condition in the thyroid. Sometimes histology may mimic a variant of anaplastic thyroid cancer.

The cause is unknown. TPOAb have been reported in about 2/3 of the patients, which could indicate autoimmune pathogenesis. Eosinophils may be present in the tissues. Inflammatory markers are often normal. Biopsy may be necessary to make a definite diagnosis.

Treatment depends on which symptoms are dominant. Glucocortico-steroids in relatively high doses, e.g. 60–100 mg prednisolone initially, have been tried and reported to give good effect in some cases, probably in patients with ongoing active inflammation. In cases that do not react to glucocorticosteroids treatment, the oestrogen antagonist tamoxifen has been tried, which, via its effects on growth factors, should inhibit proliferation of fibroblasts.

Substitution with thyroxine is given if hypothyroidism is diagnosed. This will not, however, affect the progression of the disease. Surgical resection may be necessary if symptoms of compression are present.

9.3.6 Acute Bacterial Thyroiditis

Even though the thyroid is well-vascularised, it is seldom the site of infections by bacteria or fungi. It is believed that high blood flow is a contributing factor, as well as iodine content and natural encapsulation against the environment.

If the normal anatomical boundaries are defective, such as in persistent open paths from the embryonal development of the thyroid, the risk of bacterial infection can be greater. Entry points to the thyroid from the pharyngeal pouches, thyroglossal duct or the piriform sinus in the neck, are thought to be possible reasons why focal bacterial thyroiditis may occur. These problems can sometimes not be resolved without surgical intervention.

Hematogenous spread is, however, considered to be the most common cause in these rarely occurring infections in the thyroid. Cystic processes can comprise a focal basis. Immunosuppressed patients are a risk group (see also Chap. 25).

Chapter 9: Thyroiditis and Pathogenesis

Thyroiditis – Pathogenesis

- Inflammatory conditions in the thyroid, thyroiditis, can have many different causes, autoimmune or nonautoimmune
- An initial phase with leakage of hormone from the thyroid and toxic symptoms is common for many forms of thyroiditis, which can later result in hypothyroidism and can be permanent if the cause is autoimmune
- In the initial toxic phase with inflammation, the follicle cells do not take up iodine, which explains why during I-131 uptake tests, low iodine uptake is observed. This can be used for diagnosis in ambiguous cases
- Autoimmune thyroiditis can present with different clinical pictures which, in the short or long term, all involve a risk of permanent hypothyroidism
- Among nonautoimmune causes of thyroiditis, subacute thyroiditis is common with a typical biphasic course including a pronounced toxic phase, but rarely permanent hypothyroidism

10 Causes of Hypothyroidism

Globally, deficiency of iodine and the often concomitant deficiency of selenium are major causes of hypothyroidism in adults. In this wider perspective, the main focus is on the effects of iodine deficiency during pregnancy, both for the mother and child. Iodine deficiency and the significance of certain foodstuffs which affect iodine uptake, goitrogens, are discussed separately (see Chaps. 6 and 33).

Hypothyroidism can exist at birth, congenital hypothyroidism, due to effects on foetal development. Because of the potentially serious consequences of undiagnosed congenital hypothyroidism, TSH is analysed in newborns in most countries.

10.1 Primary Hypothyroidism and Chronic Autoimmune Thyroiditis

When a previously healthy adult falls ill with primary hypothyroidism, the cause is nearly always an autoimmune process. Autoimmune thyroid disease is more common in areas with high iodine intake and the prevalence of autoimmune hypothyroidism increases in a country after introduction of iodine supplementation.

10.2 Epidemiology

The risk of developing hypothyroidism is 4–8 times higher for women than men. It is particularly high in the postpartum period (see Chap. 31) and during menopause, after which the risk increases with increasing age (Fig. 10.1). The prevalence of diagnosed hypothyroidism in this latter group is 2–3%. The prevalence of undiagnosed hypothyroidism in the female population is probably relatively high (around 0.5%). According to the literature, the incidence of hypothyroidism is 350/100,000/year in woman and 80/100,000/year in men.

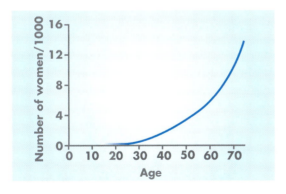

Fig. 10.1 Annual risk for hypothyroidism

E. Nyström, G.E.B. Berg, S.K.G. Jansson, O. Törring, S.V. Valdemarsson (Eds.),
Thyroid Disease in Adults,
DOI: 10.1007/978-3-642-13262-9_10, © Springer-Verlag Berlin Heidelberg 2011

Hypothyroidism even occurs in dogs, and it is estimated that in Sweden several thousand of our four-footed friends receive thyroxine. Because of their rapid metabolism, their daily dose is about 4–5 times higher than that for humans.

10.3 Hypothyroidism After Treatment for Hyperthyroidism

Autoimmune hyperthyroidism and hypothyroidism are closely related pathological conditions, and about 15% of patients with toxic diffuse goitre who have been treated with antithyroid drugs develop persistent hypothyroidism after the thyrotoxic phase is over. This may occur within a few years or after a much longer period.

Patients who undergo surgery for hyperthyroidism caused by Graves' disease or toxic multinodular goitre usually have such extensive resection of the thyroid that they intentionally become hypothyroid postoperatively. The reason for more extensive surgery such as total thyroidectomy, is to reduce the risk of recurrence.

If Graves' disease is treated with radioiodine therapy, the doses used today are often so high that the treatment rapidly results in underactivity of the thyroid. The reason for this is to achieve a cure as quickly as possible, and to give only one treatment session without the need for repeated sessions. Radioiodine therapy thus almost always results in permanent hypothyroidism in the end, and a requirement for thyroxine substitution.

If such a low radioiodine dose has been given that the patient does not require thyroxine substitution afterwards, there is a high risk of later developing hypothyroidism. This risk remains for the rest of their life and it is therefore necessary to follow-up with these patients. If there is a long latency period between the treatment for thyrotoxicosis and symptom onset of hypothyroidism, there is a risk that neither the patient nor the treating doctor will associate these problems to the earlier cured disease.

10.4 Hypothyroidism After Surgery for Nontoxic Multinodular Goitre

Previously, patients who underwent surgery for nontoxic goitre normally had a hemithyroidectomy and did not require thyroxine after the operation (even though thyroxine was often given postoperatively to reduce the risk of recurrence). Nowadays, more extensive resection is often performed and thus the patient requires thyroxine substitution to a greater extent. Sometimes however, residual thyroid tissue can grow in spite of thyroxine treatment, and hormone production can become so high that, after a time, the requirement for thyroxine drops or is no longer necessary.

10.5 Hypothyroidism After Surgery for Thyroid Cancer

In most cases of thyroid cancer, total thyroidectomy is carried out. The patient therefore requires lifelong substitution with thyroxine. Guidelines for thyroxine treatment in thyroid cancer are discussed in Chap. 30.

10.6 Central Hypothyroidism

An unusual cause of hypothyroidism is impaired TSH secretion, which can be due to pituitary disease, defective function of the hypothalamus or overlying structures with a resultant reduction in TRH stimulation of the pituitary. Causes include a pituitary tumour, infiltrative disease, infectious processes, and traumatic brain injuries. If the patient has received external radiation therapy that includes central areas of the brain, the symptoms may not appear until many years later. A loss of TSH is nearly always combined with a loss of other hormones, but an isolated TSH deficiency can occur in rare cases and the diagnosis can be easily missed, especially in mild cases.

10.7 Iodine-Induced Hypothyroidism

Iodine supplementation affects the thyroid in various ways and can induce both hypothyroidism and thyrotoxicosis, primarily in patients predisposed to this.

Some patients with autoimmune thyroiditis have an increased risk of iodine-induced hypothyroidism due to malfunction of the escape mechanism. Even the immature thyroid tissue in the foetus can react in this way. This highly complicated interaction between iodine and the thyroid is discussed in Chap. 6. Large quantities of iodine can be taken up from iodine-rich health supplements such as algae capsules (now banned in Sweden) and iodine-containing medicines such as amiodarone, contrast media and wound dressings.

The blocking effect of iodine on the thyroid is still sometimes used as preoperative treatment in cases of adverse reaction to antithyroid drugs or in cases of extremely severe thyrotoxicosis/thyrotoxic crisis. Iodine is then administered as a 5% iodine-potassium iodide solution (Lugol's iodine) daily for 7–10 days before surgery (see Chap. 17 and 24). Note that the blocking effect is temporary.

10.8 Iatrogenic (Medicine-Induced) Hypothyroidism

Several medicines can induce hypothyroidism and a detailed description can be found in Chap. 33. A brief overview is included here.

- *Antithyroid drugs* Thiamazol and propylthiouracil inhibit synthesis of the thyroid hormones. Propylthiouracil also inhibits the peripheral conversion of T4 to T3
- *Lithium salts* Inhibits synthesis via several mechanisms
- *Dopamine* In rare cases, medication in acute conditions (primarily dopamine-related pharmaceuticals, which are given parenterally during intensive care) affects thyroid function via central inhibition of TSH secretion

- *Interferon*   Treatment with interferon can probably affect the development of autoimmune thyroiditis. The presence of TPOAb at the start of treatment appears to be associated with an increased risk
- *Amiodarone*   Can inhibit hormone release from the thyroid due to the high iodine content. If medication is continued, there is also a risk of developing thyrotoxicosis

10.9 Hypothyroidism After External Radiation of the Head and Neck Regions

In addition to the risk of developing thyroid cancer and hyperparathyroidism in the long-term after external radiation of the neck, there is also a high risk of developing underactivity of the thyroid. This underactivity can develop several years after the radiation treatment, when the patient is otherwise judged to be cured of the cancer. It is therefore important that patients who have received external radiation therapy of the neck region are regularly followed-up with respect to thyroid function.

10.10 Other Causes of Hypothyroidism

In rare cases, lymphoma and collagenosis can cause hypothyroidism due to destruction of the hormone producing tissue.

> **Most Common Causes of Hypothyroidism in Adults**
>
> - From a global perspective: iodine deficiency
> - Autoimmune thyroiditis in countries with adequate iodine availability
> - Surgery or radioiodine therapy for hyperthyroidism or thyroid cancer
> - Medicines (antithyroid drugs, lithium, interferon, amiodarone)

11 Symptoms of Hypothyroidism

11.1 Autoimmune Thyroiditis – Natural Progression

In many cases of early autoimmune thyroiditis, thyroid function is not affected. The patient remains symptom-free with normal concentrations of serum TSH and thyroid hormones but with elevated TPOAb. When thyroid function is affected, there is a slow drop in T4 secretion during development of the disease.

TSH secretion increases due to the hypothalamus–pituitary–thyroid feedback system and the impaired functional capacity of the thyroid gland is partly compensated by the increasing TSH concentration (Fig. 11.1). However, the elevated TSH concentration most probably always corresponds to a lower than normal T4 concentration for the individual.

A patient with elevated TSH and falling concentrations of T4 can display symptoms of hypothyroidism, even though the concentration of free T4 still lies within the normal reference range. This is partly counteracted by the increased conversion of T4 to the biologically active hormone T3, which occurs when the serum concentration of T4 drops.

This condition with elevated TSH, but T4 and T3 levels within the population reference range, is referred to as subclinical hypothyroidism, and is discussed in more detail in Chap. 13.

The clinical symptoms in the early stages of hypothyroidism are nonspecific. The symptoms become easier to interpret as the concentration of thyroid hormones drops and the classic case of hypothyroidism emerges. Autoimmune thyroid disease can develop slowly following the pattern illustrated in Figs. 11.2, 11.3, 11.4 and 11.5.

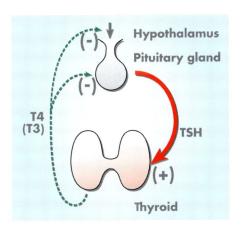

Fig. 11.1 Hypothalamus–pituitary–thyroid feedback

E. Nyström, G.E.B. Berg, S.K.G. Jansson, O. Törring, S.V. Valdemarsson (Eds.),
Thyroid Disease in Adults,
DOI: 10.1007/978-3-642-13262-9_11, © Springer-Verlag Berlin Heidelberg 2011

Chapter 11: Symptoms of Hypothyroidism

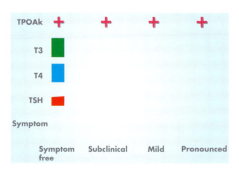

Fig. 11.2 Autoimmune symptom-free thyroid disease. High concentration of antibodies against thyroid tissue, particularly TPOAb, normal hormone concentrations of TSH, T4 and T3, no symptoms

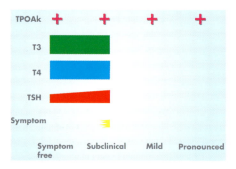

Fig. 11.3 Subclinical hypothyroidism. TSH concentration elevated but T3 and T4 within reference range, possibly nonspecific symptoms

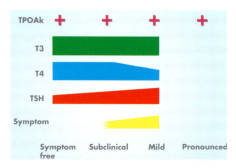

Fig. 11.4 Mild hypothyroidism. T3 within reference range, lowered T4, elevated TSH, mild symptoms

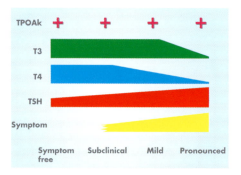

Fig. 11.5 Pronounced hypothyroidism. Lowered T4, if extreme T4 drop, also lowered T3, elevated TSH and classic clinical symptoms

11.2 Organ-Related Symptoms

A lack of thyroid hormone exhibits symptoms in most organs and affects many metabolic processes. The most common symptoms associated with various organs are summarized in this chapter in Sect. 11.3.

Symptoms can vary from case to case, which means that patients with hypothyroidism can be referred to a variety of specialists. As emphasized earlier, symptoms in autoimmune hypothyroidism develop gradually.

Characteristic of the early phase is that the patient does not notice any specific symptoms. Deterioration can occur so slowly that the symptoms can be quite pronounced before the patient visits the doctor and is diagnosed. In early stages of the disease, the patient can present with relatively nonspecific symptoms, such as tiredness, depression, dry skin, hair loss, weight gain or simply the feeling that things are not as they should be.

In patients with pronounced hypothyroidism, classic symptoms emerge such as coldness, constipation, hoarseness, reduced sweating, general swelling of the hands and face, particularly periorbitally (Fig. 11.6). The most prominent symptom can differ between patients.

The lowered metabolism caused by lack of thyroid hormone makes the patient sweat less and prefer warmer surroundings. Weight gain, which is seen occasionally, is caused partly by the reduced energy requirements and the accumulation of fluids and mucopolysaccharides in the tissues, resulting in swelling of the skin and face (myxoedema). In severe cases, effects on the larynx as voice alteration are observed as well as narrowing of nerve passages.

The term myxoedema is used to describe both the swelling in tissues, primarily in the face, seen in pronounced hypothyroidism (see Chap. 14), and the local swelling which can occur primarily frontally on the tibia (pretibial myxoedema) in Graves' disease. The pathogenesis of the two conditions is most probably different.

Slower metabolism lowers the basal body temperature and the demands on circulation. A typical sign is a decreased heart rate. A changed cardiac load is reflected in a

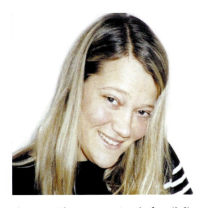
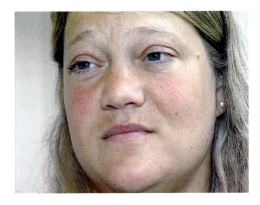

Fig. 11.6 The same patient before (*left*) and after (*right*) developing hypothyroidism

so-called low voltage in ECG, in which there is also a change in the ST-T segment in pronounced hypothyroidism. These ECG changes are reversible with treatment.

Hypothyroidism is thought to be associated with an increased occurrence of coronary sclerosis. This was first demonstrated in postmortem studies in the 1960s, in which increased coronary sclerosis was found in hypothyroid patients who, in addition, had hypertension. Later studies have also proposed a connection between autoimmune thyroid disease and arteriosclerosis.

In hypothyroidism, there is a disturbance in lipoprotein metabolism with a pronounced increase in the cholesterol-rich LDL fraction as the prominent finding. This disturbance can be mostly explained by the effects of thyroid hormone on key enzymes in lipoprotein metabolism and on the function of the LDL receptor. This effect on lipoprotein metabolism is reversible.

Occasionally, individuals with primary hypothyroidism can present with an increase in serum prolactin, because the increase in TRH release not only stimulates secretion of TSH, but also prolactin. In these cases, prolactin levels rarely exceed 60 µg/L (2,000 mIU/L). Because pronounced hypothyroidism can result in an enlargement of the pituitary and also of the sella turcica, primary hypothyroidism can, in these cases, give incorrect suspicion of a prolactin-producing pituitary adenoma.

11.3 Symptoms and Findings in Hypothyroidism

11.3.1 Neurological
- Paresthesis, peripheral nerve compression, for example carpal tunnel syndrome
- Impaired coordination, ataxia
- Slow tendon reflexes (relaxation phase)
- Hearing impairment
- Impaired sense of taste
- Headaches
- Dizziness
- Effects on the pituitary (hyperplasia with or without sella enlargement)

11.3.2 Mental
- Tiredness
- Apathy, anxiety, restlessness, irritability
- Impaired memory, concentration difficulties
- Depression
- Disorientation, pseudodementia, paranoid symptoms, myxoedema madness
- Alcohol intolerance

11.3.3 Gastrointestinal
- Enlarged tongue, dysphagia
- Slow intestinal movement, constipation
- Ascites in severe cases
- Gallstone formation

11.3.4 Musculoskeletal
- Reduced length in children due to slow skeletal growth
- Incomplete closure of the epiphyses in children
- Arthralgia, bursitis
- Muscle swelling
- Stiffness, aches, pains, cramps and muscular weakness

11.3.5 Dermatological
- Dry, cool, pale skin
- Itching
- Dry hair
- Hair loss
- Sparse eyebrows laterally
- Brittle nails
- Swelling (myxoedema in the face, eyelids, back of hands, and other places)
- Fragile blood vessels, bruising in severe cases

11.3.6 Ear, Nose and Throat
- Deeper and hoarser voice
- Hearing impairment
- Swelling of the mucous membranes
- Swallowing difficulties

11.3.7 Gynecological and Andrological
- Late pubertal development
- Amenorrhea, menorrhagia
- Galactorrhea
- Impotence
- Impaired fertility
- Impaired libido
- Dry mucous membranes

11.3.8 Heart and Blood Vessels
- Bradycardia
- Low-voltage ECG, AV-block
- Blood pressure changes (increase in blood pressure)
- Coronary sclerosis
- Ventricular septal hypertrophy
- Mitral valve prolapse
- Dyspnoea
- Pericardial exudate in severe cases

11.3.9 Hematological
- Anaemia
- Viscous aspirate at bone marrow aspiration
- Impaired thrombocyte function
- Bleeding tendencies, petechiae, bruises

11.3.10 Respiratory
- Hypoventilation, in severe cases resulting in hypoxia, hypercapnia
- Dyspnoea, upper respiratory tract obstruction, pleural effusion

11.3.11 Renal and Urological
- Impaired glomerular filtration, increased creatinine
- Bladder hypotonia

11.3.12 Electrolyte Balance, Intermediary Metabolism
- Hyponatraemia, hypoglycemia, hyperuricemia

11.3.13 Changes in Lipid Metabolism
- Hypercholesterolemia
- Increase in LDL cholesterol

11.4 Central Hypothyroidism

The clinical symptoms of central (secondary) hypothyroidism, for example due to a pituitary tumour, often appear relatively late. The patient is typically found to have a T4 level immediately below or within the lower limit of the reference range with inappropriate TSH levels. Because there is an overlap between the concentration range for euthyroid patients and those with mild thyroid hormone deficiency, diagnosis is difficult. Determination of TSH is not useful.

In fact, the TSH concentration can be low, lie within the reference range, or be slightly raised. This is because the pituitary, in the absence of hypothalamic effect via TRH, releases a small amount of low-glycosylated TSH. This form of TSH has a longer half-life, which contributes to the higher serum levels. This TSH is not biologically active, but can be codetermined using immunological routine methods for analysis of TSH.

In the TRH stimulation test, a slow increase in TSH is observed, most probably resulting from the release of low-glycosylated TSH molecules, which due to their long half-life, cause a prolonged increase in TSH.

In certain cases, pituitary insufficiency is detected because at analysis of thyroid samples the profile typical for secondary hypothyroidism (low free T4 without increase in TSH) is found. The degree of pituitary insufficiency is often relatively advanced and the function of other hormonal systems is also impaired. In these patients, the symptoms observed for hypothyroidism are the same as those for primary hypothyroidism, both clinically and metabolically.

Previously, it was thought that secondary/central hypothyroidism could be distinguished from primary hypothyroidism as it did not result in lipid disturbances. However, this is not the case: secondary hypothyroidism also results in the typical hypercholesterolemia seen in primary hypothyroidism when the thyroid hormone deficit is so severe that not only T4 but also T3 levels drop.

The diagnosis of central hypothyroidism can thus be difficult to make, particularly in mild cases, and if there is only a deficit of TSH and not of the other pituitary hormones (isolated TSH deficiency). Currently, there is a lack of generally accepted diagnostic criteria in borderline cases of serum TSH concentrations. It is, however, important to keep this condition in mind, not least if other clinical data support a hypothalamic–pituitary effect, such as previous encephalitis, head trauma, or symptoms suggestive of effects on the pituitary (headaches, disturbed vision and absence of other pituitary hormones).

Central Hypothyroidism

- In most cases caused by hypothalamic and pituitary processes
- Symptoms often dominated by absence of other hormones
- Total or free T4 is low, or in lower part of the reference range
- TSH low, normal, or slightly elevated
- Total or free T3 normal in mild cases

12 Treatment of Hypothyroidism

12.1 Primary Hypothyroidism

The symptoms in hypothyroidism are caused by a deficiency of thyroid hormone in the tissues and the consequences of this on the function of various organs or metabolic processes. Therapy is simple with thyroid hormone substitution.

The goal of treatment for hypothyroidism is to normalize metabolism without adverse effects. During continued therapy, which is nearly always lifelong, the patient must be followed-up regularly to monitor possible dose adjustment, compliance and the onset of associated pathological conditions. The thyroxine dose is based on symptomatic relief and guided by the concentration of TSH. The goal should be to achieve TSH levels that lie between the range 0.4–2.0 mIU/L.

In connection with the first consultation, all patients with manifest primary hypothyroidism must be informed that treatment will be lifelong. Women of child-bearing age should also be informed that they should undertake contraceptive measures until their hormone levels are normalized (see Chap. 31). If a woman becomes pregnant in the future, they should contact their doctor immediately to check their hormone levels. They must under no circumstances interrupt their thyroxine treatment, and should be informed that thyroxine treatment poses no problems for pregnancy or breastfeeding.

Substitution treatment should be initiated gradually except if hypothyroidism is diagnosed during pregnancy, when full-dose thyroxine is administered from the start. The dosage should take into account the severity of the disease and duration, the age of the patient and whether other diseases, primarily cardiac disease, are present. In young patients with mild hypothyroidism, an initial dose of 50 µg/day with a dose increase every fourth week should be appropriate, while more care should be exercised in older

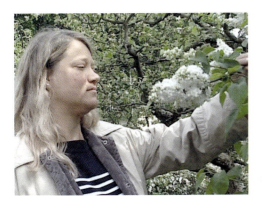

Fig. 12.1 A woman suffering from hypothyroidism

E. Nyström, G.E.B. Berg, S.K.G. Jansson, O. Törring, S.V. Valdemarsson (Eds.),
Thyroid Disease in Adults,
DOI: 10.1007/978-3-642-13262-9_12, © Springer-Verlag Berlin Heidelberg 2011

Chapter 12: Treatment of Hypothyroidism

patients and in more pronounced disease. In these cases, a starting dose of 25 µg each or every other day would be appropriate, with a dose increase every fourth to sixth week. In older patients with extreme hypothyroidism, the patient should perhaps be hospitalized at the start of treatment, particularly if cardiac conditions are present. If there is a clinical suspicion of Addison's disease (low blood pressure, pigmentation) or secondary adrenal failure, serum cortisol (morning sample) should be checked and adequate therapy instituted before substitution with thyroxine is started.

Patients with subclinical hypothyroidism often require only a low dose of thyroxine, e.g. 25–50 µg initially. It is also wise in these cases to proceed with caution when starting thyroxine, as some of these patients experience palpitations if started abruptly.

Previously, fully substituted patients received up to 400–500 µg thyroxine/day. Current laboratory methods for follow-up treatment have shown that these substitution doses were too high. Today, most patients are treated with 50–200 µg thyroxine/day. The average daily requirement for patients with primary hypothyroidism is 125 µg.

At uptitration of the thyroxine dose, changes at close time intervals should be avoided because it takes at last 6 weeks before the pituitary thyroid axis achieves a new steady state after an increase in dose. This means that there should be at least a 6-week delay before checking TSH. During the initial phase of substitution treatment, a falling TSH level reflects the effect of treatment, and is inversely proportional to increasing T4 levels. Often only a small change in the thyroxine dose is required for fine adjustment (25 µg, 12.5 µg or even 6.25 µg). Assessing the correct thyroxine dose for a patient who presents with pronounced hypothyroidism may, in some cases, not be possible until a year later, because absorption of thyroxine can improve gradually as the intestinal function is restituted.

In patients with severe hypothyroidism, a continued clinical improvement is observed even after normalization of the TSH concentration. It has been shown, for example, that neurophysiological tests, lipid metabolism and physical performance are not normalized until several months after TSH has reached a normal level.

It is important to assure the patient that it can take time before he/she is back to normal, sometimes 6–12 months in pronounced hypothyroidism. Many patients feel tired and "up and down" during the convalescence period and may become depressed in spite of normal hormone concentrations (including TSH). A rapid increase in dose or an initial overdose of thyroxine will not result in elimination of the symptoms more quickly. Instead, the risk is that the patient will experience intolerance symptoms.

At clinical check-up, it should be noted whether the symptoms have receded, and whether any signs of intolerance symptoms have appeared as an expression of overdose. A single clinical assessment is insufficient for thyroxine-substituted patients. Regular laboratory checks of thyroid function must be performed. It should be pointed out that not all patients feel that they are optimally substituted when their TSH concentration lies within the range desired. The situation and negative effects of slight over- and undersubstitution should in these cases be discussed with the patient.

It should be remembered that in many such cases there may be a physiological reality behind the opinion of the patient regarding his or her optimal hormone level. It should also be remembered that depression is fairly common in connection with thyroid dysfunction during the initial therapy period and that the symptom can be a result of this depression and not thyroid disease. If the depressive symptoms are judged to require treatment, follow normal guidelines. At check-ups, attention should be paid to presence of other autoimmuno-related diseases, primarily diabetes mellitus, adrenal insufficiency and pernicious anaemia.

12.2 Laboratory Tests – Special Aspects

As presented above, thyroxine substitution is guided using TSH determination. Because thyroxine hormone levels are not stable until about 6 h after intake of thyroxine, samples should be drawn in the morning before taking the tablet. Checking TPOAb levels is not indicated during substitution treatment with thyroxine for autoimmune hypothyroidism because this does not add any additional clinical information.

After treatment for thyrotoxicosis, TSH secretion can be suppressed for 3 to 6 months. In those patients who receive thyroxine treatment after therapy for hyperthyroidism, treatment is managed by determination of T4 and T3 until TSH secretion returns to normal and can be used as a substitution guide.

At check-up of thyroxine substitution in patients with central hypothyroidism, T4 and T3 are usually analysed to help pinpoint the dosage. In these cases, TSH can not be used to check thyroxine substitution, but the target should be that free T4 and T3 lie within the reference range.

Patients receiving thyroxine substitution for autoimmune thyroid disease should undergo annual thyroid tests. In addition, haemoglobin, electrolytes, fasting blood sugar and cobalamines may be considered at the start of therapy and later as indicated.

12.3 Special Problems

Patients with coronary sclerosis, angina pectoris and heart failure need special attention. For these patient categories, particular care must be exercised at the start of substitution with thyroxine. One risk is that latent angina pectoris can be demasked when higher myocardial performance is required. In pronounced cases, cardiac failure can progress. In such cases, it may be impossible to achieve full substitution. Cardiac symptoms must be given priority and thyroxine undersubstitution temporarily accepted.

The patient should be given antianginal treatment when indicated. Prompt care is essential if the problems are severe. Surgery can be performed in hypothyroid patients with only minor risk. It is important, however, to consider the slow metabolism of sedatives and other drugs.

Initiation of thyroxine treatment should be withheld in a hypothyroid patient with untreated Addison's disease or pituitary insufficiency, since it could result in triggering acute symptoms of cortisol failure.

Hypothyroidism entails an increased risk of insulin sensitivity in diabetics. After starting treatment with thyroxine, normal sensitivity returns.

12.4 Resorption of Thyroxine

Resorption of thyroxine takes place in the jejunum and ileum. Because the sodium salt of thyroxine is difficult to resolve in water, particle size is important for resorption. This is why thyroxine preparations from different pharmaceutical manufacturers do not always give the same tissue concentration curve at administration of identical amounts of compounds. Thus, if one thyroxine preparation is replaced with another pharmaceutical preparation additional checks of TSH levels must be carried out.

Patients with malabsorption have reduced resorption of thyroxine. Increased thyroxine requirements can be an indication of development of this condition. Fibre-rich food and soy-based products can also affect resorption of thyroxine. For reliable absorption, thyroxine is best taken on an empty stomach, e.g. 15–20 min before breakfast.

Several medicines can inhibit intestinal resorption of thyroxine. The medicines listed below should be taken at least 4 h before or after thyroxine:
- Iron containing compounds (primarily in patients with impaired acid production in the stomach, i.e. atrophic gastritis)
- Preparations containing calcium
- Antacids based on aluminium hydroxide or sucralfate
- Resins (synthetic organic polymers) such as cholestyramine, cholestipol and sodium polystyrenesulphate
- Imatinib mesylate (used for treatment of chronic myeloid leukaemia and gastrointestinal stromal cell tumours) and other tyrosine kinase inhibiting drugs
- Raloxifene

Disturbed resorption of thyroxine has also been noted in patients on proton pump inhibitors and undergoing eradication treatment for a helicobacter pylori infection.

12.5 Pharmaceutical Interaction in Thyroxine Treatment

Hypothyroid patients may have a prolonged elimination of medicines. This should be kept in mind when treating with sedatives, anaesthetics and anticoagulants. After substitution with thyroxine, increased metabolism and faster elimination of medicines (insulin, etc.) can be assumed and the patient needs to be followed-up after initiation of thyroxine treatment.

12.6 Oestrogens and Hypothyroidism

Oestrogen increases the concentration of thyroxine binding globulin (TBG). This explains why treatment with oestrogen containing contraceptive pills raises the concentration of total T4 and T3. During pregnancy, TBG increases, which results in an increased thyroxine requirement in those patients whose thyroid function is completely or almost completely lost. This is shown early in pregnancy. In certain cases an increase of up to 50% in the thyroxine dose may be necessary in order to keep a normal TSH. After delivery, the TBG concentration falls and the thyroxine dose can be decreased to the former level. This is discussed in more detail in Chap. 31.

In women who have started oestrogen treatment, the effect on TBG can result in an increased thyroxine requirement during a transition period (a few years). This has been demonstrated in women who receive oestrogen due to deficiency symptoms during menopause, but probably also applies to women who take oestrogen-containing contraceptive pills and tamoxifen.

12.7 Do All Patients Tolerate Thyroxine?

Some patients on thyroxine medication may experience symptoms they interpret as side effects. These are nearly always a reaction to the pharmacological effect of the preparation, such as palpitations and restlessness. A temporary reduction in dosage and reassuring words solves the problem in most cases.

Very few cases of genuine oversensitivity reactions to thyroxine supplement have been reported. On the other hand, it is not unusual for the patient at the start of treatment or at a dose increase to report itching, muscular aches or mild erythematous skin changes. In the event of skin reactions when starting treatment with thyroxine preparations, one should also consider reactions against other components of the tablet. It should also be noted that many thyroxine preparations contain a small amount of lactose which, in rare cases, can cause problems in people with lactose intolerance.

12.8 Treatment with Triiodothyronine

In recent years, a number of studies have been performed with a combination of thyroxine and triiodothyronine for substitution treatment of hypothyroidism. This is theoretically interesting, because physiologically, the thyroid releases a small amount of triiodothyronine in addition to thyroxine, while in the ordinary substitution therapy, only thyroxine is given. Randomized prospective studies have not been able to show any clear positive effect of the treatment with combination of thyroxine and triiodothyronine.

Some patients may benefit from this combination treatment. Triiodothyronine should then be given in a low dose, at most 10 µg/day, and thyroxine should be given in a lower dose than if given alone. In some countries, preparations are still available which contain both thyroxine and triiodothyronine, either in a synthetic form or as an extract of animal thyroid.

Temporary treatment with triiodothyronine, instead of thyroxine, has been routine for follow-up of radioiodine investigations and treatment with I-131 in patients who have undergone surgery for thyroid cancer. Because of the considerably shorter half-life of T3 (1 day) compared with T4 (7–8 days), it is only necessary to interrupt the triiodothyronine medication for about 2 weeks before the radioiodine administration to make the patient hypothyroidic. A TSH above 30 mIU/L is necessary for the radioiodine investigations/treatment to be effective.

During recent years, this routine has been replaced in some centres by the use of recombinant human TSH. Using recombinant TSH, the patient retains their thyroxine dose and therefore has normal T4 and T3 levels. The desired TSH stimulated increase of isotope uptake in residual thyroid tissue, both benign and malignant, still can be achieved.

Treatment with triiodothyronine has been discussed within intensive care as an attempt to counteract the low concentrations of T3 that arise due to reduced conversion of T4 to T3 in connection with severe general disease (see Sect. 2.10). However, there is no agreement on the extent to which these peripherally measured low T3 values really have an adverse effect on the patient. There is a risk that treatment with triiodothyronine in these cases can lead to an increased catabolism or increased risk of arrhythmia.

Another aspect has been improvement of myocardium performance, partly through a direct effect of triiodothyronine on the myocardium, partly through the vasodilating effect of triiodothyronine, but there is no clear consensus. Today, triiodothyronine has no documented place in intensive care.

12.9 Parenteral Treatment with Thyroid Hormone

Both thyroxine and triiodothyronine are available in injectable form. For some patients who are substituted with thyroxine, it can be necessary to administer the hormone parenterally, for example in connection with long-term care in the intensive ward.

Because the half-life of thyroxine is about 7 days, a temporary interruption of thyroxine for a few days in connection with surgery has no practical significance. If the interruption lasts a week or longer, thyroxine should be given parenterally. Levothyroxine can be given in injectable form. Parenteral treatment requires about 75% of the dose given perorally. Thyroxine injection can also be used for treatment of patients with myxoedema coma (see Chap. 14). Another option is to administer thyroxine in tablet form via a stomach tube.

12.10 Overdosing with Thyroxine and Triiodothyronine

In adults who take high doses of thyroxine, the symptoms are often not pronounced (mild thyrotoxicosis) and in most cases only tachycardia and restlessness are noted. Laboratory studies reveal elevated free T4, while the increase in T3 is less pronounced due to reduced conversion of T4 to T3. The more severe symptoms (tachycardia, fever, muscle cramps) are generally noted only in children who take high doses of thyroxine.

An overdose of triiodothyronine or thyroid extract (contains both thyroxine and triiodothyronine), the clinical symptoms are more pronounced because the patient will be exposed to the active hormone triiodothyronine directly.

Radioiodine uptake is, of course, blocked in these cases with extremely high thyroxine/triiodothyronine intake. The serum concentration of thyroglobulin is low during the acute phase in patients overdosed with thyroxine or triiodothyronine.

In many cases, it is satisfactory to temporarily withdraw thyroxine treatment. Beta blockers may be used in tachycardia. Early in the process, the patient can be given activated carbon. For severe overdose, plasmapheresis has been used, but the result of this treatment is uncertain due to the extensive protein binding of the thyroid hormones. In patients on TSH suppressive dose of thyroxine after treatment for thyroid cancer, beta blockers are appropriate to counteract increased heart rate and palpitations.

12.11 Compliance

Patients are sometimes seen with TSH at inappropriately high even though the patient says thyroxine has been taken as prescribed. Laboratory tests with slightly elevated TSH and free T4 values within the reference range indicate that in these cases the patient, for whatever reason, has not received the thyroxine as prescribed, but complied with the prescription for a few weeks prior to the test. In these cases, it is important to ensure that the patient has not also taken a preparation which could affect the resorption of thyroxine from the intestines or developed malabsorption. Sometimes, doubt can arise as to whether the patient really resorbs thyroxine. In these cases, it may be helpful to measure free T4 a few hours after taking the tablet, in which case an increase in free T4 demonstrates resorption.

In certain lack of compliance cases, a successful treatment can be achieved by administration of thyroxine once a week (under supervision) and in a dose which corresponds to the weekly requirements.

12.12 Temporary Treatment with Thyroxine

Once in a while, the question is raised whether thyroxine treatment can be stopped, for example in transient hypothyroidism after subacute thyroiditis or postpartum thyroiditis, or if the original treatment indication is later considered to be doubtful. In these cases, thyroxine can be stopped completely and immediately, and the patient recalled after 2–4 weeks for a check-up. If the TSH concentration is elevated, the thyroxine treatment should continue. Often it is more practical to give 50% of the original dose and recall the patient for a check-up after 1–2 months.

Analysis of TPOAb can be informative at suspicion of autoimmune thyroiditis, and if there is doubt about the indication for starting treatment. An elevated concentration supports the probability that the thyroxine has been initiated correctly.

The thyroxin dose should be reduced or the treatment stopped if there are signs of autonomous thyroid function. Such patients display suppressed TSH, and often elevated free and total T3, while the concentration of free T4 may lie within the upper part of the reference range. This can be seen in patients who, during an earlier stage, started thyroxine treatment because of multinodular goitre.

Earlier, thyroxine was administered with the aim of reducing the volume of the goitre or after partial thyroid resection, an indication which is now questionable. In these cases, the thyroxine dose should be reduced gradually while checking TSH levels. The thyroxine substitution can often in these cases eventually be terminated. Persistent TSH suppression is further evaluated using thyroid scintigraphy.

12.13 Central (Secondary) Hypothyroidism

As previously mentioned, pituitary insufficiency with an isolated lack of TSH occurs very rarely. In case of concomitant secondary adrenal insufficiency, it is important to first treat cortisol deficiency and thereafter start thyroxine substitution using the same principles as for primary hypothyroidism substitution therapy.

Treatment of Hypothyroidism

- Uncomplicated cases are managed by the primary health care services
- Young patients with mild hypothyroidism: Thyroxine, initial dose 50 µg; dose increase 25–50 µg every 4–6 weeks
- Older patients with pronounced hypothyroidism: Thyroxine, initial dose 25 µg daily or every other day; dose increase 25 µg every 4–8 weeks
- Problems with coronary disease:
  – Slow increase in thyroxine dose in cooperation with cardiologist
  – Incomplete substitution may be accepted
- Addison's disease or pituitary failure need to be evaluated before initiating thyroxine
- Adjust thyroxine guided by the TSH level and the patient's sense of well-being
- Treatment goal TSH 0.4–2.0 mIU/L
- Long term (up to 6–12 months) before complete full recovery
- Medication, malabsorption and food can interfere with thyroxine absorption (e.g. Al-containing antacids, Fe-preparations, calcium preparations and fibre-rich food)
- For final calibrating of the dose, 6–8 weeks needs to pass to allow the body to fully adapt to the latest dose adjustment
- Well-substituted patients are checked once a year

13 Subclinical Hypothyroidism

13.1 Introduction

The term subclinical hypothyroidism has been in use for a long time to describe the condition where TSH is elevated, and the concentrations of T4 and T3 are within their reference ranges. Subclinical hypothyroidism frequently occurs as an early stage in the development of autoimmune clinical hypothyroidism with classic textbook symptoms. Longstanding subclinical hypothyroidism can also be observed after surgery in which a significant part of the thyroid has been removed, or after radioiodine therapy.

The designation subclinical hypothyroidism is unfortunate, because many investigations demonstrate that individuals with subclinical hypothyroidism often have symptoms, i.e. non-subclinical. Although designations such as mild hypothyroidism have been proposed and are now used more frequently, the name subclinical hypothyroidism still predominates.

This definition is also problematic because it is based only on biochemical analyses. The relationship between the reference range used for these analyses (the normal range) and the normal range for the individual in question is not clarified satisfactorily (see Chap. 3).

13.2 Prevalence

Subclinical hypothyroidism is more common in young to middle-aged women than in men of the same age. The prevalence in the female population is probably 2–3%. The prevalence increases with increasing age to about 10% at 70 years of age, when the condition becomes just as common in men.

Subclinical hypothyroidism is found:
- In autoimmune thyroid disease
- After recent parturition
- After thyroid resection
- After radioiodine therapy

Other conditions which predispose to development of subclinical hypothyroidism are:
- Radiation therapy targeting the thyroid
- Treatment with or intake of iodine-containing medicines and preparations
- Treatment with certain drugs such as interferon or lithium
- Other autoimmune disorders, e.g. diabetes mellitus type 1 or Addison's disease

13.3 Substitution Treatment with Thyroxine in Subclinical Hypothyroidism

Investigations demonstrate that a TSH value which exceeds 2.5 mIU/L increases the risk of later development of the classic symptoms of hypothyroidism and that this risk is greater if TPOAb are present. The combination of elevated TSH and presence of antibodies gives a 4–5% annual risk of developing hypothyroidism. If TSH >10 mIU/L, the risk of developing symptoms is so high that consensus is for immediate initiation of thyroxine substitution. As emphasized in several sections of this book, a clinical decision on substitution should not be based solely on one isolated analysis of TSH. In the clinical situation, the analysis should be repeated after a few weeks to months and supplemented with analysis of TPOAb before thyroxine therapy begins. Meanwhile, iodine supplementation (150 μg) may be considered if the dietary intake of iodine is judged to be insufficient. This double check rules out a temporary compensatory TSH increase (Fig. 2.14).

A number of studies have shown that the pituitary is probably not alone in reacting promptly to falling serum concentrations of thyroid hormone (by increasing the production of TSH). It is possible to trace subtle changes, for example in lipid metabolism, cardiopulmonary, muscle and also CNS function very early in the development of subclinical hypothyroidism. There is no threshold value for TSH or for the start of these gradually occurring signs and symptoms. An attempt should be made to evaluate the clinical significance of observed changes in each individual case.

Symptoms of thyroxine deficiency that can be linked to subclinical hypothyroidism disappear at substitution therapy. These symptoms are frequently nonspecific and often occur relatively frequently in euthyroid patients making a clinical diagnosis and decision of treatment difficult.

Possible symptoms due to subclinical hypothyroidism include:
- Tiredness
- Lowered quality of life
- Mild depression
- Dry skin
- Hair loss
- Reduced work capacity
- Menstrual disturbance
- Infertility (due to anovulatory cycle)
- Misscarriage

In addition, biochemical investigations reveal slightly raised concentrations of cholesterol and LDL cholesterol, which subsequently fall upon substitution with thyroxine.

Population studies have revealed that about one in four patients with subclinical hypothyroidism may have clinically significant symptoms. Advanced studies have been conducted to highlight how the various organs and organ functions are affected in subclinical hypothyroidism, including changes in lipid metabolism, cardiac function, muscle function, oxygen uptake and cognitive function. In many cases, these studies have been conducted on small patient groups and with insufficient controls.

This has resulted in a proposal for a mass screening program for subclinical hypothyroidism, but there is no scientific evidence today to support this. However, a discussion of screening programs for certain subpopulations, such as pregnant women and patients with diabetes type 1, appears relevant.

It must be emphasized that the clinical situation is different when a patient contacts a doctor because he/she does not feel well, than if a slightly elevated TSH level is found at a general health care screening. If, in the former situation, a slightly elevated TSH value is found, in particular in the presence of TPOAb, the symptoms may very well be related to subclinical hypothyroidism. The higher the TSH value, and/or if there are cases of autoimmune thyroid disease or type I diabetes, vitiligo or other manifestations of autoimmune polyglandular syndrome (APS) in the family, the higher the probability.

Subclinical hypothyroidism should always be suspected in certain clinical situations, especially if the patient is a woman more than 40–45 years of age:
- If the patient has other autoimmune diseases
- If autoimmune thyroid disease exists in the family
- If the patient has a goitre

As pointed out above, the symptoms alone should not form the basis for the diagnosis, because the nonspecific symptoms found at subclinical hypothyroidism are also highly prevalent in an euthyroid population.

Initially, thyroxine is given at approximately 25–50 µg/day (depending on TSH and clinical findings). Follow-up every 6 weeks. The goal is to achieve TSH levels within the range 0.4–2.0 mIU/L. A practical target value of TSH is ~1 mIU/L. Women who are considering pregnancy and pregnant women should always receive thyroxine in cases of diagnosed subclinical hypothyroidism, or if TPOAb are present and TSH is > 2,5 mIE/L (see Chap 31). Elevated serum cholesterol and the presence of goitre give further support for treatment. Subclinical hypothyroidism may lead to infertility due to anovulatory menstrual cycle. An increase in spontaneous miscarriage has been reported.

Check the thyroid function promptly at confirmed pregnancy in women at risk of thyroid disease. Pregnancy involves an increased load on thyroid function which, even early in pregnancy, can result in falling hormone concentrations in a woman with subclinical hypothyroidism and thus increase the risk for negative influence on CNS development in the foetus (see Chap. 31).

Proposed Diagnostic Procedure and Treatment in Subclinical Hypothyroidism

- Repeat TSH and free T4 after 4 weeks, supplemented by TPOAb
- If TSH >10 mIU/L: Always substitute with thyroxine
- If TSH from upper reference limit to 10 mIU/L:
  - If no symptoms, check TSH and free T4 after 6 months. Elevated TPOAb strengthens the need for follow-up and the indication for substitution
  - If symptoms present (including nonspecific symptoms; goitre): Substitution with thyroxine, with biochemical and clinical assessment after 6 months
- Pregnant women must always receive treatment
- Women with fertility problems should receive treatment

14 Myxoedema Coma

Myxoedema coma is an uncommon condition that primarily affects patients with known hypothyroidism who, for some reason, have stopped taking their thyroxine medication. Other causes are longstanding undiagnosed hypothyroidism due to Hashimoto's thyroiditis or previous treatment with radioiodine for which the patient has stopped attending follow-up. Triggering causes are infections, cerebrovascular insult (CVI), surgery, treatment with sedatives or other psychopharmaceuticals. Frequently, these are elderly patients. The condition is life threatening.

Myxoedema coma does not necessarily involve unconsciousness or coma. Pathophysiologically, progression to myxoedema coma can be regarded as a loss of the regulatory mechanisms initiated to counteract consequences of severe hypothyroidism. This applies particularly to peripheral vasoconstriction, the purpose of which is to maintain body temperature. The triggering factor interrupts this mechanism with resultant circulatory problems and the patient declines further.

14.1 Symptoms

Patients with myxoedema coma often present pronounced clinical signs of hypothyroidism:
- Cold, rough, and dry skin
- Eyelid oedema
- Bradycardia
- Swelling of the face and tongue
- Effects on the sensory system, psychomotor activity and reflexes
- Occasionally, ascites, pericardial exudate and congestive heart failure

Not infrequently, the following divergences are also observed:
- Hyponatraemia
- Hypoglycemia
- Impaired renal function (increased creatinine levels)
- Respiratory insufficiency with CO_2 retention
- Low blood pressure amplitude
- Impaired bone marrow functions

Typical signs for diagnosis also include:
- Changed mental state (disorientation, confusion, psychosis)
- Defective thermoregulation (hypothermia)
- Presence of triggering factors

14.2 Diagnostic Tests

Free T4 is low and often lower than the detection limit. In these cases, the deficit of T4 is so great that T3 is also extremely low or nondetectable. If the cause is primary hypothyroidism, as is normally the case, TSH is high. However, there is not always a pronounced elevation of TSH because the pituitary cells may have an impaired capacity in synthesizing TSH when the deficit of thyroxine is severe.

If myxoedema coma is suspected, free T4 and TSH should be the first analyses conducted. In addition, routine analyses should be performed including blood and coagulation status, electrolytes, creatinine and liver function tests. Serum cortisol and also ACTH should be analysed because primary adrenal insufficiency can be present. In addition, diagnosis/exclusion of infection should be included in the primary series of investigations.

Arterial blood gas analysis should be performed because oxygen saturation can be difficult to measure using a pulsoxymeter due to the slow peripheral blood flow.

The biochemical tests are supplemented with pulmonary X-ray, ECG and, if possible, with echocardiography. Continued care must take place in the intensive care unit, preferably in consultation with an endocrinologist or other specialist.

14.3 Treatment

14.3.1 Thyroid Hormone
Thyroxine treatment must be initiated without delay:
- First 24 h: 200 µg thyroxine given intravenously twice with an interval of 12 h. If an injectable form of thyroxine is not available, 400 µg can be given via a stomach tube on the first day. Parenteral administration is, however, safer because these patients normally have reduced gastrointestinal motility and often impaired absorption of thyroxine.
- Following days: 25–75 µg thyroxine daily is given intravenously, depending on the condition of the patient. A lower dose is preferred in patients with high age and latent cardiac insufficiency. Increasing temperature indicates an adequate effect
- Daily analyses of free T4 should also be performed
- After about 1 week: thyroxine can usually be given orally, 25–50 µg daily, with gradual dose increase depending on the free T4 and TSH levels and the clinical condition

14.3.2 Hydrocortisone
The ability of the adrenals to synthesize steroid hormone is impaired in severe hypothyroidism. This impairment may partly be due to simultaneous adrenal failure. Futhermore, there is an increased need for cortisol when thyroxine treatment is initiated. After sampling (serum cortisol), hydrocortisone is given initially as 100 mg intravenously, and then as 50–100 mg 3–4 times during the first 24 h, and 50 mg 3–4 times during the following 24 h for up to a week.

14.3.3 Monitoring Respiration
Check oxygenation and free airways. Assisted ventilation may be necessary due to risk of hypoventilation with hypoxia and hypercapnia.

14.3.4 Monitoring Circulation
Because circulatory problems can arise and there is a risk of retention of body fluids, the patient should be monitored, if possible, by measuring the central venous pressure. Be aware of the risks for bradyarrhythmia, hypotension, myocardial insufficiency and pericardial effusion.

14.3.5 Temperature Regulation
Body temperature rises (often before the heart rate) as an expression of initial effect of therapy. External warming should be avoided because of the risk of vasodilation and blood pressure drop. Avoid loss of heat from the skin by using reflecting blankets.

14.3.6 Fluids and Electrolyte Treatment
Fluids are given cautiously due to the risk of fluid retention and congestive heart failure. Hyponatraemia (with or without ADH activation) often occurs and care should therefore be exercised when giving diuretics. Erythrocyte transfusion should be given in cases of anemia and low EVF.

14.3.7 Infection
Antibiotics are always administered due to the risk of infection (reduced bone marrow function and reduced leukocyte function in severe hypothyroidism). Patients with pronounced hypothyroidism and an infection do not frequently react with fever due to defective thermoregulation.

14.3.8 Coagulation
Reduced thrombocyte function may be observed in hypothyroidism. May respond to vasopressin.

14.3.9 Miscellaneous
Remember that medicines metabolize slowly. If thyroxine is not available for injection, it can be supplied as tablets via a gastric tube. Injection of triiodothyronine is not recommended. Administration of triiodothyronine has been reported to increase the risk of cardiovascular complications.

Myxoedema Coma

- Unusual condition with a high mortality rate
- Mostly seen with undiagnosed or inadequately treated hypothyroidism
- Can be triggered by infection, stroke, surgery, sedatives, etc.
- Typical hypothyroid symptoms include altered mental status and defective thermoregulation
- Low free T4 and elevated TSH (primary hypothyroidism) or low TSH (central hypothyroidism)
- Requires intensive care nursing (respiration, circulation, infection management, slow metabolism of medicines, risk of fluid retention and myocardial insufficiency)
- Initially treated with thyroxine intravenously, later perorally
- Hydrocortisone
- Antibiotics
- Restricted fluids
- Rising body temperature indicates good therapeutic response

15 Causes of Thyrotoxicosis – an Overview

Hyperthyroidism and thyrotoxicosis are used by many as synonymous terms. However, thyrotoxicosis describes the clinical condition that covers symptoms following high concentrations of the thyroid hormones, T4 and T3, in extrathyroidal tissues, but without regard to the origin of these elevated hormone concentrations.

Hyperthyroidism on the other hand is used to denote hyperactivity in the entire or part of the thyroid that results in synthesis and release of thyroid hormones in excess of that required by the body to maintain euthyroidism.

Hyperthyroidism is the dominating cause of thyrotoxicosis. Thyrotoxicosis, however, can occur even when the elevated hormone levels are due to other disturbances in the thyroid, e.g. hormone leakage, as in various forms of thyroiditis, or administration of inappropriate high doses of thyroxine or triiodothyronine.

On the other hand, in thyroid hormone resistance (see Chap. 34), a state of hyperthyroidism is outbalanced by decreased effects of T3 at the cellular level in most organs, leaving the patient euthyroid in major aspects.

It is of major importance with regards to treatment to clarify whether the thyrotoxic condition is the result of overproduction of thyroid hormone (hyperthyroidism) or due to other causes. In hyperthyroidism, the uptake and turnover of iodine and/or diagnostic isotopes is often raised throughout the entire or parts of the gland.

The various causes of hyperthyroidism and thyrotoxicosis are summarized in Table 15.1, which also presents the expected results at scintigraphy/uptake measurements.

Overall, the incidence of hyperthyroidism is estimated to be 50–80/100,000/year and 10/100,000/year/ for females and males, respectively. There is a considerable geographic variation.

The most common causes of hyperthyroidism are toxic diffuse goitre, toxic nodular goitre, and toxic autonomous adenoma. The risk of developing Graves' disease is several times higher for women than men.

In older patients, toxic nodular goitre is a more common cause of hyperthyroidism. Autonomous adenoma is the cause of hyperthyroidism in less than 10% of cases. In autonomous adenoma, activating mutations have been demonstrated in the gene for the TSH receptor protein. In unusual cases, mutations in the TSH receptor have been the cause of a general hyperactivity of the thyroid.

Various types of inflammation of the thyroid are the most common cause of thyrotoxicosis without hyperthyroidism. The inflammatory reaction causes leakage of hormone from the follicle to the blood. This results in a transient thyrotoxic condition, which is seen typically in the initial stages of both subacute thyroiditis (see Chap. 26) and autoimmune thyroiditis (see Chaps. 9 and 25).

During the first months of pregnancy, hCG from the placenta can stimulate TSH receptors, occasionally resulting in a more or less pronounced hyperactivity of the gland. The mechanism is similar to that for hyperthyroidism due to gestational trophoblastic tumour.

Chapter 15: Causes of Thyrotoxicosis – an Overview

Table 15.1 Causes of thyrotoxicosis

Cause	I-131 uptake	Radionuclide distribution at scintigraphy
Diffuse toxic goitre; Graves'/Basedows*	Increased	Evenly
Nodular toxic goitre; Plummer's disease*	Increased, normal	(Increased) locally in nodules
Toxic autonomous adenoma*	Increased, normal	(Increased) locally in the adenoma
Subacute thyroiditis	Undetectable, low	Rarely detectable
Silent thyroiditis Postpartum thyroiditis	Undetectable, low	Rarely detectable
High-iodine supplement	Low, (normal)	Irregular (if detectable)
hCG-induced (gestational) thyrotoxicosis*	Should not be performed	Should not be evaluated
TSH-producing pituitary adenoma*	Increased	Evenly
Ectopic/ovarian goitre	Low in the thyroid	Extrathyroidal
Exogenous (factitia, nutritional)	Undetectable	Not detectable
Secondary to trauma	Low	Rarely detectable

* Hyperthyroidism (increased synthesis and release/secretion of thyroid hormones)

A TSH-producing pituitary adenoma is an unusual cause of hyperthyroidism and can be difficult to diagnose because the patient can have normal or elevated TSH levels combined with a high concentration of T4 and T3. A similar laboratory profile can be seen in patients with thyroid hormone resistance. This latter patient group exhibits increased synthesis and release of thyroid hormones but only occasionally symptoms of thyrotoxicosis from selected organs.

Ectopic production of thyroid hormone can occur subsequently in ovarian tumours that contain thyroid follicles. In such cases the thyroid is inhibited, which leads to a low uptake of isotope at the same time as scintigraphy of the abdomen can demonstrate isotope uptake at the position of the ovary or tumour.

Self administration of high doses of thyroid hormone, thyrotoxicosis factitia (see Chap. 27), is a further example of the occurrence of thyrotoxicosis without hyperthyroidism. The patient can have consumed, intentionally or accidentally, high doses of thyroid hormone. Thyrotoxicosis has also been described when people have eaten food, such as hamburgers, containing thyroid tissue. This has been the cause of several outbreaks of otherwise inexplicable thyrotoxicosis.

Thyroid cancer (with hormone-producing metastases) can rarely cause thyrotoxicosis.

Iodine supplements in larger quantities than the daily requirements can, in some circumstances, cause thyrotoxicosis. This is seen most typically in individuals with multinodular goitre with autonomous areas, and in autonomous adenomas. In patients with Graves' disease, increased availability of iodine can result in more severe hyperthyroidism, especially in areas of endemic iodine deficiency.

16 Symptoms of Thyrotoxicosis

In patients with thyrotoxicosis, the symptoms can be partly due to the effects of elevated concentrations of thyroid hormones and partly to the underlying thyroid pathology. Patients with thyrotoxicosis sometimes have an enlarged thyroid, which can give local symptoms in the neck and even affect the trachea and other adjacent organs, primarily in toxic nodular goitre.

Graves' disease, in addition to symptoms due to thyrotoxicosis and goitre, also presents with symptoms caused by extrathyroidal manifestations of the immunological disturbance of this disease, i.e. ophthalmopathy and dermopathy. Here, only the general symptoms of thyrotoxicosis associated with elevated concentrations of T4 and T3 are discussed.

16.1 Weight Loss and Energy Metabolism

Thyroid hormone is critical for metabolic processes and the energy expenditure of the cell. The cellular mechanism of the calorigenic effect of thyroid hormone has not been mapped in detail. However, it is generally accepted that elevated concentrations of T4 and T3 result not only in increased aerobic metabolism, but most probably also increases anaerobic metabolism.

In most cases, increased energy expenditure results in utilization of body energy reserves and consequent weight loss. Typically, there is weight loss in spite of a good appetite. The increased metabolic activity releases nonutilized energy which is eliminated as heat. This explains why the patient feels constantly warm and sweaty, has difficulty in hot environments and dresses lightly. Reattaining the capacity to feel cold is a sign of normalized metabolic rate when treating the disease. It must be pointed out that some patients (2%) are paradoxically affected by a weight gain when they develop hyperthyroidism. It is also important to recognize that in some patients the thyrotoxic condition is associated with a general feeling of illness with lack of appetite and sometimes nausea, which further exacerbates the catabolic situation.

The increased blood flow through the skin, which is necessary for heat dissipation, also results in moist, soft and warm skin. Body temperature is normal. Fever is thus not typical in thyrotoxicosis unless the disease is accompanied by infection or a thyrotoxic crisis, or is caused by subacute thyroiditis.

16.2 Mental Problems

Tiredness is a very common symptom in thyrotoxicosis. Changes in mood with irritability and mild aggression are not uncommon, as are problems with concentration and sleeping. Such effects can affect the patient's working and family situation. Many patients, not least the elderly, may be depressed. More serious mental disorders can occur, particularly in connection with thyrotoxic crisis.

16.3 Muscle Weakness

The increased consumption of the energy reserves of the body can be critical in muscle function. Muscle effects are mostly noted in the large, proximal muscle groups in the arms and legs. Patients feel generally tired and weak, and can have great difficulty getting up from a squatting position (proximal muscle weakness), walking up stairs or performing other physical activities. Part of the explanation for the patient's weight loss is reduced muscle mass. Follow-up of patients after treatment for thyrotoxicosis has shown that the muscle mass increases as soon as the patient becomes euthyroid. This occurs before the fat reserves are restored.

The effects of elevated thyroid hormones on muscle function and circulation result in a general reduction of the patient's physical performance. Patients with thyrotoxicosis often experience increased tiredness and a clear decline in fitness.

Thyrotoxic periodic paralysis is an uncommon condition most often affecting patients with Asian ancestors. Its clinical manifestation is a localized or general muscular weakness, which is caused by increased transport of potassium into the cells, and can occur in patients with thyrotoxicosis. The condition can be triggered by extreme stress, high intake of carbohydrates, alcohol or insulin administration. The potassium concentration in plasma is often, but not always, lowered during attacks but normal in between. The attacks disappear when the patient becomes euthyroid.

16.4 Cardiac Arrhythmia and Cardiac Insufficiency

Increased catabolism and an increased requirement for elimination of thermal energy put demands on circulation. The cardiac/minute volume increases via increased heart rate. In younger patients, this presents as a regular tachycardia, often with perceived palpitations (Fig. 16.1a). Flow-dependent cardiac bruits are common.

Thyrotoxicosis can trigger atrial fibrillation in older people and even in younger people with no prior history of heart problems (Fig. 16.1b). In patients with impaired heart function, thyrotoxicosis can exacerbate the condition and result in heart failure, particularly if associated with atrial fibrillation. Atrial fibrillation results in an increased risk of arterial embolism, particularly in patients who are already at risk for this. Treatment with anticoagulants should be considered. Thyroid function must always be monitored in patients with new-onset atrial fibrillation. Treatment for hyperthyroidism should be started and euthyroidism achieved before electroconversion.

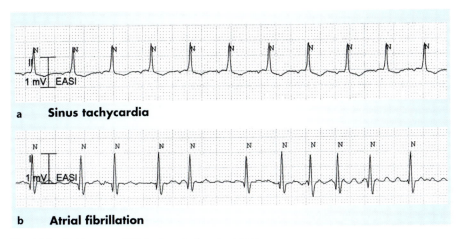

Fig. 16.1 a, b Common ECG findings in thyrotoxicosis

This procedure is seldom successful until the patient is euthyroid. In many patients there is a spontaneous conversion from atrial fibrillation to sinus rhythm when thyroid function is normalized. Oedema in the lower legs and ankles commonly occurs in thyrotoxic individuals with no prior heart disease

16.5 Sympathetic Nervous System

There is an interaction between thyroid hormone and the function of the sympathetic nervous system. The concentration of catecholamines does not increase in hyperthyroidism, but the sensitivity to catecholamines appears to increase, not least in the heart and CNS. This contributes to tachycardia, and also explains the typical tremor that patients can experience.

Increased sympathetic activity can, in addition, contribute to anxiety in many patients. This increase in activity also explains the tendency for retraction of the eyelid, the so-called lid retraction, which results in a staring gaze and reduced ability to lower the upper eye lid (Graefe's sign). This must not be confused with the eye symptoms caused by the autoimmune process associated with Graves' disease (thyroid-associated ophthalmopathy, see Chap. 19).

The effects on the autonomous nerve functions can also explain the increased intestinal movement that can occur. The patient may experience more rapid stomach emptying and resorption of foods. The passage of food through the intestines is faster, causing the patients to have more frequent defecations.

16.6 Dermatological Symptoms

The quality of nails and hair is affected. The distal part of the nail can loosen from the nail bed (onycholysis). The hair feels softer and looses its natural wave. An increased number of hair follicles are activated, which results in a more rapid turnover of hair. Increased hair loss is noticed particularly in the months after a patient has become euthyroid. This is completely reversible; the hair loss decreases when the patient has been euthyroid for a time and the number of active hair follicles drops again.

16.7 Reduced Glucose Tolerance and Effects on Blood Lipids

The increased energy turnover associated with elevated concentrations of thyroid hormones affects the metabolism of carbohydrates, lipids and proteins. Glucose metabolism is affected and impaired glucose tolerance or even diabetes mellitus may occur temporarily in connection with thyrotoxicosis. In diabetics, hyperthyroidism, via various mechanisms, results in impaired metabolic regulation with fluctuating blood glucose levels and increased insulin requirements.

The metabolism of lipids and lipoproteins is affected in a typical manner. The concentration of total cholesterol drops, mostly due to increased elimination of the LDL fraction, which is therefore lower than normal for the individual person, as is the HDL fraction. Changes in concentration of triglycerides are less pronounced and not completely clarified.

16.8 Fertility

The gonadal function is often affected by thyrotoxicosis. Fertility is, however, most often preserved. Oligomenorrhea and anovulation may occur. The duration of menstruation often becomes shorter. These functions are restituted quickly after initiation of treatment and the patient has become euthyroid.

16.9 Bones and Calcium

High concentrations of thyroid hormones result in increased bone turnover and a negative bone tissue balance. The mineral content of bones decrease during long-term thyrotoxicosis, which increases the risk of osteoporosis and fractures of the vertebrae. Fractures are seen in osteopenic patients but is rarely a clinical problem in younger patients.

Hypercalcaemia is frequently observed in pronounced thyrotoxicosis and develops if renal clearance of calcium can not cope with the increased release of calcium from bones into the blood due to the enhanced turnover of bone tissue in the hyperthyroid state. In these cases, the concentration of parathyroid hormone is lowered. Hypercalcaemia is corrected spontaneously when the patient becomes euthyroid.

Thyrotoxicosis

- **Metabolic effects**
  Increased basal metabolism, increased bone turnover with hypercalciuria, occasionally hypercalcaemia and decreased BMD. Enzyme induction: elevated concentrations of ASAT, ALAT, ALP (both bone and hepatic phosphatases) and GT. Lowered serum cholesterol, impaired glucose tolerance and diabetic control with increased insulin requirements.
- **Symptoms**
  Weight loss, palpitations, tiredness, muscular weakness, tremor, increased appetite, sweating, nervousness and restlessness, emotional lability, heat intolerance, rapid intestinal passage, sleep disturbance, and hyperactivity.
  Occasionally nausea, loss of appetite, apathy, passivity, and tiredness (apathetic hyperthyroidism in older patients).
- **Clinical findings**
  Emaciated patient, psychomotor restlessness, wide open eyes, fine tremors, goitre (not obligatory), soft, moist, warm skin, tachycardia/atrial fibrillation, hyperreflexia, onycholysis, blood flow bruits over the thyroid and ankle oedema.

17 Hyperthyroidism Treatment Options – an Overview

Three treatment options are available for patients with hyperthyroidism: antithyroid drugs, surgery and radioiodine therapy. For patients with Graves' disease all three options can be applied. For patients with toxic nodular goitre or toxic adenoma, treatment with antithyroid drugs is only indicated for a limited time, prior to definitive therapy with one of the other two methods.

Treatment routines vary between clinics and countries, most markedly for Graves' disease. In Europe, for example, the preferred method of treatment for this disease is medical therapy, while in the USA, radioiodine is the preferred method. This variation reflects the difference in therapeutic traditions and other factors, such as local legislation governing radiation exposure. The variation in therapy also reflects the fact that no single therapy is considered to be outright superior to another. In several countries radioiodine therapy has gained increasing acceptance due to the relatively low risk of complications and also the cost effectiveness.

17.1 General Considerations

The patient should, as far as possible, be informed of the available therapies and the patient's own viewpoint should be taken into account when choosing therapy. At the same time, they should also be informed about the typical disease symptoms. Frequently, the patient is found to have more thyrotoxic symptoms than they had noticed themselves.

Patients with pronounced thyrotoxicosis can experience a lower threshold for stress ("short fuse"), asthenia and depression and frequently be involved in conflicts and experience problems in social relations both at home and work. A reassurance that the

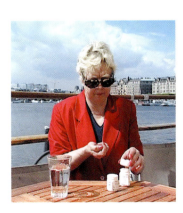

Fig. 17.1 Medical treatment of Graves' disease

E. Nyström, G.E.B. Berg, S.K.G. Jansson, O. Tørring, S.V. Valdemarsson (Eds.),
Thyroid Disease in Adults,
DOI: 10.1007/978-3-642-13262-9_17, © Springer-Verlag Berlin Heidelberg 2011

Chapter 17: Hyperthyroidism Treatment Options – an Overview

problems may be linked to the disease, that they are transitory and will resolve when the disease has been treated, can be a relief for both the patient and others involved in a difficult situation. The patient should also be informed that the problems can persist for several months after successful therapy through normalization of hormone levels.

It is not unusual for the patient to quickly regain weight once treatment has been initiated and in some cases continue with further weight increase. The patient should therefore receive appropriate dietary advice at quite an early stage. Because many patients loose muscle mass, it is advisable to provide individually tailored exercise advice when the patient becomes euthyroid.

As in many other diseases, it is important that patients adjust their lifestyle to the situation. The importance of adequate sleep must be emphasized to the patient and similarly the importance of planning the day and adjusting demands and expectations.

17.2 Medical Treatment

Medical treatment of hyperthyroidism can be used for patients of all ages. The most commonly used medical treatment is antithyroid drugs, which have a direct effect on hormone synthesis by the thyroid cells. Medical treatment also includes beta blockers.

Beta blockers (propranolol 20–40 mg × 3 or metoprolol as depot tablet 50–100 mg × 1–2) can be given to relieve symptoms while the patient is waiting for further investigation and before hormone levels have normalized and symptoms have receded. Beta blockers alleviate adrenergic symptoms such as palpitations, tremor and to a certain extent restlessness, while the elevated metabolism is not affected. In contrast to patients treated with antithyroid drugs, patients who only receive beta blockers do not regain muscle mass and body weight.

Beta blockers in higher doses are used at certain institutions as treatment prior to and during surgery for mild hyperthyroidism. Treatment with stable iodine is reserved for presurgery for patients who react negatively to antithyroid drugs or develop toxic crisis.

17.2.1 Antithyroid Drugs

Antithyroid drugs block the capacity of the thyroid gland to synthesize the hormones T3 and T4. Commonly used medicines are thiamazol, carbimazole (less commonly) and propylthiouracil. The half-life of thiamazol is longer and is therefore given in two daily doses (Table 17.1). Propylthiouracil is normally given in three doses. Thiamazol and propylthiouracil have similar mechanisms of action in the thyroid, but propylthiouracil can also inhibit the peripheral conversion of T4 to T3. Propylthiouracil is commonly recommended when treating hyperthyroidism during pregnancy, lactation or thyrotoxic crisis.

Table.17.1 Antithyroid drugs

Drug	Initial dose
Thiamazol (5 mg)	10–15 mg, two times daily
Propylthiouracil (50 mg)	50–100 mg, three times daily

After starting therapy the patient experiences an improvement after 1 to 2 weeks and hormone levels are often normalized after 2 to 4 weeks.

> Antithyroid drugs most probably exert their effect by interaction with TPO, which plays an important role in iodination of tyrosine in the thyroglobulin molecule and in coupling of iodinated tyrosine residues to T4 and T3 (Fig. 2.8). Uptake of iodide across the basal membrane is not thought to be directly inhibited by antithyroid drugs. This uptake can, however, be blocked by perchlorate ions, which is exploited for treatment of amiodarone-induced hyperthyroidism.

Antithyroid drugs primarily have a place in treatment of patients whose disease has an underlying immunological cause (Graves' disease). This category of patients is commonly treated for 12–18 months and in some cases even longer. It is presupposed that the immunological activity abates and the disease then goes into remission during treatment. Antithyroid drugs may also have a mild modulating effect on the immunological process. Stable and normal hormone levels likely have a significant positive effect. If the patient has a more severe disease with high T4/T3 values at the outset of disease and a large goitre, the probability of recurrence is high after discontinuation of antithyroid drug therapy (see Chap. 18).

In patients with nodular toxic goitre or toxic adenoma, antithyroid drugs have an inhibitory effect on synthesis of thyroid hormone during treatment, but a persistent cure should not be expected. Hormone synthesis and release will increase again when the treatment is stopped. In these cases, treatment with antithyroid drugs is therefore not the preferred final choice. In the very elderly it is not always possible to operate or make use of radioiodine therapy. In these cases, patients can receive antithyroid drugs at low doses for the rest of their lives.

In patients with thyrotoxicosis due to thyroiditis, such as subacute thyroiditis, there is no benefit of antithyroid drugs. In patients who have hyperthyroidism as a consequence of high iodine intake, for example in amiodarone-induced hyperthyroidism, antithyroid drugs have a limited effect. In amiodarone induced hyperthyroidism antithyroid drugs are given in higher doses, sometimes with concomitant treatment such as potassium perchlorate (see page 276).

Two different treatment models can be applied. Either the patient is treated only with antithyroid drugs, given as the lowest dose that controls the patient's hyperthyroidism, or antithyroid drugs are given in higher doses throughout the entire treatment period in combination with thyroxine. This is discussed in more detail in Chap. 18.

The most important side effects of antithyroid drugs are:
- Effects on bone marrow
- Rashes
- Itching
- Arthralgia

- Fever
- Hepatotoxicity (hepatocellular) and cholestatic events
- Metallic taste

The most serious adverse effect of treatment with both thiamazol and propylthiouracil is effects on the bone marrow with a risk of agranulocytosis. Blood status should be checked before the treatment starts. Checks should be performed during the first visit after initiating therapy with antithyroid drugs. A white blood cell count does not have any predictive value for predicting agranulocytosis. However, a decreasing number of neutrophiles in the blood count is an important observation, since it may precede a more pronounced adverse impact with leucopenia/agranulocytosis. Decreasing neutrophiles should thus stop further antithyroid drug treatment.

Effects on bone marrow (primarily agranulocytosis) affects 0.1–0.4% of treated patients, often appearing within 3 months after starting treatment and usually has an acute onset, less than 24–48 h.

The most common symptoms in agranulocytosis are fever and sore throat. Patients who are treated with antithyroid drugs must receive written information instructing them to stop therapy and seek medical advice immediately if any such symptoms occur or if they experience other signs that could indicate leucopenia. A patient who experiences effects on the white blood cell count with one antithyroid drug must not be treated with any other antithyroid drug due to the high risk of cross reaction.

Skin reactions are relatively common and often associated with itching and can sometimes cause rashes. The rash often has the appearance of a slightly raised, somewhat scaly erythema, which disappears when treatment is stopped. If this type of reaction occurs during treatment with thiamazol, the patient can switch to propylthiouracil and vice versa. The risk of developing skin reactions appears to be dose dependent.

Arthralgia without inflammatory reaction abates when the dose is reduced. Cholestatic icterus, hepatocellular toxic cell damage, angioneurotic oedema and a SLE-like syndrome with severe pain in the joints are other serious but rare side effects that necessitate prompt cessation of treatment.

Another unusual side effect of antithyroid drugs is anosmia or metallic taste in the mouth. If this symptom occurs, treatment must be stopped promptly. As a rule, restitution normally takes place, but this can take several months.

17.2.2 Treatment with Stable Iodine

Iodine has long been used to block thyroid hormone release and was the first medical therapy for hyperthyroidism. Iodide blocking is now rarely used, but is still very useful when given preoperatively in cases where a rapid effect is desired. If iodine is continuously administered to patients with hyperthyroidism, the blocking effect falls after 7–10 days. A subsequent rapid increase in release of hormone involves a risk that the severity of thyrotoxicosis increases. Preoperative treatment with iodine thus necessitates surgery within 10 days. Iodine uptake is down-regulated over a longer time which makes radioiodine treatment impossible.

Iodine solutions are available for oral use: Iodine-potassium iodide; 5% solution (iodine 5; potassium iodide 10, aq. dest. 85) contains about 2.2 mg iodine per drop. Initially, 5 drops (11 mg) iodine are given 3 times a day, and thereafter increased if necessary to 10 drops or more, 3 times daily until the symptoms are under control and the pulse <90/min. Surgical intervention must take place at most 10 days from start of treatment.

The main indications for medical treatment are:
- First onset of diffuse toxic goitre in younger and middle-aged patients with moderately elevated thyroid hormone values and without pronounced thyroid enlargement
- Hyperthyroidism during pregnancy, lactation
- Before surgical treatment
- Before radioiodine treatment
- Graves' disease with TAO
- Hyperthyroidism in the elderly (also toxic nodular goitre and toxic adenoma), for which other treatments are not possible

17.2.3 Treatment with Radioiodine

Radioiodine treatment has been used for more than 60 years and there is extensive experience with this treatment modality. The method is simple and cheap, but requires access to special equipment for isotope therapy.

17.2.3.1 Aspects of Radiation

The patients may be afraid of radiation with radioiodine treatment and may worry that the treatment carries an increased risk of cancer. However, many extensive follow-up studies have been completed since the 1940s without demonstrating any clear increase in the incidence of malignancy.

Experiences from the nuclear power plant accident in Chernobyl have nevertheless demonstrated that children exposed to radioactive isotopes released at the accident were at risk of developing thyroid cancer. Cancer in the thyroid developed primarily in children younger than 10 years old at the time of exposure.

With respect to radiation risk, it is now accepted that radioiodine treatment can be given to all adult patients. There may however be other factors that would suggest other forms of treatment in younger adults such as the problems of radiation protection in families with small children. An additional risk is an increase in antibodies (TRAb), which in pregnancy may cross the placenta and affect the foetus. However, in realty, foetal thyrotoxicosis due to maternal TRAb is quite rare.

The treatment can be given on an outpatient basis. In most countries there is a limit of permissible maximal radioactivity given for outpatient treatment. In Sweden this limit is now individualized according to the circumstances, but for practical work, it is about 600 MBq.

From the point of view of radiation safety, treatment with radioiodine has no effect on later pregnancies. The radiation dose received by the ovaries is about the same as that received at urography (7 mSv). The patient is nevertheless recommended to postpone pregnancy until 6 months after treatment. The most important reason for this recommendation is that it takes about 6 months before the desired effect has been achieved and pregnancy can be completed while the mother is free from persistent or rapidly recurring hyperthyroidism. Sexual intercourse should be avoided in the time immediately following treatment (a couple of weeks), primarily to protect the partner against undesired effects of radiation.

Chapter 17: Hyperthyroidism Treatment Options – an Overview

The radiation received at radioiodine treatment does not cause hair loss, something which patients are occasionally anxious about. However, temporary hair loss can sometimes be seen due to the changes in thyroid hormone levels caused by the disease.

Iodine allergy in the patient does not contraindicate treatment.

17.2.3.2 Dosage Calculation and Therapy

The dose can be calculated for each patient before radioiodine treatment. This involves determining iodine uptake and retention of a test dose after the 24 h I-131 uptake test and/or at a later time point (4–6 days). The effective half-life can be calculated from the isotope's biological half-life and physical half-life and thus has importance for the residence time of radionuclide in the gland.

Preparations before treatment can also include thyroid scintigraphy to assess the underlying cause for hyperthyroidism and the volume of thyroid iodine-absorbing tissue.

The radiation dosage required for the thyroid tissue is then decided (normally 90–120 Gy for Graves' disease and multinodular toxic goitre, and 200–300 Gy for toxic adenoma). Next, the activity in MBq necessary to achieve the treatment objective is calculated. This calculation must take into account the size of the gland, the radioiodine uptake and the effective half-life. Both the test dose and the treatment dose is given perorally as a solution with a neutral taste or as a capsule (Fig. 17.2).

In some centres fixed activities of radioiodine are used. However, in order to be able to give as low a dose as achievable, and avoid repeated treatments, dose calculation is highly recommended.

Uptake of radioiodine also occurs to a very limited extent in the salivary glands, the mucous membranes of the stomach, the choroid plexus and the mammary glands. However, iodine only binds to proteins in the thyroid, which is why persistent tissue damage most probably only occurs in the thyroid gland at the concentrations used in treatment of hyperthyroidism.

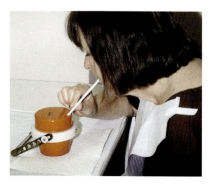

Fig. 17.2 Radioiodine administration

17.2 Medical Treatment

The patient rarely experiences any acute side effects of the treatment. If the administered dose is large, a certain amount of soreness may be experienced in the throat, similar to that with a cold. However, this passes quickly.

17.2.3.3 Radiation Safety After Radioiodine Treatment

At higher concentrations, the patient must remain in a radiation-proof room in the hospital until the activity has dropped. Because a large proportion of the administered dose is excreted in the urine, additional precautionary measures must be taken when treating incontinent patients. Guidelines are given by the local radiation safety officer.

Any person in the proximity of the patient must be protected from radiation in accordance with current radiation safety guidelines. The foetus and/or children of close family and friends must not be exposed to more than 1 mSv. For adults up to the age of 60, the limit is 3 mSv and for adults above the age of 60 the limit is 15 mSv. For anyone else, stricter restrictions apply, with a limit of 0.3 mSv. In practice, this is achieved by maintaining a distance of 3 m in the first week after treatment. The most important factor is to avoid close contact with small children and pregnant women.

17.2.3.4 Consequences of Radioiodine Treatment

There is always a risk of developing hypothyroidism after radioiodine treatment. It is therefore of utmost importance that patients who receive radioiodine treatment, and who do not immediately receive thyroxine, are followed-up regularly (at least once a year) for the rest of their lives.

Development of hypothyroidism after radioiodine treatment for Graves' disease normally occurs within 2 years, but may also appear years later. In many centres today, the standard objective for radioiodine treatment of Graves' disease is to achieve permanent hypothyroidism. Thyroxine substitution is initiated 2–3 weeks after I-131 therapy so that the patient never experiences symptoms of thyroid hormone deficiency.

Patients with nodular toxic goitre who receive radioiodine treatment do not always develop hypothyroidism. These patients should nevertheless be followed-up regularly because there is a risk of recurrent hyperthyroidism.

A rise in TRAb is frequently observed after radioiodine treatment of patients with Graves' disease (Fig. 18.6). Even in patients with Graves' disease or toxic nodular goitre, who did not have TRAb before treatment, can have these antibodies develop after treatment. Because this may be associated with the development of ophthalmopathy, attempts are sometimes made to counteract it by giving concomitant steroid treatment with the radioiodine therapy in Graves' hyperthyroidism.

In certain cases, a radiation-induced, thyroiditis-like reaction can occur some weeks after treatment. This can result in a period with elevated hormone levels before onset of underactivity. The symptoms are primarily thyrotoxic with palpitations, tremors, sweating and restlessness. The patient is treated symptomatically with beta blockers until the symptoms decline.

Because underactivity can occur fairly rapidly after treatment of patients with Graves' disease, T4 should be closely monitored in patients not receiving thyroxine. To distinguish between persistent hyperthyroidism and an acute radiation reaction in Graves' patients, an I-131 iodine uptake test can be conducted about 10 weeks after treatment. If uptake at this point is low, rapid development of hypothyroidism can be expected. If uptake is high, this indicates that there is persistent autonomous activity in the tissues and it may be necessary to repeat the radioiodine treatment.

For patients with nodular toxic goitre, repeat treatments may be necessary because parts of the gland can have low uptake during the first treatment. Normally, this decision is made after about 4 months.

The primary indications for radioiodine therapy are:
- Diffuse toxic goitre (Graves' disease) in patients without clinically significant ophthalmopathy
- Nodular toxic goitre in patients without pressure symptoms from the goitre
- Toxic adenoma (alternative to surgery)
- Recurrence after previous surgery

17.2.4 Surgery

A prerequisite for uncomplicated surgery of hyperthyroidism is that the symptoms are under control. This can be achieved by using preoperative antithyroid drugs until the patient is euthyroid and/or controlling the symptoms using beta blockers. After adequate pretreatment, the patient is admitted to the hospital and surgery is performed under general anaesthesia.

Surgery for hyperthyroidism can sometimes be technically demanding and should be carried out by an experienced surgeon. The principles for surgical treatment of hyperthyroidism vary between different centres. Some surgeons prefer to resect nearly all thyroid tissue and immediately place the patient on thyroid substitution, while others perform a less extensive resection in the hope that the patient will become euthyroid without the requirement for thyroxine substitution.

The requirement for postoperative treatment with thyroxine is based on how much thyroid tissue has been removed and on the results of thyroid hormone analyses. Patients with thyroid-associated ophthalmopathy should always receive thyroxine substitution to avoid development of postoperative hypothyroidism.

17.2.4.1 Surgical Routines

In conventional surgery, the thyroid gland is exposed through so-called Kocher collar incision. The incision is made two to three finger widths above the jugulum aiming at an optimal cosmetic result (Fig. 17.3). The surgeon exposes the thyroid and identifies the parathyroid glands and recurrent nerve before resection of the thyroid tissue.

Nowadays, minimally invasive techniques using different approaches are used at some clinics. The principles for surgical resection are the same as in open surgery, but these techniques leave minimal scars (Fig. 17.4).

Postoperative follow-up should include determination of serum calcium during the first days to detect and treat any disturbance. If the patient is affected by unexplained hoarseness or respiratory problems, the motility of the vocal cords should be checked.

Normally, the patient can eat and drink the day after the operation. If there are no complications during the operation and postoperative period, the patient can generally be discharged after 1 or 2 days. Infection in the wound is uncommon, and wound healing is normally straightforward, leaving only a small scar, which seldom leads to any cosmetic concerns. The patient should be advised to cover the scar and avoid pro-

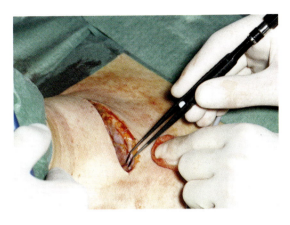

Fig. 17.3 Kocher incision for surgical exposure of the thyroid gland. Bipolar diathermia is used for hemostasis

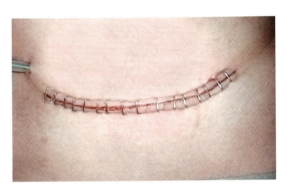

Fig. 17.4 Skin-incision is closed using staples

nounced sunshine exposure directly on the scar tissue during the first 4–6 months. After uncomplicated surgery, a patient will require about 1–2 weeks sick leave.

17.2.4.2 Indications for Surgical Treatment

Surgical treatment of hyperthyroidism is suitable for both Graves' disease and nodular toxic goitre and toxic autonomous nodules.

Surgical treatment is preferred, especially in young patients with Graves' disease and if the patient has pronounced hyperthyroidism and a large goitre at the onset of disease. The reason is that the chance for persistent remission after conclusion of medical treatment is lower. At certain institutions, surgical treatment is performed early in the course of the illness if the patient has severe ophthalmopathy. Surgery may also be preferred for those cases in which medical treatment does not maintain good control.

The choice at treatment of toxic multinodular goitre and toxic autonomous nodules lies often between radioiodine therapy and surgery. One advantage with surgery is that there is a rapid reduction in the size of the goitre and thus alleviation of local pressure symptoms.

Surgical treatment of hyperthyroidism is an alternative to medical treatment during pregnancy. The operation should be performed during the second trimester.

At reoperation after previous subtotal thyroidectomy, the risk of complications increases. Patients with recurring hyperthyroidism after surgical treatment should therefore preferably be offered treatment with radioiodine or antithyroid drugs.

The main indications for surgical treatment are:
- Younger patients with Graves' disease, particularly with pronounced goitre
- Recurrence or insufficient effect of medical treatment in Graves' disease
- Multinodular toxic goitre with local symptoms
- Multinodular toxic goitre for which radioiodine treatment is difficult to employ due to low iodine uptake
- Toxic autonomous adenoma with local symptoms
- Patients with a large goitre regardless of age
- Treatment option during pregnancy
- Patient, regardless of age, with Graves' disease and pronounced ophthalmopathy
- At suspected malignancy
- Recurrence after repeated radioiodine treatment
- Medically intractable amiodarone induced thyrotoxicosis

17.3 Laboratory Checks After Treatment for Hyperthyroidism

After treatment for thyrotoxicosis, TSH secretion can be suppressed for 3–6 months. In these cases, determination of T4 should be used to diagnose hypothyroidism and for controlling treatment with thyroxine until suppression of TSH is released (Fig. 17.5).

Determination of total or free T3 is particularly valuable for demonstrating persistent or recurring autonomous hormone secretion. This can be of particular value at suspicion of recurrence in a patient who has received thyroxine after treatment for hyperthyroidism.

It should always be kept in mind that patients who have undergone surgery with partial thyroid resection or treated with radioiodine to achieve euthyroidism and who do not receive thyroxine, run a great risk later on of developing hypothyroidism. Neither should it be forgotten that about 10%–15% of patients treated only with antithyroid drugs for Graves' disease gradually develop hypothyroidism.

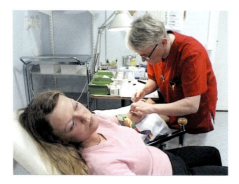

Fig. 17.5 Laboratory check-up after treatment

18 Graves' Disease

In iodine sufficient countries, Graves' disease is the predominant cause of hyperthyroidism in young and middle-aged patients. The incidence is about 30–50/100,000 inhabitants per year. Graves' disease can affect all ages, but is most common in people between 20 and 50 years of age. Graves' disease also occurs in elderly individuals, for whom toxic nodular goitre is another common cause of hyperthyroidism.

18.1 Pathophysiology

Graves' disease is caused by specific IgG antibodies (TRAb) that bind to and stimulate the TSH receptor. There is an increased lymphocyte count in the thyroid that most probably also has pathophysiological significance. The reason for immune system activation is not known, but is considered to be multifactorial, with both endogenous and exogenous elements affecting certain genetically predisposed individuals (see Chap. 7).

Patients with Graves' disease also frequently have antibodies against other antigens, for example thyroid peroxidase (TPO). This is an additional expression of the autoimmune process targeting the thyroid.

Autoimmune thyroid disease may occur in several members of the same family, in which one person may have Graves' disease and another chronic thyroiditis. Graves' disease can be the only manifestation, or one of several in a person with a multiorgan specific syndrome (autoimmune polyglandular syndrome, see Chap. 7). Chapter 7 also covers the effects of smoking, stress, etc. on the onset of Graves' disease.

In certain cases, exposure to iodine is thought to have a triggering effect that might operate via disturbances in the autoregulation of iodine metabolism in the follicle cells.

The reason for the female predominance in Graves' disease (Fig. 18.1) is uncertain, but is considered to be the result of a possible modulating effect of oestrogen on autoimmune reactivity. Such mechanisms could also explain the increased incidence in women after pregnancy.

18.2 Symptoms Specific to Graves' Disease

The general symptoms of thyrotoxicosis due to Graves' disease are often pronounced. The most important clinical findings that favour the diagnose of Graves' disease are the presence of thyrotoxic symptoms for longer than 4–6 weeks and the presence of other immunologically mediated symptoms, primarily ophthalmopathy, but also (rarely) pretibial myxoedema (Fig. 18.2) and thyroid-associated acropachy (Fig. 18.3).

Pretibial myxoedema is seen in a few patients with Graves' disease. This is a localized accumulation of glycosaminoglycans distinct from the generalized increase seen in se-

Chapter 18: Graves' Disease

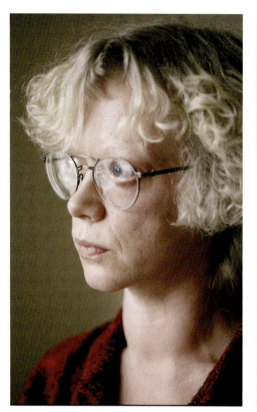

Fig. 18.1 Woman with Graves´ disease

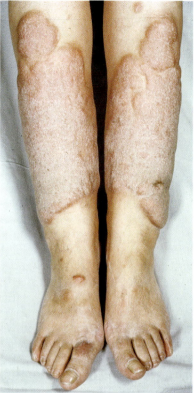

Fig. 18.2 Pretibial myxoedema

vere hypothyroidism and myxoedema, and is often localized to the front of the lower leg. Thus, pretibial myxoedema has become the accepted name (Fig. 18.2).

Thyroid-associated acropachy (Figs. 18.3 and 18.4) is an extremely rare painless swelling of the soft tissues similar to that observed in pretibial myxoedema. The swelling is generally localized to the hands (fingers) and feet. The skin often becomes hyperkeratotic and pigmented, and increased subperiostal bone formation can be seen in X-ray investigations, primarily in the middle and distal phalanges. Subcutaneous autoimmune storage of glycosaminoglycans can also be seen.

Graves' disease has the following characteristics:
- Immunologically mediated hyperthyroidism
- Presence of TRAb and commonly TPOAb
- Extrathyroidal immunological manifestations
  - Thyroid-associated ophthalmopathy (TAO)
  - Pretibial myxoedema,
  - Thyroid-associated acropachy (rarely)
  - Cardiac effects (including myxoedemous valves, mitral prolapse)

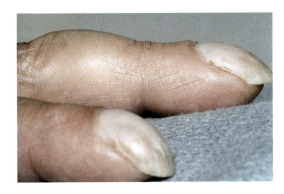

Fig. 18.3 Thyroid-associated acropachy

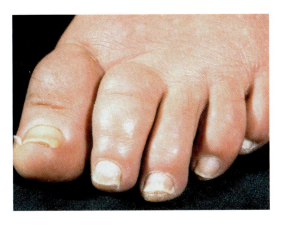

Fig. 18.4 Thyroid-associated acropachy. Swelling of soft tissues similar to pretibial myxoedema

- Goitre (diffuse) is common but not a prerequisite
- Women develop the disease 5–10 times more frequently than men
- Relapse is common

18.3 Diagnosis

Graves' disease is the predominant cause of hyperthyroidism in younger people, but it is important to know that elderly people also can be affected. If the classic symptoms of thyrotoxicosis and signs of ophthalmopathy (TAO) are present, the patient most probably has Graves' disease. In some cases, thyrotoxicosis due to pathophysiological mechanisms similar to those seen in Graves' disease develops after radioiodine therapy for toxic nodular goitre.

If the patient does not have eye symptoms, the thyrotoxic symptoms might be associated with the initial phase of thyroiditis. In these conditions, the thyrotoxic symptoms are mild and transient and disappear spontaneously within a few weeks, an observation that helps differentiate Graves' disease.

Clinical examination in most cases of Graves' disease will reveal a diffusely enlarged gland. Asymmetric diffuse goitre does occur and can be misleading. However, it is not uncommon for the patient to have a normal sized (not necessarily palpable) or only slightly to moderately enlarged thyroid.

The diagnosis of thyrotoxicosis is confirmed biochemically by suppressed TSH, which can not be otherwise explained by, for example, nonthyroidal illness (NTI) or the intake of certain medicines. Elevated levels of T4 and/or T3 reinforce the diagnosis and also provide information on the severity of the thyrotoxic condition. However, clinically significant thyrotoxicosis can be present even if the concentration of T4 is only slightly elevated or within the upper normal reference range, particularly in elderly patients. A typical clinical picture supports the diagnosis.

In some patients with thyrotoxicosis, a relatively larger increase in T3 than in T4 may be seen. Determination of free T3 can thus sometimes be more sensitive than free T4 for assessment of the severity of the disease and, in addition, is a valuable tool for identifying recurrence in a patient who has received thyroxine substitution after previous therapy (surgery or radioiodine) for hyperthyroidism.

The I-131 uptake is increased and scintigraphy reveals a uniform uptake throughout the entire thyroid. Scintigraphy is thus helpful in the differential diagnosis of conditions with increased levels of thyroid hormones, not least with respect to silent thyroiditis which, based on palpation findings, can be very similar to Graves' disease. Here, isotope uptake is low or completely absent. I-131 uptake is also low in iodine-induced hyperthyroidism. Scintigraphy and/or uptake measurements should always be considered in cases that can not otherwise be confirmed as Graves' disease.

Analysis of TRAb reveals the presence of antibodies in about 95–99% of cases.

18.4 Treatment

There is currently no treatment that directly affects the underlying immunological disorder. Instead, treatment is aimed at reducing the ability of the thyroid to produce hormone.

Antithyroid drugs, radioiodine therapy and surgery can all be used for treatment of Graves' disease. The choice of method varies between centres and also depends on local experience and resources (Table 18.1). Treating a patient with Graves' disease frequently involves long-term measures that require experience and insight into the different manifestations and progress of the disease. General knowledge has increased in recent years, consistent with the increased insight into the immunological mechanisms involved.

18.4.1 Medical Treatment

Medical treatment follows the guidelines given in the general treatment principles in Chap. 17. The greatest disadvantage of antithyroid drugs is the relatively high risk of recurrence (40–60%).

Medical treatment is primarily suitable for younger and middle-aged patients with first time onset of Graves' disease with moderately pronounced hyperthyroidism and without a large goitre. In these cases, the chances of persistent remission are high. On

Table 18.1 Factors that affect Graves' disease treatment choice and ranking of each choice as either the preferred choice (+++), an option that can be used (++), an option, but not a preferred choice (+) and not recommended (–)*

	Surgery	I-131	Medical treatment
Low age	++	+	+++
High age	+	+++	++
Large goitre	+++	++	+
Significant TAO	+++	–	+++
Pregnancy	+	–	+++
Recurrence after surgery	+	+++	++
Recurrence after I-131	++	+++	++
Recurrence after medical treatment	+++	+++	+

*This is a schematic representation. An individual assessment must be made in which the doctor takes into account the patient's own preferences.

the other hand, low age at onset of disease and the presence of a large goitre, high levels of T4/T3, and high concentrations of TRAb at diagnosis, can indicate a higher risk for nonpersistent remission after conclusion of medical treatment. In the event of recurrence, both surgery and radioiodine therapy are appropriate choices for treatment.

Pregnancy has a modulating effect on immunological activity, including that directed towards the thyroid. Patients who suffer from Graves' disease during pregnancy often achieve a spontaneous remission. In these cases, temporary treatment with antithyroid drugs is therefore a suitable alternative during the toxic phase.

The choice of therapy for hyperthyroidism in patients with Graves' disease varies, but should result in euthyroidism without the risk of triggering or exacerbating ophthalmopathy. Because medical treatment may have an immune-modulating effect, it is theoretically possible that treatment with antithyroid drugs offers an advantage in these cases. There are two antithyroid drug treatment models to choose between in hyperthyroidism.

The first involves only the administration of antithyroid drugs, monotherapy, which starts with thiamazol (10 mg twice/day) or propylthiouracil (100 mg 3 times/day). Lower doses can be given in milder hyperthyroidism. An effect is normally achieved within 2–4 weeks, when the patient will notice an improvement. The dose is gradually tapered and adjusted guided by analysis of T4 and/or T3 so that the patient is kept euthyroid. This treatment is based on administrating the lowest dose of antithyroid drugs that maintains the patient in a euthyroid state.

In the majority of patients, the concentrations of T4 and T3 are normalized within 3–4 weeks after starting therapy. TSH remains suppressed in the following weeks to months after the patient has become euthyroid, which is the reason for following the effect of therapy by determining T4 and T3 during this time.

The second form of therapy, called block and replace therapy or combination therapy, retains the antithyroid drug at full dose during the entire treatment period so that synthesis of thyroid hormone is blocked. After 2–4 weeks, the antithyroid drug is supplemented with thyroxine, 50–75 µg daily, with an increase to 100–150 µg daily at around 4 weeks from start with the antithyroid drug. Initially, the dose of thyroxine is adjusted guided by analysis of T4 and/or T3 so that the patient remains euthyroid. The patient continues with block and replace treatment during the entire treatment period (12–18 months) with regular blood tests every third month.

Block and replace treatment (Fig. 18.5) normally provides good control of the symptoms without the risk of hypothyroidism. Furthermore, lab checks can probably occur at longer intervals. Block and replace therapy is the preferred treatment prior to surgery. In patients with ophthalmopathy, the block and replace regimen gives the best option for stable control. Continuous fluctuations in hormone levels are thought to increase the risk of activation or exacerbation of the ophthalmopathy. The disadvantage of combination treatment is that larger doses of antithyroid drugs are given throughout the treatment period compared to monotherapy, with the accompanying risk of adverse effects.

The choice between thiamazol or propylthiouracil is often dependent on local tradition. Studies indicate that thiamazol might give more rapid normalization of T3/T4 concentrations and perhaps a slightly lower risk of adverse events, which are dose-dependent to a lesser extent for thiamazol than for propylthiouracil. One advantage of thiamazol is the longer half-life, and the possibility of dose administration twice or even only once a day.

Propylthiouracil is often preferred in pregnant women because of its shorter half-life, and also because it appears less likely to cause developmental anomalies than thiamazol. However, severe hepatic adverse reactions have been reported more frequently with propylthiouracil.

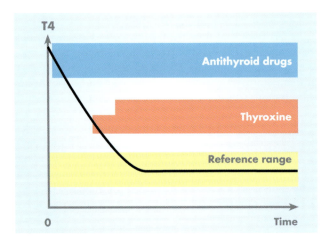

Fig. 18.5 Principles of block and replace therapy

Generally, the recommended treatment period with antithyroid drugs is 12–18 months for Graves' disease. There is no evidence to suggest that a longer treatment period increases the chance of persistent remission. It has not been possible to prove that block and replace therapy gives a better chance to achieve permanent remission than monotherapy.

It is difficult to predict whether a patient will remain euthyroid after completion of medical treatment. Often, falling TRAb levels are seen in patients who respond well to medical treatment. Persistently high T4 levels, and especially T3 levels, are observed in spite of treatment, when the thyroid is not adequately blocked. If this is the case, the dose of antithyroid drugs should be increased. Reduction of the thyroxine dose should then also be considered. Occasionally surgery or radioiodine treatment have to be considered in patients who are difficult to control using antithyroid drugs.

Falling TRAb values, or most importantly, absence of TRAb, may indicate that the immunological activity is in the process of declining, but is no guarantee that persistent remission will be achieved. Persistently high TRAb levels, on the other hand, indicates that exacerbation of the hyperthyroid state can be expected after discontinuation of antithyroid drugs. In most cases, increasing TRAb values after conclusion of medical therapy precede recurrence.

One advantage of medical therapy is that it does not cause persistent hypothyroidism. On the other hand, there is a risk of adverse effects, and in some cases treatment can not be completed because of this. As presented above, another disadvantage is the risk of relapse. The incidence of recurrence can be as high as 40–60% after 12 and 48 months in a nonselected series of patients, independently of whether monotherapy or block and replace treatment is used. The risk of recurrence is greater in younger patients, who prior to treatment, have high T3 levels, high TRAb levels and a large goitre. These factors also underpin the importance of planning alternative therapies early in the course of the disease.

Smoking is thought to counteract the possibility of remission after medical treatment and patients should be advised to stop smoking.

In persistent hyperthyroidism or recurrence after completion of medical treatment, surgery or radioiodine should be considered.

18.4.2 Radioiodine Treatment

For Graves' disease, the current objective in many centres is to give only one course of radioiodine. It may, however, be necessary to repeat the radioiodine treatment if the initial treatment had an inadequate effect. After treatment, there is slow improvement of symptoms, which may be evident after about 3 weeks or longer. Persistent disease activity is occasionally seen up to 3–4 months and repeated treatment may then be necessary. Occasionally, immediately after treatment, an increase in hormone levels may be observed due to radiation damage with hormone leakage. If the hormone levels are still high after 10 weeks, a new I-131 uptake test can be performed to distinguish between radiation thyroiditis (low uptake) and persistent hyperthyroidism (elevated uptake). In the elderly and patients with a heart condition, the elevated hormone levels after treatment can cause a temporary exacerbation of cardiac symptoms (see also Chap. 17).

Chapter 18: Graves' Disease

After therapy it is important that patients do not enter a phase with hypothyroidism. Many institutions now start treatment with thyroxine early, often 2 weeks after radioiodine therapy, and without first evaluating whether the treatment has resulted in hypothyroidism. The thyroxine dose is adjusted gradually, guided by T4, T3 and subsequently by TSH. It is thus of major importance to avoid even transient hypothyroid conditions since this may increase the risk for ophthalmopathy.

During the first years after treatment for Graves' disease with radioiodine, the concentration of TRAb rises (Fig. 18.6). What role this plays in the progress of the disease after treatment, or for development of TAO, is not presently clarified. In prospective studies, a higher risk of debut or exacerbation of ophthalmopathy, has however been documented after treatment with radioiodine than after medical or surgical treatment.

When Graves' disease is complicated by more than mild TAO, radioiodine treatment should not be the treatment of choice and if still chosen should only be used after careful consideration. If radioiodine is to be administered to patients mild TAO, concomitant administration of steroids has been reported to reduce the risk of developing or worsening ophthalmopathy. Starting the day before radioiodine treatment, 30–40 mg prednisolone is administered daily and gradually tapered over a period of 2–3 months.

In patients with overt thyrotoxic symptoms or with, for example, a cardiac condition, it is advisable to modify thyroid hyperfunction during a period of time before radioiodine therapy by administering antithyroid drugs up until about 1 week before

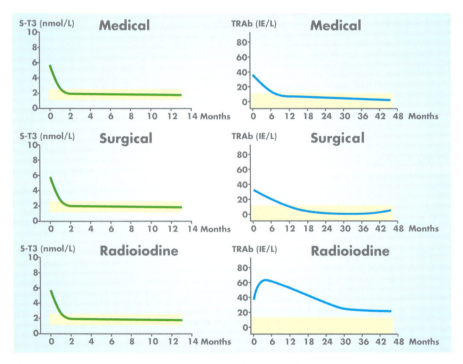

Fig. 18.6 Changes in T3 and TRAb after treatment for Graves' disease

treatment starts. Also in these cases, increased release of hormone is observed after radioiodine therapy, but it is less pronounced. Whether this procedure reduces the effect of radioiodine has been discussed, but there is no evidence that suggests this is the case when using thiamazol. It is, however, important to calculate the absorbed dose precisely because pretreatment with antithyroid drugs may reduce the biological half-life of radioiodine.

18.4.3 Surgical Treatment

The target group for surgical treatment of Graves' disease is primarily younger patients with high hormone levels, pronounced symptoms and a large goitre. Surgery should also be recommended in those cases where concomitant tumour in the thyroid is suspected. Surgery in the second trimester is an alternative if the patient is pregnant, although treatment with antithyroid drugs is the preferred choice (see also Chap. 17).

18.4.3.1 Preoperative Treatment

Patients with Graves' disease who undergo surgery must receive preoperative medical treatment. Most commonly, antithyroid drugs are given. When the patient has become clinically and biochemically euthyroid, antithyroid drugs are combined with thyroxine to maintain the patient's euthyroid state up until surgery. The block and replace treatment is also believed to reduce vascularization in the gland, which facilitates the surgical procedure.

Preoperative treatment of patient symptoms with beta blockers alone has been shown in many studies to be a suitable alternative. It must be pointed out that patients with thyrotoxicosis metabolize beta blockers faster than normal, and thus high doses (e.g. propranolol 40–80 mg × 4) must be used. Beta blockers should be continued during at least 1 week postoperatively in order to avoid the risk of thyroid storm. The advantage of beta blockers is the relatively short preoperative treatment period of 1–2 weeks that is sufficient to get the symptoms under control. Biochemically, however, the patient continues to be thyrotoxic. Many surgeons, therefore, avoid beta blockers as the sole preoperative medication in severe hyperthyroidism.

Previously, the classic preoperative treatment in Graves' disease was iodine blocking using stable iodine solution for oral use. This treatment continues to be used when it is necessary to quickly achieve a euthyroid state in the patient, especially if the patient has shown adverse reaction to antithyroid drugs. An additional benefit of iodine is that it seems to reduce the high vascularization of the gland accompanying the hyperthyroid state. The preoperative stable iodine treatment time must be limited to a maximum of 10 days because the effect on hormone release then rapidly declines (see also Chap. 17).

18.4.3.2 The Surgical Technique

The traditional surgical method for Graves' disease is bilateral subtotal resection followed by thyroxine replacement. The volume of residual thyroid tissue varies from centre to centre. Some surgeons consider that 2–3 g on either side is optimal, offering the patient a reasonable chance of becoming euthyroid without making the patient hypothyroid.

In recent years, an increasing number of surgeons favour a more radical resection and only leave 0.5–1.0 g of tissue on each side (near total thyroidectomy). The aim is to cure the patient and minimize the risk of recurrence, but with the knowledge that the patient will require thyroxine substitution postoperatively. Even total thyroidectomy is used and advocated by some surgeons. The risk of surgical complications such as injury to the laryngeal and recurrent nerve and hypoparathyroidism increases with more extensive surgery, in particular if total thyroidectomy is performed, but can still be kept at an acceptably low incidence in the hands of an experienced surgeon.

Many speak in favour of surgical treatment in patients with TAO, but there is no evidence that this has long-term advantages over medical treatment, except for lower recurrence rate. Neither has total thyroidectomy been proven to be superior to subtotal resection with respect to improvement in TAO, even though this has been claimed by some.

18.4.3.3 Postoperative Treatment and Follow-Up

After surgical treatment in Graves' disease, antithyroid drug therapy can normally be stopped immediately. Postoperatively, more or less pronounced hypocalcaemia will be occasionally recorded, which may be related to the degree of thyrotoxicosis. The reason for this temporary hypocalcaemia could be hypoparathyroidism. Another possible explanation is that the skeleton of the patient has been exposed to demineralization and hungry bone syndrome occurs, i.e. the elevated release of calcium that occurs during thyrotoxicosis, ceases, while the uptake of calcium in bone tissue continues.

In patients with TAO, it is important that thyroxine is given early after surgery in order to avoid even short episodes of hypothyroidism. In most cases, patients require postoperative thyroxine substitution immediately. An appropriate dose of thyroxine is 125–150 µg, adjusted by T4 and, later, by TSH (0.4–2.0 mIU/L). After surgery, TRAb often drops gradually (Fig. 18.6).

18.4.3.4 Recurrence

The risk of recurrence depends on factors such as the extent of resection, the degree of lymphocyte infiltration and TRAb levels. Recurrence occurs in 5–15% of cases after bilateral subtotal resection. After total thyroidectomy the risk for recurrence is minimized. Recurrence after surgical treatment of Graves' disease is normally seen within the first years after surgery but may also appear later. Reoperation after a previous bilateral resection is associated with a significantly higher risk of complications than a primary intervention and should thus be avoided if possible. Instead, these cases should be treated with antithyroid drugs and/or radioiodine.

18.5 Quality of Life

Graves' disease often results in a lowered quality of life. Several studies have demonstrated that the quality of life worsens during the first years after diagnosis.

18.5.1 Neuropsychiatric Symptoms
In addition to the symptoms thought to be due to increased metabolism, patients with Graves' disease often experience neuropsychiatric symptoms such as:
- Impaired memory
- Emotional lability
- Irritability
- Depressive or hypomanic symptoms
- Anxiety problems
- Sleep disturbances

18.5.2 Quality of Life Studies
Some studies have demonstrated that a significant number of these patients have persistent neuropsychiatric problems in spite of successful treatment of thyrotoxicosis. These symptoms occur with an increased incidence of cognitive symptoms, for example, in patients who several years previously had Graves' disease. In one study, an impairment in neuropsychiatric tests were found in 43% of individuals who had previously had Graves' disease compared to 10% in the control population.

In a randomized study that compared medical, surgical and radioiodine treatment, the number of days of sick leave was about the same independent of the choice of treatment. The study found that 96% of the patients were satisfied with the treatment they received. In spite of this, nearly every third patient stated that relationships with family or work mates had been negatively affected. For many patients, it took more than a year before they felt they were fully recovered, independent of treatment type. After almost 3 years, 20% did not feel completely well in spite of successful treatment of the thyrotoxicosis and achievement of euthyroidism.

Every third patient with TAO experienced their eye symptoms as greater than the problems associated with their thyrotoxic condition/disease. In a long-term follow-up (14–20 years) of the same study population, no difference between the three treatment methods could be demonstrated with respect to physical and mental quality of life. On the other hand, all treatment groups displayed lower vitality than the normal population.

In particular, patients with TAO reported a significantly lowered health-related quality of life for many years after the onset of the disease.

Chapter 18: Graves' Disease

Graves' Disease

- Immunologically mediated through TSH receptor-stimulating antibodies (TRAb)
- Common cause of hyperthyroidism
- Occurs sporadically and in families predisposed to autoimmune thyroid disease
- Women develop the disease 5–10 times more frequently than men
- Diffuse goitre, thyroid-associated ophthalmopathy and pretibial myxoedema are characteristic
- Goitre and eye and skin symptoms may, however, be absent
- Suppressed TSH, elevated T4 and T3 as well as the presence of TRAb are typical findings
- Treated with thyrostatic drugs, radioiodine or surgery
- Recurrence occurs frequently and is dependent on treatment given
- Associated with other autoimmune conditions

19 Thyroid-Associated Ophthalmopathy

Eye symptoms are a common feature of Graves' disease, where the symptoms have an underlying immunological cause. Several designations have been used: endocrine ophthalmopathy, dysthyroid orbitopathy, dysthyroid ophthalmopathy, orbitopathy, infiltrative ophthalmopathy and thyroid-associated ophthalmopathy (TAO).

TAO has gradually gained favour among thyroidologists internationally. We therefore use this expression for the most part. The advantage of this term is that it indicates a direct association with the thyroid gland. In addition to Graves' disease, TAO can also be seen in chronic autoimmune thyroiditis, even though this is far less common.

19.1 General Eye Symptoms in Thyrotoxicosis

Clinically observable signs in the eyes are present in 40–50% of all patients with thyrotoxicosis. Retraction of the eyelid is caused by increased activity in the sympathetic nervous system in thyrotoxicosis, and can therefore occur regardless of etiology. The consequence is an increased tone in the levator muscle of the upper eyelid, which can result in a closing defect when the gaze is directed downwards and is called lid lag (lagophthalmus or von Graefe's sign). Sympathetic activity also contributes to the staring gaze that is often observed. Sometimes, a persistent upper eyelid retraction is a consequence of TAO, clinically most evident if unilateral. Convergence insufficiency (Moebius' sign) and a higher blinking frequency (Stellwag's sign) are other typical symptoms. When the hormone levels are normalized these symptoms disappear.

19.2 Eye Symptoms Specific to Graves' Disease

TAO gives considerable problems in 10–20% of all patients with Graves' disease. Early stages of TAO often improve when the function of the thyroid has been normalized, but TAO can also have a distinct, prolonged, unpredictable and difficult-to-treat progression. In very severe cases, treatment with high doses of steroid and/or orbital decompression are necessary to avoid compression of the optical nerve.

TAO is normally linked with Graves' disease, but the same form of ophthalmopathy sometimes occurs in chronic autoimmune thyroiditis. Although less common, the progress of TAO is generally more problematic in males.

19.3 Risk Factors and Pathophysiology

The cause of TAO is not known, but several factors are thought to play a role in the development and progression. In patients who have previously undergone surgery or received radioiodine therapy for Graves' disease, an activation or reactivation of ophthalmopathy can be observed if they develop hypothyroidism or if the substitution dose of thyroxine is abruptly reduced. Another triggering factor is inadequate control of the disease with fluctuating hormone levels.

The risk for a patient developing or exacerbating TAO is greater after radioiodine therapy compared to surgery or medical therapy (Fig. 19.1). In the study on which this figure is based, the radioiodine-treated patients did not receive thyroxine until they showed signs of hypothyroidism. A recent 3 year randomized study where the radioiodine group was kept euthyroid confirmed the increased risk for TAO by radioiodine treatment. Currently, most institutions give thyroxine a few weeks after radioiodine treatment in an attempt to avoid rapid changes in the hormone balance. Even if hypothyroidism is thereby avoided, this routine does not, however, eliminate the risk of developing TAO after radioiodine treatment. Sometimes development of ophthalmopathy is observed after I-131 treatment of toxic nodular goitre or autonomous nodule.

High/increasing concentrations of TRAb seems to be associated with exacerbation of ophthalmopathy. It can therefore be assumed that TSH receptors in the orbital tissue play a role in the development and progression of TAO.

In TAO, an inflammatory reaction occurs in the eye socket with fibroblast infiltration with effect on the muscles of the eye and on the orbital adipose tissue. Examination with MR, computer tomography or ultrasound reveals an increase in volume in one or more muscles. Occasionally, an increased volume can be seen in the retrobulbar fat. Secondary to the swelling, shortening and stiffness of the muscles can occur resulting in eye muscle dysfunction and diplopia. The increase in the volume of the orbital tissue can result in forward displacement of the eye (proptosis) and disturbance of the venous flow with consequent eyelid oedema. In addition, there is a risk that the optical nerve can be compressed, which can result in optic neuropathy. In severe proptosis, there is an increased risk of a closing defect and corneal lesions.

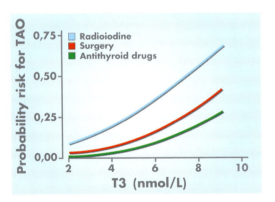

Fig. 19.1 Probability of developing or worsening TAO in relation to T3 levels and treatment given for Graves' disease

It is not entirely clear whether the inflammatory reaction is directed towards the muscle cells or the cells in the connective tissue. Histologically the muscle cells are intact, however, and the inflammatory cells are found in the connective tissue. Increased synthesis of glycosaminoglycans occurs, primarily hyaluronic acid, which binds fluid and results in a volume increase in the eye muscles.

19.4 Symptoms and Diagnosis

In most cases, TAO occurs concomitantly with development of hyperthyroidism. Onset of the condition can, however, occur before development of Graves' disease or a long time after treatment has been initiated. In principle, ophthalmopathy is a bilateral condition, but can occur unilaterally. In such cases, a retrobulbar tumour must be excluded. The diagnosis of TAO is initially founded on clinical examination. Further investigations include computer tomography, MR or ultrasound of the orbit to demonstrate thickening of one or more eye muscles.

Many patients display mild eye signs or symptoms without developing clinically significant TAO. Early symptoms are sensations of grit in the eye, increased tear production and a feeling of pressure behind and above the eye. The disturbed venous flow results in increased vascularity (redness), oedema and swelling of conjunctiva (chemosis) and contributes to proptosis, eye muscle dysfunction and visual impairment (Figs. 19.2, 19.3). The function of the eye muscles is often affected early in the course of the disease. In the beginning, the patient can be affected by intermittent diplopia, particularly when tired. A characteristic sign in many patients with TAO is a decrease in eye movement. This can best be observed when the patient looks to the side and then tries to raise the gaze. In milder cases, this may be experienced only as an oppressive feeling behind the eye bulbs.

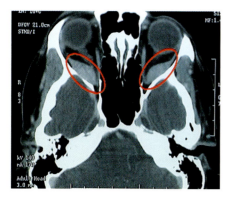

Fig. 19.2 Eye muscle thickening in TAO

The more pronounced the dysfunction of the eye muscles, the greater the effect on the movement of the eye, with diplopia in most sight directions and, in very severe cases, almost total inhibition of eye movement. After a few or several months with increasing diplopia, the inflammation can progress to fibrotization of the eye muscle. This often results in a progressive and gradually permanent diplopia. At the same time, the patient can experience worsening gritty sensations, increased tear production and an extremely problematic and painful sensitivity to light (photophobia).

In late stages of the disease, fibrotic changes in the eye muscles can result in a total inability to lift the gaze, for which the patient compensates by holding the head tilted slightly backwards. An attempt to elevate the gaze under these circumstances is often followed by a further retraction of the upper eyelid, enforcing the impression of a staring gaze.

Patients with proptosis can have particular problems closing their eyes while asleep. The exposed cornea can thereby get dry with a resultant risk of corneal lesions and infections. Proptosis also increases exposure of the eye to wind and sunlight and to the risk of repeated injury to the cornea.

The degree of exophthalmos/proptosis does not always reflect the severity of the disease. An apparently mild ophthalmopathy without exophthalmos can hide a condition with high intraorbital pressure and compression of the optical nerve. In these patients, a pronounced characteristic periorbital swelling, conjunctival blood vessel markings and chemosis are observed. Careful eye check-ups are necessary because there is a risk that the optical nerve may be damaged permanently as a result of the intraorbital process in TAO.

Impaired colour vision is a sensitive test of optic neuropathy. Impaired vision, visual field defects and fixed pupils are serious signs of threatening optic compression and risk for permanent damage.

In pronounced ophthalmopathy, orthoptists should accurately map the eye muscle dysfunction. The conditions in the orbit (muscles, effects on optic nerve, retrobulbar fat) can be examined using MR or CT (Fig. 19.4).

The degree of exophthalmos/proptosis can be assessed using an ophthalmometer (Hertel or Krahn, Fig. 19.5). These measure the axial distance between the lateral orbit front edge and the proximal point of the cornea. Most often this distance is less than 20–22 mm, but there is large individual variation. Hertel or Krahn measurements are most useful for following progression of the disease in a patient by performing repeated measurements. Patients with TAO of different severity are presented in Figs. 19.6–19.11.

Important clinical findings in TAO:
- Eyelid retraction
- Conjunctival redness and oedema (chemosis)
- Swelling and erythema of the eyelid
- Eye muscle dysfunction, diplopia
- Exophthalmos/proptosis
- Corneal lesions
- Impairment of visual acuity and colour vision
- Visual field defects due to compression of the optical nerve

19.4 Symptoms and Diagnosis

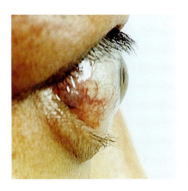

Fig. 19.3 A Patient with TAO. Note upper lid retraction, proptosis, chemosis and hypervascularisation

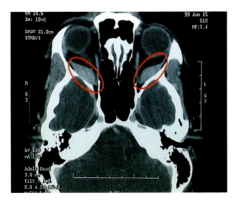

Fig. 19.4 CT scan from a patient with TAO showing bilateral thickening of the lateral eye muscle (red circles)

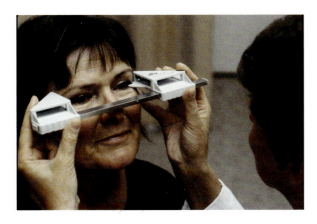

Fig. 19.5 Assessment of proptosis using an ophthalmometer

Chapter 19: Thyroid-Associated Ophthalmopathy

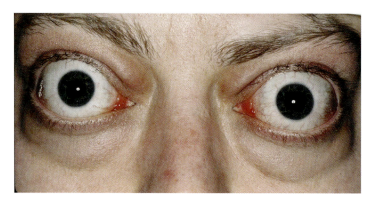

Fig. 19.6 TAO: Patient with exophthalmos/ proptosis and eyelid retraction

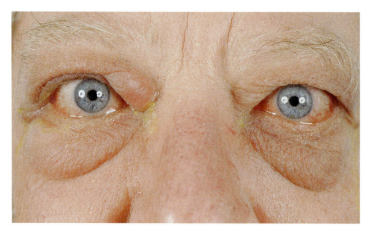

Fig. 19.7 TAO: Swelling and redness of conjunctiva and eyelids

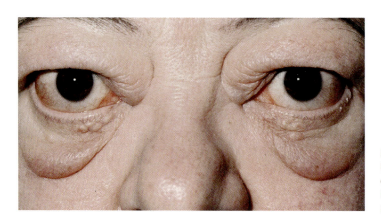

Fig. 19.8 TAO: Pronounced eyelid oedema in an elderly patient

19.4 Symptoms and Diagnosis

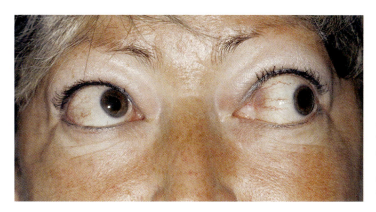

Fig. 19.9 TAO: Gaze direction to the left and upwards. Reduced elevation of left eye

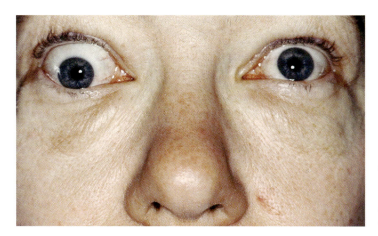

Fig. 19.10 TAO: Gaze direction upwards. Impaired elevation right eye

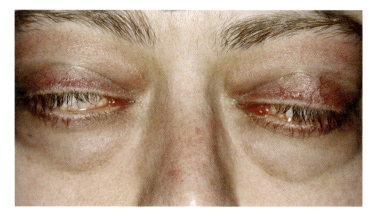

Fig. 19.11 TAO: Difficulty in closing the eyelids

19.5 Practical Management

Clinical examinations are the basis of the diagnosis. CT/MR is recommended if the diagnosis is unclear (thickened eye muscles indicate TAO), if compression of the optic nerve is suspected and if there is unilateral exophthalmos/proptosis (in order to exclude a retrobulbar tumour).

Because TAO can develop later in the course of the disease and is often gradual, it is important that the first consultation for Graves' disease includes a full medical history and eye examination with the results noted in the medical records.

The following questions should always be asked:
- Is your vision impaired?
- Do your eyes feel irritated?
- Do you suffer from increased tear flow?
- Does it feel as though you have grit or dirt in your eyes?
- Are you sensitive to light?
- Do you feel pain behind your eye globes?

During clinical examination, the following should be particularly noted:
- Are the conjunctiva red or oedemous (chemosis)?
- Are there blood vessel markings in the eye muscle fixtures?
- Is there oedema or erythema in the upper/lower eyelid or periorbitally?
- Are the eye muscles affected? This is easily tested by having the patient follow the investigator's finger with their eyes while drawing an "H", i.e. laterally up and down, to both sides and then inwards (for convergence disorders)
- If possible measurement of proptosis with an ophthalmometer (Hertel/Krahn)
- Investigate visual acuity and colour vision in special cases

A form for systematic assessment of the patient (clinical activity score) is presented later in this chapter. General irritation of the eyes, increased tear flow, sensations of grit and increased light sensitivity are common symptoms which often abate when euthyroidism is re-established. Special examination or treatment by an ophthalmologist is thus seldom necessary in patients with these mild symptoms.

Symptoms and findings that indicate the need for referral to an ophthalmologist:
- Lack of improvement or progression of symptoms
- Episodes with double vision/diplopia
- Eye muscles with reduced eye movements (intermittent or consistent)
- Continuous pain behind the eyes
- Unilateral proptosis

Symptoms which indicate the need for *prompt* referral to an ophthalmologist:
- Unexplainable impairment of vision (compression of the optic nerve)
- Changed colour vision (compression of the optic nerve)
- Pronounced proptosis with closing defect and suspicion of corneal lesion
- Rapidly developed and pronounced disturbance of eye motility

19.6 Clinical Activity Score

Euthyroid patients with suspected TAO and patients with hypothyroidism and TAO, should be referred to an endocrinologist or other specialist for evaluation of the eye symptoms.

19.6 Clinical Activity Score

In recent years, the clinical activity score (CAS) has gained widespread acceptance. CAS is a validated estimation of clinical activity and is a method for assessing improvement or progression of eye symptoms. In contrast to NOSPECS (Sect. 19.7), CAS also includes certain significant subjective symptoms.

A proposed assessment template for the investigation of patients with TAO is provided in Table 19.1.

Each point/class is scored with 0 or 1, i.e. is absent or present. The number of positive findings are compared with previous assessment as a estimation of activity.

Classes 1–7 reflect the activity of the disease: an increase or decrease of at least two units indicates changed activity. Classes 8–11 reflect the severity of the disease. Positive findings indicate the need for assessment by an ophthalmologist.

Table 19.1 A simple modified clinical activity score sheet

Class	Symptom
	Pain
1	Painful, oppressive feeling on or behind the globe during the last 4 weeks
2	Pain when looking up, aside or down during the last 4 weeks
	Redness
3	Erythema of the eyelids
4	Redness covering at least ¼ of the conjunctiva
	Swelling
5	Inflammatory swelling of the eyelid
6	Conjunctival oedema (chemosis)
7	Swelling of the caruncle or plicae in the nasal angle between the eye lids
8	Proptosis (ophthalmometer measurement). Individual variation. ≥ 23 mm or progress of 2 mm between measurements support TAO
	Impaired function
9	Reduced eye motility in any direction more than 8 degrees for 1–3 months
10	Double vision (intermittent or constant)
11	Effects on the optic nerve with reduced visual acuity and/or impaired colour vision

Table 19.2 The ATA classification system (NOSPECS)

Class	Symptom
0	**N**o symptoms or clinical signs
1	**O**nly upper eyelid retraction and staring gaze with or without solitary proptosis and no subjective symptoms
2	**S**oft tissue involvement (tear production, sensation of grit, retrobulbar pressure, oedema, conjunctival blood vessel markings, chemosis)
3	**P**roptosis
4	**E**xtraocular muscle involvement (normally diplopia)
5	**C**orneal involvement (ulceration, necrosis, perforation)
6	**S**ight loss (pale pupils, defective field of vision, blindness)

19.7 The ATA Classification

The following classification system (Table 19.2) was introduced by the American Thyroid Association (ATA Classification or NOSPECS, from the first letter of classes 0–6). ATA classification includes those changes seen in TAO with increasing severity graded from *no symptoms or objective signs* (0) to *vision impairment* (6), but without consideration given to the chronological order in which the symptoms occurs.

NOSPECS grades of 0 or 1: no need for referral to an ophthalmologist.
NOSPECS grade of 2 or 3: referral to an ophthalmologist should be considered.
NOSPECS grades of 4–6: referral to an ophthalmologist strongly recommended.

19.8 TAO in Autoimmune Chronic Thyroiditis

TAO can occasionally develop in patients with autoimmune chronic thyroiditis and hypothyroidism. In these cases, distinction must be made between TAO and the periorbital oedema, which can be seen in patients with pronounced hypothyroidism and which disappears after treatment and when the patient resumes euthyroidism. The clinical picture is the same as that observed in Graves' disease, but is often less active and can be persistent for a long time. The condition may well improve with thyroxine substitution.

19.9 Euthyroid TAO

TAO can occur without any clear laboratory indication of a disturbance in thyroid function and is referred to as euthyroid TAO. In euthyroid TAO, the concentrations of TSH and thyroid hormones are thus normal.

Demonstration of immunological activity against the thyroid (TRAb, and/or TPOAb) supports this diagnosis. In the diagnosis of euthyroid TAO, eyelid retraction is considered to be an obligatory finding which must be present together with at least one other symptom, such as proptosis, eye muscle dysfunction or effects on the optic nerve (colour vision, visual acuity and/or effects on visual fields).

19.10 Choice of Therapy for Hyperthyroidism in Patients with Ophthalmopathy

The choice of treatment for hyperthyroidism in patients with Graves' disease and TAO is a subject of intense discussion. At many institutions, the preferred treatment for patients diagnosed with TAO is antithyroid drugs combined with thyroxine. In these cases, treatment may need to be continued for a longer time compared to medical treatment in uncomplicated Graves' disease.

Studies have shown an increased risk for development or worsening of TAO after radioiodine treatment. In most cases the effect of radioiodine can be prevented by performing the treatment under steroid protection. Radioiodine treatment should not be carried out in individuals with severe TAO.

In recent years, patients with severe ophthalmopathy has to a wider extent undergone total or near total thyroidectomy followed by thyroxine replacement. Total thyroidectomy is associated with a slightly increased risk of complications. The objective of this intervention is to eliminate antigen structures in the thyroid, which may have an impact on the immunological process. In addition, a more stable control of thyroid hormone concentrations is achieved, which is also a positive factor with respect to progression of the ophthalmopathy (see also Chap. 18).

Surgical treatment is preferred by most treatment centres rather than radioiodine treatment if a patient with pronounced TAO does not comply with or does not tolerate antithyroid drugs.

19.11 Treatment Considerations

19.11.1 Practical Aspects

In cases of pronounced light sensitivity, sunglasses or darkened glasses with side protection, if necessary, can be used. In cases of dryness or feeling of grit, a tear substitute can be used. Periorbital oedema can sometimes be counteracted if the patient sleeps with their head high. Eye ointments can be applied at night to prevent corneal lesions.

In cases with corneal ulceration, antibiotic ointments are applied. If the lid closure is incomplete at night, the patient could be supplied with a humidified chamber covering the eye or in long-term cases, lateral sutures (tarsoraphy) applied.

Alternatively, minor upper eyelid surgery can be used, to prolong the levator palpebrae muscle so as to reduce the closing defect. This can also temporarily be achieved in selected cases with botulinum toxin injections, an effect which persists 4–6 weeks. Problematic diplopia can often be corrected with prismatic spectacles.

Because smokers with TAO are affected particularly badly, the importance of quitting smoking should be particularly stressed in this group of patients.

19.11.2 Specific Precautions

It is important to get the hyperthyroid condition under control and to avoid fluctuations in T3 and T4 levels. It must be emphasized that the patient must be kept stable and euthyroid. This also applies to treatment of TAO in hypothyroidism.

Experience shows that it can be an advantage if the thyroid function is regulated so that TSH lies below or in the lower part of the normal range. Being a sensitive indicator, T3 must on the other hand be normal, as a marker that the hyperthyroid condition is well-controlled. Hypothyroidism must be avoided.

Euthyroidism often results in an improvement of TAO, but often symptomatic and anti-inflammatory treatments are also necessary. Corticosteroids continue to be the anti-inflammatory agent that provides the best results.

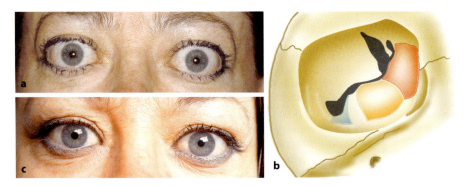

Fig. 19.12 a–c **a** Before orbital decompression. **b** Marked bone walls are removed at decompression. **c** After orbital decompression surgery

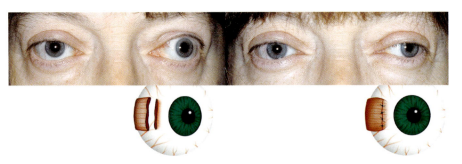

Fig. 19.13 Muscle corrective surgery after earlier orbital decompression

One absolute indication for steroid treatment is signs of compression of the optic nerve. Early signs can be registered by testing visual fields and acuity plus colour vision. If effects on the optic nerve persist for more than a number of days, there is a risk that damage to vision could be permanent.

Steroid treatment should be utilized at the early stages of severe forms of the disease, for example in new onset ophthalmopathy with dysfunction of the eye muscles. This can be evaluated by estimating the ability to elevate the eye. At this early stage, treatment with steroids can reduce the inflammatory reaction so that later development of fibrotic tissue in the muscles is avoided or less pronounced. Often a relatively high oral steroid dose is required, equivalent to at least 45–60 mg prednisolone daily. The initial dose should be high and thereafter tapered slowly. A risk of adverse side effects of the steroid, including osteoporosis and diabetes, is present and should be monitored. Treatment may be longer than 6 months. After this time, the possibility of further effect is relatively small with respect to restitution of eye muscle function.

In recent years, intravenous pulse treatment with high doses of methyl-prednisolone has been increasingly used in patients with progressive ophthalmopathy. One frequently used regimen is 0.5 g methyl prednisolone intravenously once a week for 6 weeks, followed by 0.25 g once a week for 6 weeks (adapted from Kahaly G et al. (2005) J Clin Endocrinol Metabol 90:5234–40). Glucose, blood pressure, etc., should be monitored during treatment. Proton pump inhibitors should be considered for patients who are receiving concomitant treatment with NSAID preparations. Because treatment with high doses of steroids has been shown to induce hepatitis, liver enzymes should be monitored.
New immunomodulating agents have been tested as a complement or substitute for existing steroid treatments, but without predictable reassuring effects.

Retrobulbar radiation treatment of the orbit can be used successfully in more difficult cases. The treatment, which must be initiated in collaboration with an ophthalmologist, is combined with concomitant steroid therapy. Treatment is given as 10–20 Gy, distributed over 10 occasions. The effect is first apparent after several months, but can provide a good foundation for reducing the steroid dose without exacerbating the eye symptoms.

In cases with rapidly developing disease with optic nerve compression not responding to medical treatment, an orbital decompression (Fig. 19.12) must be considered. This technique removes parts of the bone boundaries of the orbit with the purpose of enlarging the retrobulbar cavity. Thus, the pressure on the optic nerve is reduced and thereby the risk of permanent damage to the nerve. The reduced retrobulbar pressure may also result in a reduction in the inflammatory reaction in the tissues, and sometimes even the degree of proptosis.

The patient must anticipate that orbital decompression can sometimes disturb the position of the eyeball and corrective surgery for double vision may be necessary at a later stage (Fig. 19.13).

Diplopia which persists after treatment has been completed can be corrected by surgery. This should not be performed until all inflammatory activity has been quiescent for at least 6 months. Corrective surgery of eyelids and cosmetic surgery are also performed late.

19.12 Follow-Up

TAO is a long-term condition. In difficult cases, treatment duration can last several years before a definite regress of the condition and corrective eye surgery has been performed. Management of severe ophthalmopathy demands cooperation between specialists in endocrinology and ophthalmologists, and extreme patience both from the patient and the treating team. Experience shows that it is extremely important that the patient remains euthyroid and has stable thyroid values, specifically avoiding increased TSH. In certain patients, TAO can persist for a very long time, sometimes life-long. The patients may need to look for support and understanding and to be able to discuss their symptoms with other patients with similar problems. Patient support associations can be of great benefit.

Thyroid-Associated Ophthalmopathy (TAO)

- Can develop before, during or after onset of Graves´ disease
- More common if the activity of Graves´ disease is high or the treatment/control of the disease is inadequate
- Important that the thyroid function is brought to stable euthyroidism
- Can be triggered or exacerbated by radioiodine treatment
- Can be triggered by rapid fluctuations in thyroid hormone levels
- Increased tear flow, sensations of grit, conjunctival redness and oedema are early symptoms
- Volume increase of eye muscles and retrobulbar fat leads to proptosis and risk of closing defect with corneal lesion
- Eye muscle function can be affected with subsequent diplopia
- Swollen eye muscles can affect the optic nerve with a risk of atrophy and sight impairment
- Topical treatment (tear substitute) in mild TAO
- High dose steroids (intravenous/oral) may be necessary
- Surgical intervention may be required (orbital decompression or, in later stages, eye muscle correction)
- In rare cases, TAO can be seen in euthyroid patients as well as in chronic autoimmune thyroiditis with hypothyroidism

20 Autonomous Adenoma

20.1 Definition and Prevalence

An autonomous adenoma (Fig. 20.1) is a genuine neoplastic process in the thyroid. An autonomous nodule, on the other hand, is a local area with follicular hyperplasia forming a nodule within the thyroid. It retains normal thyroid gland structure but lacks the histopathological characteristics of a neoplastic process. Normally, the autonomous nodule is a part of a multinodular goitre that has begun to develop hyperactive areas. From a clinical viewpoint, these conditions may appear similar. The designations autonomous adenoma and nodule are well-established in clinical procedures. We have chosen the designation autonomous adenoma for a hyperactive well-defined palpable lump in the thyroid. For further information on the pathogenesis of autonomous nodule, please refer to Chap. 21, which deals with toxic multinodular goitre.

Some characteristics of autonomous adenoma and autonomous nodule include:
- An autonomous functioning palpable lump that releases thyroid hormone independently of TSH and comprises either an autonomous adenoma or an autonomous nodule
- An autonomous adenoma is a benign neoplasm that is separated from the surrounding normal thyroid tissue by a fibrous capsule
- An autonomous nodule is a palpable lump in the thyroid comprised of a hyperplastic follicular epithelium, which retains the capacity to synthesize and release thyroid hormone
- The only certain way to diagnose an adenoma is by examination under a microscope
- A dominating autonomous functioning nodule in a multinodular goitre can be clinically similar to a solitary autonomous adenoma

In a cohort of more than 900 patients from six European countries, autonomous adenoma was the cause of thyrotoxicosis in 9% of the patients. In a Swedish study, the annual incidence of toxic adenoma was 4.8/100,000 individuals, and was most common in women older than 50 years.

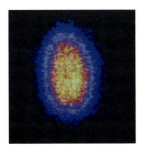

Fig. 20.1 Scintigraphic image of an autonomous adenoma

E. Nyström, G.E.B. Berg, S.K.G. Jansson, O. Tørring, S.V. Valdemarsson (Eds.),
Thyroid Disease in Adults,
DOI: 10.1007/978-3-642-13262-9_20, © Springer-Verlag Berlin Heidelberg 2011

20.2 Pathophysiology

An autonomous adenoma releases thyroid hormone independently of TSH. Increased secretion of hormone results in suppression of TSH and, secondary to this, a decreased function of the other parts of the thyroid. Consequently, a scintigram reveals a high uptake in the autonomous adenoma and a more or less absent uptake in the other normal parts of the thyroid tissue. An isotope-uptaking adenoma is called hot or warm. It is distinct from nonisotope uptaking, or cold, adenoma.

In autonomous adenoma, activating mutations have been demonstrated for the protein of the TSH receptor (TSH-R). The frequency, however, varies considerably between the various reported series that may be explained by geographic variations and different patient populations, but also because different regions of the TSH-R were studied. Depending on these factors, the incidence of TSH-R mutations reported vary between 10–80% in autonomous adenoma.
Activating TSH-R mutations have also been reported in abnormal hyperactive follicular thyroid carcinoma.

20.3 Specific Symptoms

As in nodular goitre, there are two types of symptoms that result in the diagnosis of autonomous adenoma: firstly, local symptoms in the neck due to the size of the adenoma, and secondly, the consequences of the autonomous, often increased, release of thyroid hormones.

An autonomous adenoma is often discovered when the patient notices a lump (Fig. 20.2), or in connection with a medical examination. Furthermore, a finding of suppressed or nondetectable TSH in cases of suspected hyperthyroidism can lead to the diagnosis.

Palpation normally reveals a well-separated lump, which is displaceable in relation to the surrounding tissues and entirely nontender. Sometimes, an autonomous adenoma comprises a larger part of one of the thyroid lobes, and can then be difficult to distinguish at palpation from a multinodular, unilateral goitre.

The degree of hyperactivity in the adenoma decides to what extent the patient experiences toxic symptoms. It is therefore possible to find euthyroid patients as well as patients with typical symptoms of thyrotoxicosis. Because an autonomous adenoma often develops slowly, the patient does not normally exhibit rapid development of symptoms. The thyrotoxic symptoms can therefore be moderate, not so obvious, and therefore not experienced by the patient as abnormal.

Often, there are nonspecific symptoms such as anxiety, restlessness and intermittent problems with palpitations. In a longer time perspective, the adenoma can increase in size with an increased risk of developing hyperthyroidism. This should be considered when deciding treatment in those patients who do not already exhibit symptoms of thyrotoxicosis.

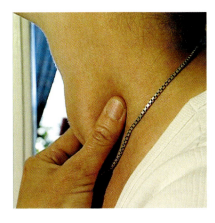

Fig. 20.2 The patient notices a lump in the neck

20.4 Diagnosis

Thyroid function is assessed using common laboratory analyses: TSH, T3 and T4. Experience has shown that an autonomous adenoma often releases relatively more T3 than T4. TRAb can also be valuable in excluding Graves' hyperthyroidism. The concentrations of T3 and T4 normally lie around the upper reference range or clearly higher. If the autonomous condition is limited to a slight increase in thyroid hormone production, T3 and T4 levels remain within the reference interval, but the TSH concentration is suppressed (subclinical thyrotoxicosis, see Chap. 22). This condition may have a continuous transition to a state with increased T3 and T4 levels and clinically apparent thyrotoxicosis.

A gamma camera (scintigraphy) investigation will confirm uptake in the adenoma and also demonstrate suppression in other parts of the thyroid.

An autonomous adenoma demonstrated by scintigraphy has often been considered to be equivalent to a benign process. In some cases, however, a highly differentiated thyroid cancer has the capacity to synthesize and release thyroid hormone and thereby imitate a benign autonomous adenoma. Therefore, fine-needle biopsy might also be considered in scintigraphically hot nodules.

20.5 Treatment – General Considerations

The indication for treatment of autonomous processes is guided by the TSH level. Earlier, a nondetectable TSH was considered treatment indication. It has, however, become more and more evident that when TSH drops below the reference range, i.e. is suppressed but still demonstrable, the treatment indication is more relative and can be decided individually depending on the clinical situation. In particular, elderly people can have clinically significant symptoms from even subclinical/mild hyperthyroidism. In addition, the size of the palpable lump can be significant for the progression of the disease. The finding of an autonomous functioning lump with a diameter >3 cm can indicate treatment.

Treatment with antithyroid drugs inhibits hormone synthesis by the autonomous adenoma and results in euthyroidism for as long as treatment continues. A persistent effect is not achieved however because the cause is not autoimmune but probably a constitutional receptor mutation. Antithyroid drugs are therefore normally not used as permanent treatment. On the other hand, it could be useful in certain cases as pretreatment before definitive surgical treatment. Surgery or radioiodine treatment are the established curative treatment alternatives currently available.

20.6 Surgical Treatment

The advantage of surgical treatment (Fig. 20.3) in autonomous adenoma is that the patient is quickly cured from hyperthyroidism and the lump in the thyroid and the local problems are eliminated. A considerable additional advantage is that a histopathological diagnosis can be made. If the patient is clinically euthyroid, there is no requirement for preoperative drug treatment. If hyperthyroidism is present, the patient should be given beta blockers and/or antithyroid drugs prior to surgery.

A solitary autonomous adenoma is normally situated in one of the thyroid lobes. The recommended surgical procedure is then unilateral lobectomy which involves the lump and surrounding thyroid tissue (Fig. 20.3). The reason for avoiding smaller resection is that the risk of complications is significantly raised if reoperation is necessary. Reoperation could be necessary if the surgery is not complete and histopathological investigation demonstrates that malignancy is present in the lump. Another reason for routinely attempting total lobectomy is that any residual adenoma tissue can regrow, which would make a new surgical intervention necessary on the same site.

Patients who undergo unilateral lobectomy and have a normal remaining thyroid lobe, in most cases manage without thyroxine substitution. The suppressed tissue in the remaining lobe recovers gradually, and can, when thyroid hormone levels return to normal, compensate for the lack of production of thyroid hormone in the tissue that has been removed.

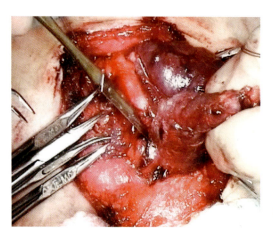

Fig. 20.3 Surgical resection of an autonomous adenoma

20.7 Radioiodine Treatment

Radioiodine treatment of an autonomous adenoma is preferred in older patients, in patients with a small lump, and if the patient does not experience any local or cosmetic problems. If cytology reveals suspicion of follicular neoplasia, the patient shall not be treated with radioiodine, but surgically.

In autonomous adenoma, the patient is administered radioiodine which is selectively taken up in the autonomous adenoma. The patient is given an amount of I-131 (Bq) which is calculated to give a relatively high absorbed dose (above 200 Gy). The healthy but suppressed residual tissue normally recovers completely. Often the adenoma gradually gets smaller after radioiodine treatment and softer with time.

The radioiodine therapy very often results in the patient becoming euthyroid with no need for thyroxine. There are, however, patients who may develop hypothyroidism and a need for substitution. In larger adenomas, the treatment dose is higher and thus exposure of healthy thyroid tissue to radiation increased.

Follow-up after radioiodine treatment involves analysis of thyroid hormones. Suppression of TSH often vanishes after treatment but can persist for a time (several months). The clinical picture and analysis of T4 and T3 are therefore important in the assessment.

Autonomous Adenoma

- Well-defined benign tumour in the thyroid with autonomous hormone production
- Scintigraphy demonstrates uptake of isotope in the lump
- Suppressed uptake in other parts of the thyroid, partial or total
- Hot nodules should be considered for fine-needle biopsy
- Always treated if TSH is not demonstrable. Concentrations of T3 and T4 are thereby often elevated
- Commonly treated if TSH is suppressed and even if the concentration of thyroid hormone is normal
- Treatment with surgery or radioiodine
- Antithyroid drugs can be used as pretreatment prior to surgery, but not for curative therapy

21 Toxic Multinodular Goitre

21.1 Development of Toxic Nodular Goitre

Toxic multinodular goitre can develop from a nontoxic multinodular goitre, which frequently arises in a thyroid that has enlarged due to hyperplasia of the follicular epithelium. The best known cause of multinodular goitre is iodine deficiency. Consequently, from a global perspective, this form of goitre is more prevalent in iodine-deficient regions. Multinodular goitre is, however, also common in areas with good availability of iodine. In these cases, the cause is more difficult to understand, but genetic mechanisms may have a role to play, as illustrated by the familial occurrence of the disease.

The causes of thyroid growth and goitre development are discussed in detail in Chaps. 8 and 28. In summary, there appears to be a difference between various follicles and follicular cells with respect to growth and capacity to secrete hormones (Fig. 21.1).

Follicle cells with greater growth potential (*yellow* in Fig. 21.1) can bud off and form new follicles, each with an ability for growth and the capacity to produce and release hormones independently of TSH (autonomous function). Other follicle cells with lower hormone production capacity (*blue* cells in Fig. 21.1) also form new follicles, but with lower follicular cell epithelium and a larger accumulation of colloid in the lumen.

Depending on the properties of the newly formed follicles and on which type dominates, the growing goitre can either remain nontoxic but still cause problems due to its size, or transform into a toxic nodular goitre with increasing synthesis and release of hormone.

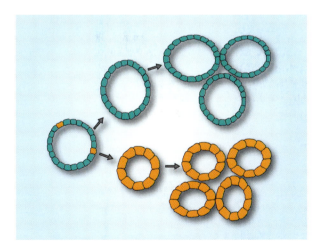

Fig. 21.1 Clones of follicle cells with autonomous potential develop from independent cells with greater growth capability

E. Nyström, G.E.B. Berg, S.K.G. Jansson, O. Tørring, S.V. Valdemarsson (Eds.),
Thyroid Disease in Adults,
DOI: 10.1007/978-3-642-13262-9_21, © Springer-Verlag Berlin Heidelberg 2011

21.2 Specific Symptoms and Clinical Picture

21.2.1 Nontoxic Multinodular Goitre

A small nodular goitre does not necessarily give any symptoms apart from a visibly enlarged thyroid gland and possibly cosmetic concerns. It is not uncommon that the patient has been aware of the goitre for many years, but never experienced any local pressure symptoms from the neck. The degree of discomfort and type of local symptoms in the neck depends partly on the size of the goitre and the position in the neck, and partly on how it extends. If the goitre expands outwards, the central structures of the neck are not affected in the same way as when the goitre is situated at the level of the jugulum, or when it grows inwards or downwards intrathoracic, in which case the airways and oesophagus are affected. The consequences of an enlarged thyroid gland are discussed in more detail in Chap. 28.

21.2.2 Transition from Nontoxic Multinodular Goitre to Toxic Multinodular Goitre

The majority of patients with nontoxic nodular goitre remain euthyroid. With time, more and larger hormone-active follicles may develop. In about 10% of cases, the autonomous hormone secretion increases to such an extent that the patient gets symptoms. This is due to the development of more and larger autonomous hormone-active follicles. The effect is counteracted to a certain extent and for a limited time through a compensatory decrease in TSH so that other TSH-dependent areas of the thyroid are less active. The initial hormone concentrations of T3 and T4 continue to remain within the reference ranges. Gradually, the autonomous secretion of hormone will progress. The consequence will be an increased concentration of T4 and T3. The nontoxic goitre thus makes the transition to a toxic multinodular goitre, known as Plummer's disease (Fig. 21.2, 21.3).

The patient gradually experiences symptoms of thyrotoxicosis such as increased heart rate, palpitations, atrial fibrillation, heart failure, tiredness, restlessness, weight loss and sleep problems. Often this occurs in older patients for whom other problems, such as latent cardiac failure, become more apparent.

In the transition from nontoxic to toxic nodular goitre, TSH is suppressed while T4 and T3 lie within the reference ranges. This condition, subclinical hyperthyroidism, is discussed in more detail in Chap. 22.

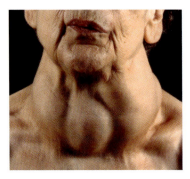

Fig. 21.2 Multinodular goitre

21.3 Diagnosis

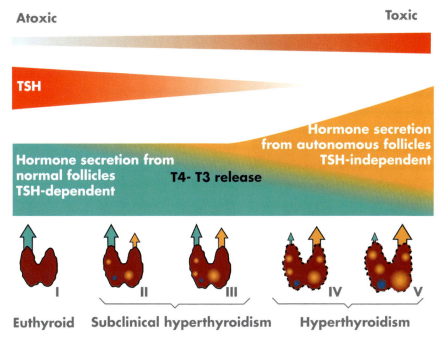

Fig. 21.3 Development of toxic nodular goitre and hormone secretion during transition from the atoxic phase. The *light blue, yellow* and *dark blue* markings refer to different developing areas within the thyroid gland (*lower*). The narrowing *red* area for TSH (*upper left*) illustrates the gradually decreased pituitary release of TSH as the autonomous centres successively increase their thyroid hormone secretion (*upper right*). Thereby, the atoxic nodular gland undergoes transition to toxic nodular goitre, as illustrated by the increase of total hormone production (*middle*)

21.3 Diagnosis

Diagnosis of toxic nodular goitre is based on medical history, clinical investigations with thyroid palpation, determination of TSH and free or total concentrations of T4 and T3, as well as the results of scintigraphy.

Many patients describe the presence of goitre within the family. As in several other thyroid diseases, women are predominantly affected. In practical clinical work, the thyroid specialist is often confronted with the question of why a patient has repeatedly low TSH values. Frequently the explanation is multinodular goitre with autonomously functioning areas. In early stages, the only biochemical abnormality might be a suppressed TSH. In these cases, further investigations should always be supplemented with scintigraphy, which often reveals one or more autonomous nodules (Fig. 21.4).

With time (months to years), a suppressed TSH level can sometimes drop to nondetectable levels. In early stages, the concentrations of T4 and T3 are often in the upper part or immediately above the reference range. Frequently, a more pronounced increase is seen in T3 than T4. In up to 15% of cases, T3 is elevated, but T4 remains normal, which is called T3 toxicosis.

In most cases, the thyroid is enlarged bilaterally, but asymmetrical enlargement does occur, as does selective unilateral enlargement, but this is less common. Multinodular goitre can thereby be difficult to distinguish from a solitary adenoma with

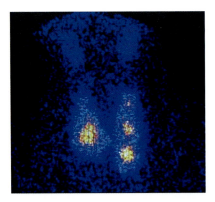

Fig. 21.4 Scintigraphic image of toxic multinodular goitre

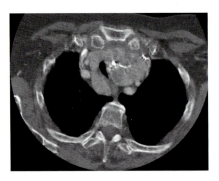

Fig. 21.5 Multinodular goitre causing compression and lateral displacement of the trachea

palpation. Otherwise, the nodular form and firm or elastic consistency, but without distinct hard lumps, is typical.

Scintigraphy reveals, in addition to an enlarged thyroid, unevenly distributed uptake of isotope between areas with concentrated uptake in autonomous or hyperactive areas and areas with reduced uptake in colloid-rich follicles (Fig. 21.4).

Ultrasound reveals enlargement of the thyroid and whether cystic, hyperplastic or solid lumps are present but, in contrast to scintigraphy, provides no information on function in the various areas of the thyroid.

CT can provide valuable information on size and extension of the goitre and any impact on, for example, the trachea (Fig. 21.5). However, one should be aware that if contrast-enhanced CT is planned, the iodine in the contrast administered at X-ray blocks uptake of iodine, so that no information can be obtained from a subsequent scintigraphy. This also excludes the option of using I-131 for treatment within the next few months. Furthermore, administered iodine can induce an increased synthesis of hormone so that the patient might be at even greater risk of developing hyperthyroidism.

The cytological picture is typical, frequently colloid-rich, with follicle epithelium and macrophages appearing as an expression of regressive events. Inflammatory events are normally scarce.

Analysis of TPOAb are not performed routinely when diagnosing toxic nodular goitre. The prevalence of elevated TPOAb are the same in these patients as in the healthy population.

Likewise, TRAb determination is not routinely performed. However, TRAb can provide valuable information as to whether a patient with multinodular goitre also has Graves' disease as the cause of hyperthyroidism. Occasionally, elevated TRAb levels are found after I-131 treatment for toxic nodular goitre.

21.4 Risk Groups/Risk Situations

Because nodular goitre develops slowly, multinodular goitre is rare in children and younger adults. The disease is more common in older patient groups, in which toxic multinodular goitre is a common cause of thyrotoxicosis.

The normal autoregulation of excess iodine in the follicle cell is put out of action in follicles with autonomous function. This means that hormone secretion is not down-regulated to the same extent as in healthy individuals at an exposure to a rapid excess of iodine in the thyroid. Instead the result is an increase in the formation and release of hormone.

Thus, when a patient with a multinodular goitre receives large amounts of iodine, for example in connection with an X-ray investigation with intravenous iodine contrast, there is a risk that the activity of autonomous nodules will increase (iodine-induced hyperthyroidism). Most often, this form of hyperthyroidism is transient, but it can cause severe thyrotoxic symptoms in predisposed individuals. Since these individuals are often elderly, even mild thyrotoxicosis can be clinically significant.

Patients with multinodular goitre also run the risk of developing hyperthyroidism if they are treated with iodine-containing medicines. In particular, amiodarone has been shown to result in difficult-to-treat hyperthyroidism (see Chap. 33). Treatment with wound dressings with a high content of iodine can also trigger hyperthyroidism.

A similar situation with increased reaction to administered iodine can occur in people who have grown up in an area with low access to iodine and move to an area with a high availability level of iodine in food. In countries that have introduced iodination of foodstuffs, an increased incidence of thyroid dysfunction has been observed in the populations.

21.5 Differential Diagnosis: Considerations

Symptoms of thyrotoxicosis are the same regardless of the mechanism causing the increased release of thyroid hormone. In contrast to Graves' disease, patients with toxic nodular goitre do not have autoimmune manifestations such as TAO. In toxic nodular goitre, a medical history of gradual development of hyperthyroidism and awareness of the goitre over a long period of time are frequent.

21.6 Treatment

Treatment of nodular goitre with autonomous production of thyroid hormones is indicated when hormone production has increased to such an extent that clinical symptoms of thyrotoxicosis are present. TSH is most often not detectable.

In milder cases, TSH is suppressed but can still be detected. In these cases, a clinical assessment decides whether the condition should be actively treated (surgery/radioiodine) or whether the patient should continue with medical check-ups. From a longer-term perspective, autonomous thyroid hormone production may result in increased morbidity in cardiovascular disease and an increased risk of osteoporosis. Indication for treatment has, in recent years, been expanded. Subclinical thyrotoxicosis is discussed in more detail in Chap. 22.

The occurrence of large goitres with local symptoms affects the choice of radioiodine or surgery. If the patient does not experience any pressure symptoms, radioiodine is the preferred treatment.

21.6.1 Radioiodine Treatment

Radioiodine treatment is a simple and, for the patient, comfortable method of treatment. One prerequisite for treating with radioiodine is, of course, that the gland has a sufficiently high uptake of isotope during an I-131 uptake test.

When treating a thyroid that has both active and nonactive areas, the administered radioactive isotope will particularily accumulate in the hot, active, nodules. This makes dose calculation more difficult, but the objective is an absorbed dose of 120–150 Gy in the hot areas.

Because the effect of the administered radiation does not reach all tissue in the gland, the posttreatment course might be unpredictable. In the most successful cases, function of the gland becomes uniform, so that euthyroidism occurs without the necessity for thyroxine substitution. Previously inactive areas can, however, be reactivated. Repeated scintigraphy confirms isotope uptake in the previously inactive nodules. This can be observed within 4–6 months after the first treatment. An additional treatment with radioiodine can then be indicated. In these cases, it may take a relatively long time after the patient has received repeated radioiodine treatment until the patient becomes euthyroid. This can be a disadvantage in certain patients, for example elderly people with heart conditions.

Occasionally after radioiodine treatment, a temporary period (1–4 weeks) may be experienced during which the release of hormone can further raise T4 and T3 levels before the aimed positive effects of treatment are experienced. This should be taken into consideration particularly in the treatment of elderly patients.

A risk of posttherapeutic hypothyroidism is present, and is dependent on the extent to which the areas between the hyperactive nodules have been exposed to radioiodine.

As in all other cases in which radioiodine is administered, follow-up must be continued for a long time. In the event of recurrence after repeated radioiodine treatment, low uptake can restrict the options for further treatment. The patient may therefore require a referral for surgery.

In some cases, a certain reduction in size of the goitre can be expected after radioiodine therapy of a toxic nodular goitre. At some institutions, I-131 treatment has been used to reduce the volume of nontoxic multinodular goitre.

21.6.2 Surgical Treatment

Surgical treatment of toxic multinodular goitre can be preferred in those cases that, in addition to hyperthyroidism, present with a large goitre with local pressure symptoms. Suspected malignancy is also an indication to chose surgery instead of radioiodine treatment. Before surgery, the patient is pretreated medically with antithyroid drugs and/or beta blockers.

Resection of the thyroid has previously been, and at many institutions still is, the most common intervention. Some thyroid tissue is left behind that has, however, the potential for further growth. In many cases, this can lead to recurrent disease after some years. In order to avoid this and the increased complication risk for reoperation, many surgeons now perform total or near-total thyroidectomy as long as this can be performed with reasonable risk, even if it results in the patient becoming dependent on thyroxine substitution. When planning the extent of thyroid resection, the age of the patient is taken into account. The younger patient has a higher risk for recurrence during lifetime and therefore a more extensive thyroid resection is recommended.

Growth of any residual thyroid tissue after surgical treatment is managed in accordance with the same principles as the primary intervention. There is, however, an increased risk of complications for repeated surgery. Radioiodine treatment, therefore, is the preferred treatment if the patient later develops signs of hyperthyroidism, provided, of course, there is high iodine uptake in the remnant.

The indication for thyroxine treatment after resection of the thyroid for toxic nodular goitre is decided by the activity of the residual tissue. Thyroxine is always given if follow-up at 6–8 weeks after surgery shows elevated TSH or low T4. If the disease progresses, and autonomous activity is resumed in the thyroid, the patient will experience thyrotoxic symptoms even if the thyroxine dose is gradually tapered. Typically, in these cases, low TSH is found with relatively high levels of T3 during administration of thyroxine.

21.6.3 Medical Treatment

Treatment with antithyroid drugs normalizes hormone production, but does not result in a permanent cure for patients with toxic nodular goitre. Antithyroid drugs are therefore, in principle, used only as pretreatment before surgery.

Long-term treatment with low doses of antithyroid drugs can be relevant in very old patients for whom radioiodine treatment is not practical, for example due to incontinence (radioactive isotopes are excreted in the urine), or who are ineligible for surgery.

Toxic Nodular Goitre

- Common cause of hyperthyroidism in the elderly
- Develops usually from nontoxic multinodular goitre
- Most frequently involves slowly increasing hormone secretion from autonomous nodules
- In early stages, TSH is often decreased while T4 and T3 lie within the reference ranges (subclinical hyperthyroidism)
- Radioiodine treatment is used in patients whose goitre does not cause local pressure symptoms
- Surgery is the appropriate treatment if the patient also experiences pressure symptoms or cosmetic problems
- Antithyroid drug treatment does not give permanent control of hormone production

22 Subclinical (Mild) Thyrotoxicosis

Subclinical thyrotoxicosis is defined as a condition with lowered (suppressed) TSH, but T4 and T3 are within their reference ranges. The designation subclinical is somewhat misleading because it has been demonstrated that many patients do in fact have thyrotoxic symptoms but in a milder form than what is in generally referred to as thyrotoxicosis. The designation mild thyrotoxicosis is therefore more frequently used. In Sweden, the prevalence is 2–4% and increases with age.

Biochemical subclinical thyrotoxicosis is often found in connection with routine determination of thyroid hormones. If the patient does not have a previously known thyroid disease or is receiving substitution treatment, the diagnosis should be confirmed by repeated measurement of TSH and free T4 after at least 4–8 weeks. The reason is that TSH suppression can occur during serious general illness and persist for a time after (Fig. 2.14). Studies in outpatients has demonstrated that suppressed TSH is normalized in 40% at follow-up after a few months in such cases. Table 22.1 summarizes the causes of subclinical thyrotoxicosis, which are also discussed below.

22.1 Nodular Goitre/Autonomous Adenoma

Most cases of mild thyrotoxicosis are seen in patients with nodular goitre, for example uninodular or multinodular goitre where autonomicity is not so pronounced that T4 and T3 exceed the reference range. In this condition fluctuating T3 levels around the upper limit of the reference range are often observed.

Table 22.1 Causes of subclinical thyrotoxicosis

Endogenous	Exogenous
Autonomicity in uni/multinodular goitre	Suppressive T4 or T3 treatment
Autonomous adenoma	Inadequately high substitution dose of thyroxine
	Iodine exposure in predisposed individuals
Graves' disease in mild form (or after incomplete surgery or I-131 treatment)	Gestational hyperthyroidism (hCG-dependent)
Graves' disease with inadequate medical treatment	
Thyroiditis in the transition phase	

E. Nyström, G.E.B. Berg, S.K.G. Jansson, O. Törring, S.V. Valdemarsson (Eds.),
Thyroid Disease in Adults,
DOI: 10.1007/978-3-642-13262-9_22, © Springer-Verlag Berlin Heidelberg 2011

22.2 Graves' Disease/Thyroiditis/hCG

A less common cause is Graves' disease, particularly after partial thyroid resection or where radioiodine treatment has been given but has not deleted activity in all thyroid tissue.

Patients with Graves' disease may in some cases have only a mild form so that this only results in subclinical thyrotoxicosis. In these cases, the disease can progress to clinical thyrotoxicosis or remit spontaneously. In the latter case, the possibility of recurrence must be kept in mind.

Subclinical thyrotoxicosis is also seen when Graves' disease is treated medically but where blocking of the thyroid is incomplete.

Thyroiditis is another cause of mild thyrotoxicosis. When subacute thyroiditis passes from the leakage phase, a period of a few weeks occurs with suppressed TSH but normal T4 and T3. The same applies in postpartum thyroiditis and in silent thyroiditis.

In early pregnancy hCG might induce a moderately increased function of the thyroid, reflected by low TSH. This is further explored in Chap. 31.

22.3 Exogenous Causes

Oversubstitution with thyroxine and/or triiodothyronine is the most common exogenous cause. American and Swedish studies demonstrate that more than 20% of patients treated with thyroxine are given too high a dose of thyroxine. In certain cases, however, a higher dose of thyroxine is intentionally given to induce suppression of TSH, for example after surgery for differentiated thyroid cancer.

Oversubstitution of primary hypothyroidism can have many other causes, which could be due to local treatment routines and to poor patient compliance. Sometimes the cause can quite simply be an age-related reduction in thyroxine requirement that has not been met with an adequate reduction of the thyroxine dose.

22.4 Suppressed TSH After Treatment for Thyrotoxicosis

Suppressed TSH that persists for 3–6 months can be observed after treatment of thyrotoxicosis, regardless of treatment type or of the underlying cause of the thyrotoxicosis. This is due to down-regulation of the gene that controls TSH synthesis in the pituitary and results from high T4 and T3 levels. It takes a long time (months) before TSH levels are normalized. The same phenomenon is seen at dose reduction of thyroxine after long-term TSH suppressive treatment.

22.5 Symptoms

The symptoms are milder manifestations of classic symptoms of thyrotoxicsis such as nervousness, restlessness, sensations of heat, and cardiac problems. Subclinical thyrotoxicosis is thus associated with an increased pulse rate and a risk of atrial arrhythmia, in particular fibrillation (Fig. 23.1). Furthermore, echocardiographic

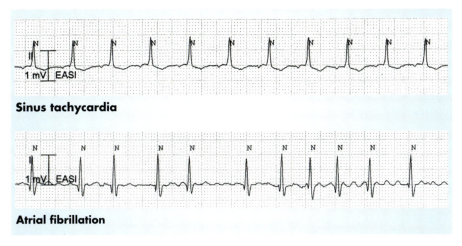

Fig. 22.1 ECG showing cardiac arrhythmia

evidence supports an increased left ventricular wall thickness, reduced relaxation phase and reduced capacity during exercise.

Symptoms vary, but are often mild, even in elderly patients. One explanation can be that the disease has progressed over several years, particularly if it is due to nodular goitre, autonomous adenoma or oversubstitution in primary hypothyroidism. The patient has more or less integrated the symptom into their personality or blames it on increasing age. This is also the reason why many patients do not admit having any symptoms. In many cases, the patients only recognize that they have had a symptomatic disease after they have resumed euthyroidism.

22.6 Cardiac Effects

It is important to diagnose and consider treatment of endogenous subclinical thyrotoxicosis and to avoid oversubstitution with thyroid hormones. The primary reason for this is that recent studies have shown that there is a two to three-fold increased mortality risk due to cardiovascular diseases. The cardiac abnormalities have been shown to be controlled by beta blockers and, in addition, reduction of the thyroxine dose.

22.7 Effects on Bone

Concerns for the skeletal system arising from oversubstitution with thyroxine have not been proven in men or premenopausal women who have been treated with suppressive doses for many years. Some studies indicate that there is an increased risk of hip fractures in postmenopausal women, but other studies have not confirmed this.

22.8 Psychological Effects

Some studies have indicated that long-term subclinical thyrotoxicosis increases the risk of cognitive disturbances. In addition, several studies reveal that patients with subclinical thyrotoxicosis often experience an impaired quality of life. This applies not only to mental (in particular cognitive) functions as previously mentioned, but also to physical performance capacity.

22.9 Clinical Recommendations

A suppressed TSH finding must always be carefully considered. Firstly, TSH and free T4 should be monitored again after at least 4 weeks, unless otherwise indicated by clinical findings. If exogenous causes are excluded, for example excessive thyroxine administration, the next step is a thyroid scintigram which is particularly relevant if autonomicity in a nodular goitre is suspected. Medically, beta blockers can be considered.

In an adult patient who has autonomicity in a nodular goitre without local compressive symptoms, the preferred treatment is radioiodine therapy. Sometimes, however, the iodine uptake is too low, making this treatment modality impossible. Then, treatment with antithyroid drugs can be an alternative.

If the cause of the suppressed TSH level is found to be an excessively high thyroxine dose, this should be gradually reduced unless the patient has been previously treated for thyroid cancer. The reduction should take place slowly with 25 µg 1–3 days a week, in order to avoid the patient experiencing symptoms interpreted as hypothyroid. After 6–8 weeks, a new assessment should be made to decide whether further dose reductions should be implemented. If the patient is on an extremely high dose, the initial reduction should take place more quickly. Some patients feel at their best when their TSH is lowered/suppressed by thyroxine administration and will not accept a reduction in dose. In these cases, bone density and cardiac function should be followed-up.

Subclinical Thyrotoxicosis

- Relatively common, particularly in middle-aged and older people with nodular goitre or in patients oversubstituted with thyroxine
- Suppressed TSH, T4 and T3 within, but often at upper regions of, the reference range
- Thyroid scintigraphy is valuable in the diagnosis of endogenous causes
- Often long-term and subtle thyrotoxic symptoms
- May result in increased cardiovascular morbidity
- Subtle cognitive disturbances

23 Thyrotoxicosis in the Elderly

Thyrotoxicosis occurs in the elderly and probably at least 30% of those who get thyrotoxicosis are older than 60. It can take a long time before a diagnosis is made, because the symptoms are frequently more discreet than in younger patients and do not always present as the classic thyrotoxicosis symptoms.

Tiredness, muscular weakness, respiratory problems, sensations of heat, weight loss and atrial fibrillation with heart failure are typical findings, but the heart rate is not always high. In a classic description from 1931, Frank Lahey drew attention to a condition in the elderly called apathetic hyperthyroidism. Here the typical patient is elderly, tired, uninterested, apathetic, has essentially a normal heart rate and no obvious goitre. In extreme physical stress, for example a severe infection, the patient can proceed to coma and succumb.

Most cases of thyrotoxicosis in the elderly are due to toxic multinodular goitre. Some patients may previously have received thyroxine in an attempt to prevent the growth of a multinodular goitre. If increasing autonomicity develops, the risk for thyrotoxicosis thereby increases. Even a slight increase in thyroid hormone levels can be of significance in the elderly.

It must also be remembered that even very old people can suffer from Graves' disease. Here, too, the symptoms are atypical. Eye symptoms can be present. A palpable enlargement of the thyroid is absent in almost half of these cases.

Other causes of thyrotoxicosis in the elderly are too high a dose of thyroxine for hypothyroidism or the presence of an autonomous adenoma. Amiodarone treatment for arrhythmia may also cause thyrotoxicosis in the elderly.

It is important to exclude the diagnosis of thyrotoxicosis in elderly patients with first onset atrial fibrillation, heart failure, weight loss, tiredness, and apathy. Analysis of thyroid hormones and palpation of the thyroid gland can be guiding. If the patient has a palpable (nodular) goitre, this is an observation but not an obligatory finding for thyrotoxicosis.

The most important analysis is the measurement of TSH. Suppressed TSH in an elderly patient must always be followed-up. Concomitant analysis of T4 can provide information as to whether the patient has mild or pronounced hyperthyroidism. It should be noted, however, that T4 often lies in the upper part of the reference range in elderly patients with mild hyperthyroidism due to toxic multinodular goitre or toxic adenoma. In these cases, T3 is also often in the upper part of the reference range or just slightly increased.

Concomitant nonthyroid illness (NTI) may affect the T3 concentration, thereby masking an increased activity of the thyroid gland. NTI can also make laboratory diagnosis of hyperthyroidism in the elderly more difficult, since they often have concomitant diseases that can affect thyroid hormone levels (see Sect. 2.10).

Thyroid scintigraphy is a highly valuable tool for demonstrating autonomous adenomas or multinodular goitres in the elderly.

E. Nyström, G.E.B. Berg, S.K.G. Jansson, O. Törring, S.V. Valdemarsson (Eds.),
Thyroid Disease in Adults,
DOI: 10.1007/978-3-642-13262-9_23, © Springer-Verlag Berlin Heidelberg 2011

The first line therapy is radioiodine treatment, which in many cases can even be given to very old people. Surgery can have a role if the goitre is very large with mechanical effects on the trachea and/or oesophagus. In the unusual case where the elderly patient is not considered suitable for surgery or radioiodine treatment, low doses of antithyroid drugs can be used. If therapy with antithyroid drugs in a patient with multinodular goitre or autonomous adenoma is terminated, the hormone levels rise once again. Antithyroid drug treatment must therefore be continued for life.

Thyrotoxicosis in the Elderly

- Normally caused by multinodular goitre, but Graves' disease and autonomous adenoma also occur
- Can be caused by inadequately high dose of thyroxine (decreasing requirements in the elderly)
- Heart failure, atrial fibrillation, weight loss, muscular weakness, tiredness and depression are common symptoms
- Apathetic hyperthyroidism: tired, uninterested, apathetic patients with essentially normal heart rate. Can develop into a serious condition if the patient is subjected to stress (infection, surgery) in unrecognized hyperthyroidism
- Most cases are treated with radioiodine therapy; surgery may be relevant if there is pronounced thyroid gland enlargement with mechanical effects on the trachea/oesophagus
- Low dose antithyroid drugs may be given long-term if none of the above therapies are suitable

24 Thyrotoxic Crisis/Thyroid Storm

Thyrotoxic crisis is an uncommon, life-threatening condition with aggravated toxic symptoms. It occurs most frequently in inadequately or untreated patients with Graves' disease, but has also been described in multinodular toxic goitre. Toxic crisis generally develops relatively rapidly and can occur in all ages and in both men and women.

It is nearly always triggered by factors such as infection, trauma or surgery. Other causes are amiodarone treatment, diabetic ketoacidosis, cerebrovascular incidents, radiation-induced thyroiditis, pre-eclampsia or parturition. A toxic crisis is rarely seen in well-controlled patients with hyperthyroidism.

24.1 Symptoms

The clinical picture is dominated by markedly elevated energy expenditure and/or pronounced signs of thyrotoxicosis.
Typical symptoms/signs are:
- Profuse sweating
- High fever
- Tachycardia
- Tachyarrythmia, in particular atrial fibrillation/flutter
- Abdominal pain, vomiting and diarrhoea
- Hypotension and circulatory failure
- Icterus
- Nervousness and restlessness
- Disorientation, psychotic symptoms
- Coma in extreme cases

24.2 Diagnosis

Various rating scales of symptoms have been proposed to reach the diagnosis more easily. The clinical picture, however, varies extensively and the rating scales are based on the fact that more severe hyperthyroid symptoms increase the likelihood for a thyroid storm. It should be kept in mind that there are no clear laboratory criteria for toxic crisis. The diagnosis is therefore often based on clinical assessment in a patient with previously unknown or inadequately treated hyperthyroidism. Importantly, high fever in a thyrotoxic patient is a warning of a possible imminent thyrotoxic crisis.
Triggering factors include:
- Infection, surgery, trauma, parturition
- Radioiodine treatment
- High iodine exposure (contrast media)
- Cerebrovascular incidents
- Diabetic ketoacidosis

E. Nyström, G.E.B. Berg, S.K.G. Jansson, O. Törring, S.V. Valdemarsson (Eds.),
Thyroid Disease in Adults,
DOI: 10.1007/978-3-642-13262-9_24, © Springer-Verlag Berlin Heidelberg 2011

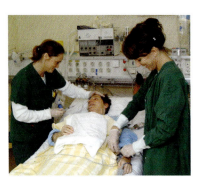

Fig. 24.1 ICU treatment of patient with thyrotoxic crisis

Some clinical characteristics are:
- Exaggerated thyrotoxic symptoms
- High fever
- Tachycardia/tachyarrythmia, cardiac failure
- Nervousness, restlessness, psychosis
- Abdominal pain, hepatic dysfunction, vomiting
- Circulatory failure

T4 and T3 levels are increased and TSH is suppressed. There is no direct relationship between thyroid hormone concentrations and the risk of thyrotoxic crisis. Patients in thyrotoxic crisis do not necessarily have extremely high hormone levels. Initiation of treatment should not be postponed while waiting for the results of tests.

The patient is nursed with appropriate intensive medical care, including tests for confirmation/exclusion of infection.

In the elderly, severe thyrotoxicosis can present as apathetic hyperthyroidism (see Chap. 23).

24.3 Treatment

In addition to possible triggering factors, treatment targets the following elements of the disease process:
- Underlying hyperthyroidism
- Adrenergic hyperactivity
- Mental and physical hyperactivity
- Fluid balance and electrolyte disturbances

Treatment should be carried out in collaboration with physicians experienced in thyroid disease.

Antithyroid drugs are given as propylthiouracil, which blocks synthesis of T4 and T3 in the thyroid and, in contrast to thiamazol, also blocks peripheral conversion of T4 to T3. Appropriate dosage is 200 mg propylthiouracil every 4 h by mouth or stomach tube.

Treatment with nonselective beta blockers should be given by mouth (or intravenously) every 4–6 h even before the diagnosis has been confirmed by the laboratory. In chronic obstructive lung disease, selective beta blockers are preferred.

Glucocorticoids are always given. The high steroid doses not only decrease hormone release from the thyroid but also inhibit the peripheral conversion of T4 to T3. Hydrocortisone (100 mg) is initially given intravenously and then every 4–6 h, or alternatively, dexamethasone (2 mg) every sixth hour.

The patient should be placed in a peaceful and quiet room, and given adequate sedative therapy with benzodiazepines. In the event of psychotic symptoms or extreme agitation, neuroleptic medicines may be needed.

It is important that the patient is kept well-hydrated with adequate electrolytes, fluid administration and nutrition.

If the above does not alleviate the condition, treatment with iodine before surgery can be considered provided that the crisis is not induced by iodine excess (i.e. amiodarone). Iodide blocks synthesis and release of thyroid hormone (iodine-potassium iodide 5% drops for oral use). Initially, 5 drops (11 mg iodine) are given three times daily. If, after 2–3 days, the pulse is above 90 bpm, the dose is increased to 10 drops three times daily. The dose may also be increased to 15 drops three times daily if the pulse remains above 90 bpm.

Treatment with iodine is reserved for severe cases of Graves' disease and is only given after the patient has received antithyroid drugs to block new synthesis of thyroid hormone. Iodine treatment must be coordinated with a scheduled thyroidectomy within 7–10 days. Iodine treatment involves a risk of thyrotoxicosis exacerbation after this time.

Peritoneal dialysis or plasmaphoresis can be performed in attempt to remove T4 and T3 from circulation. Since circulating T4 and T3 are to a large extent protein bound, only minor and transient effects are achieved.

Acetylsalicylic acid should be avoided as this drug can release protein-bound thyroxine and triiodothyronine. Paracetamol can, however, be given.

Chapter 24: Thyrotoxic Crisis/Thyroid Storm

Thyrotoxic Crisis/Thyroid Storm

- A condition where a patient with hyperthyroidism presents with exaggerated thyrotoxic symptoms, pronounced tachycardia, unexplained fever and mental disturbance
- May be triggered by infection, surgery, trauma, radioiodine treatment and parturition in patients with inadequately treated or newly onset hyperthyroidism
- Nondetectable TSH, elevated concentrations of T4 and T3. The symptoms do not necessarily correlate with thyroid hormone concentrations
- The symptoms may persist for several days despite normalized T3 and T4
- The most important elements of treatment should take care of underlying hyperthyroidism, adrenergic hyperactivity, mental and physical hyperactivity and disturbance of the electrolyte and fluid balance
- Beta blockers, propylthiouracil, glucocorticoids, fluids, sedatives and calm environment
- In difficult-to-control cases, blocking of thyroid hormone synthesis and release may be achieved by treatment with stable iodine. Thyroidectomy must then be performed within 7–10 days

25 Thyroiditis – Clinical Aspects

Thyroiditis may be due to autoimmune disease or other causes. For a general review of the different forms of thyroiditis, please refer to Chap. 9, in which additional clinical aspects are discussed.

25.1 Thyroiditis with Autoimmune Mechanism

25.1.1 Hashimoto's Disease

Autoimmune thyroiditis with goitre, Hashimoto's disease, is characterized by a more or less enlarged thyroid and, if the hormone secretion from the gland is reduced, also by symptoms of hypothyroidism. The patient may present with goitre, and/or with symptoms due to hypothyroidism. In typical cases, the patient has a painless diffuse goitre with firm consistency and without tenderness or solitary lumps. In some patients, the thyroid may be irregular with palpable nodules (Fig. 25.1).

In most cases TPOAb will be detected, which confirms the diagnosis. Fine-needle biopsy is not necessary in typical cases, but must always be performed in patients with palpable solitary lumps. Fine-needle biopsy is also performed if the thyroid is firm and irregularly enlarged.

Scintigraphy and measurement of iodine uptake are rarely indicated when investigating Hashimoto's disease. Besides, in pronounced hypothyroidism, isotope uptake is either very low or absent, in which case scintigraphy does not give any further information.

When the hormone production falls, TSH will increase, and the patient develops symptoms of hypothyroidism. Substitution with thyroxine is then initiated and is normally life-long. The inflammatory process is not specifically treated. Treatment with thyroxine is also indicated in euthyroid patients if the thyroid is enlarged. The size of the goitre is often reduced with time after thyroxine treatment.

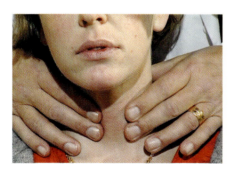

Fig. 25.1 Palpation of patient with suspected thyroiditis

E. Nyström, G.E.B. Berg, S.K.G. Jansson, O. Törring, S.V. Valdemarsson (Eds.),
Thyroid Disease in Adults,
DOI: 10.1007/978-3-642-13262-9_25, © Springer-Verlag Berlin Heidelberg 2011

In cases in which elevated TPOAb are noted, but the patient does not have a pronounced goitre or elevated TSH, the patient should be informed that there is a risk of later developing hypothyroidism. Thyroid function should be followed- up regularly.

Follow-up involves clinical assessment, palpation of the thyroid and measurement of TSH. Determination of TPOAb seldom needs to be repeated. The concentration of TPOAb can slowly diminish during treatment with thyroxine. Follow-up should also include observation for appearance of other autoimmune diseases.

25.1.2 Atrophic Autoimmune Thyroiditis

In atrophic autoimmune thyroiditis without goitre, also named, atrophic thyroiditis or primary myxoedema, development of hypothyroidism dominates the clinical picture. The thyroid is often barely palpable in these patients. Treatment is with thyroxine (see Chaps. 10–12).

25.1.3 Silent Thyroiditis and Postpartum Thyroiditis

Silent thyroiditis (painless thyroiditis) is probably similar to postpartum thyroiditis (Fig. 25.2). Symptoms of mild thyrotoxicosis are often the reason the patient seeks medical advice. The initial thyrotoxic symptoms spontaneously remit within a few weeks. Because the disease exhibits a biphasic progression, the patient sometimes first presents at a later stage with signs of hypothyroidism. In these cases, the medical history may reveal that the patient has previously experienced symptoms due to increased thyroid hormone levels.

The thyroid in patients with silent thyroiditis is rarely enlarged. On the other hand, the gland is often firm in consistency and thus easy to delimit. Sometimes the gland is smaller than normal, and feels like a horizontal string across the front of the trachea. Inflammatory markers are almost always normal.

In the early toxic phase, the destruction phase, a differential diagnosis could be a mild form of Graves' disease. TPOAb can be demonstrated in both conditions, and is thus not an indicator of value. Often, time will clarify the situation, because the patient with silent thyroiditis spontaneously recovers from the thyrotoxic state within weeks. The presence of TRAb strongly indicates Graves' disease (see Chap. 31).

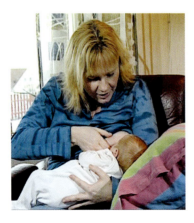

Fig. 25.2 Patient with postpartum thyroiditis

If the diagnosis is in doubt in the toxic phase, scintigraphy and/or measurement of iodine (I-131) uptake can be used if the patient is not pregnant or breastfeeding. The absence of uptake supports the diagnosis of thyroiditis. Normal or elevated iodine (I-131) uptake supports the diagnosis of Graves' disease.

Treatment with beta blockers can be given in the toxic phase of silent thyroiditis. In contrast, treatment with antithyroid drugs or I-131 has no effect, since there is no increased hormone synthesis.

Thyroxine substitution may be indicated in the hypothyroid phase. Because these patients can regain thyroid function, substitution with thyroxine may need to be reassessed. This is done simply by reducing the dose by half. If TSH rises, thyroxine substitution must be continued with the former dose.

In cases in which the inflammatory process abates and the thyroid regains its function, there is always a risk that the patient may develop hypothyroidism later in life. Follow-up is therefore necessary, particularly in connection with pregnancy.

25.1.4 Autoimmune Thyroiditis in Children and Adolescents

In children and adolescents determination of TSH, T4 and TPOAb are most often used for diagnosis, and fine-needle biopsy performed only in cases with a solitary nodule. Treatment of autoimmune thyroiditis in adolescents follows the same principles as in adults (see Chap. 32 for further details).

25.1.5 Focal Thyroiditis

Postmortem examinations have revealed that focal infiltration of lymphocytes in the thyroid is quite common in adults. In clinical work, lymphocyte infiltrates can be demonstrated by cytological examination. Demonstration of the presence of lymphocytes should result in evaluation of whether the patient has clinically significant thyroid disease with a risk of hypothyroidism.

The risk of developing hypothyroidism must be suspected if examination of tissue from resection of the thyroid performed for other indications reveals lymphocyte infiltration. Also, determination of TSH and TPOAb provides supplementary information. Follow-up of these patients is thus important not only with respect to the preoperative diagnosis.

25.1.6 Patients Receiving Interferon Treatment

Disturbances of thyroid function occur quite frequently in patients receiving treatment with interferon. In predisposed patients, i.e. TPOAb carriers, treatment with interferon can unmask an underlying autoimmune thyroid disease. The patient can develop thyrotoxic symptoms due to hormone leakage from the thyroid and in a later stage, hypothyroidism. In some cases, hyperthyroidism similar to that seen in Graves' disease will instead develop. In other cases, the clinical picture may be more similar to that in subacute thyroiditis.

The prognosis for recovery is good. The dysfunction of the thyroid is often normalized when treatment with interferon is terminated. The occurrence of TPOAb, with concomitant increased risk of being affected by thyroiditis with an autoimmune mechanism, however, should not be a cause for avoiding treatment with interferon. Neither should the appearance of thyroid dysfunction result in the termination of interferon treatment. Thyroiditis associated with medical treatment is further discussed in Chap. 33.

25.2 Thyroiditis from Other Causes

25.2.1 Subacute Thyroiditis

Subacute thyroiditis is a relatively common condition in which the patient in the majority of cases displays typical symptoms with pain over the thyroid and laboratory and clinical signs of inflammation. The thyroid is tender and characteristically firm within the inflamed areas. In some cases, local symptoms are absent. The picture can thus resemble that of silent thyroiditis or even Graves' disease, because these patients also experience a phase with hormone leakage and signs of thyrotoxicosis. Subacute thyroiditis is described in more detail in Chap. 26.

25.2.2 Radiation-Induced Thyroiditis

Radiation-induced thyroiditis with leakage of hormone may occur 4–12 weeks after treatment with radioiodine (see Chap. 10). Scintigraphy/measurement of iodine (I-131) uptake can be used to clarify whether persistent/recurrent thyrotoxicosis by this time is due to radiation-induced thyroiditis or exacerbation of thyroid hyperfunction. Low uptake of iodine (I-131) is observed in radiation-induced thyroiditis. In these cases, a gradual drop in T4 and T3 concentrations can be expected which, within a relatively short time, progresses to hypothyroidism.

Radiation-induced thyroiditis seldom produces local discomfort in the thyroid and is not indicated by the inflammatory variables. Symptomatic treatment with beta blockers can be given until the condition resolves.

25.2.3 Acute Bacterial Thyroiditis

The differential diagnosis between subacute thyroiditis and acute bacterial thyroiditis can be difficult in the acute phase. Both types can present with fluctuating fever, local tenderness over the thyroid and signs of inflammation. Fine-needle biopsy (Fig. 25.3) can often provide guidance by demonstrating the presence of copious amounts of leukocytes and occasionally pus, which indicates bacterial infection.

Almost any type of bacterial infection, including tuberculosis, can cause bacterial thyroiditis through hematogenous spread. The process is often focal, causing pronounced leukocyte infiltration with pus and signs of an abscess. Tubercular bacteria may spread diffusely within the thyroid. The diagnosis is based on the clinical picture, local symptoms, aspiration biopsy for bacteria cultivation, and laboratory tests, as determinants of infection. As pointed out, differential diagnosis versus subacute thyroiditis can be difficult.

Localized bacterial thyroiditis is considered to result only rarely in such extensive hormone leakage that the patient experiences thyrotoxic symptoms.

Treatment with appropriate antibiotics is vital. In severe cases, parenteral treatment is required. In the event of abscess formation, repeated aspiration or surgical drainage may be necessary.

As pointed out, thyroid function is rarely affected during the acute phase. Follow-up using TSH measurements is, however, always indicated because more serious damage can eventually cause (partial) hypothyroidism.

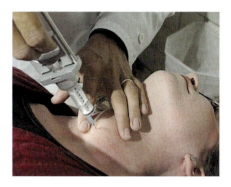

Fig. 25.3 Fine-needle biopsy

25.2.4 Fibrous (Riedel) Thyroiditis

Fibrous thyroiditis is an extremely uncommon condition that can be dominated by progressive fibrotization in and around the thyroid, sometimes associated with hypothyroidism. Clinical progression can switch between rapid growth to longer stable periods. A biopsy is often needed to give an absolute diagnosis using histological examination. It may be pointed out that a fibrous variant of anaplastic thyroid cancer with low cellularity may histologically resemble fibrous thyroiditis.

Surgery may sometimes be necessary due to compression of the surrounding tissues by the fibrosis. Medical therapy includes thyroxine substitution in hypothyroidism. Glucocorticoids may be tried. Recently, positive effects have been reported after treatment with tamoxifen.

Fibrous thyroiditis is discussed in more detail in Chap. 9.

Clinical Aspects of Thyroiditis

- Thyroiditis can have autoimmune or other origins
- Autoimmune etiology involves a risk of developing hypothyroidism
- Autoimmune thyroiditis can cause:
  - Pronounced inflammation in the thyroid with goitre and often hypothyroidism
  - Atrophy of the thyroid with hypothyroidism
  - Transient dysfunction of the thyroid (silent thyroiditis and postpartum thyroiditis)
  - Focal lymphocytic infiltration in the thyroid (focal thyroiditis)
- Characteristic for silent thyroiditis and postpartum thyroiditis as well as for subacute thyroiditis is a biphasic process initially with leakage of hormone and toxic symptoms, followed by an often transient phase with hypothyroidism
- Scintigraphy during the toxic phase reveals low or absent uptake of isotope
- In the toxic phase, symptoms can require treatment with beta blockers
- In the hypothyroid phase, thyroxine substitution should be given
- No specific treatment is given for the autoimmune inflammatory process

26 Subacute Thyroiditis
(de Quervain´s Disease/Giant-Cell Thyroiditis)

Subacute thyroiditis, or de Quervain's disease, which is sometimes called giant-cell thyroiditis or granulomatous thyroiditis, is an inflammatory thyroid disease in which nearly all cases (95%) will fully recover.

In the typical case there are inflammatory symptoms with pain over the thyroid. This form of thyroiditis is therefore often referred to in the literature as painful thyroiditis in contrast to painless, which is used for silent autoimmune thyroiditis. In addition, the patient often exhibits general symptoms.

The inflammatory process results in a temporary release of thyroid hormone because of a disruption of the integrity of the follicle cells, a destruction phase, which is followed by a period with failing hormone production before the thyroid regains its function. The consequence is thus a dynamic biphasic progression before remission.

Subacute thyroiditis is uncommon in children. It occurs most frequently in young and middle-aged people and is slightly more common in women than men.

26.1 Etiology

The etiology of subacute thyroiditis is unclear. The fact that the disease often develops 1 or 2 weeks after upper respiratory tract infection indicates a possible connection with viral infections. Several viruses have been associated, such as the adeno and coxsackie viruses. Raised titres of antibodies have been demonstrated against upper respiratory tract viruses, but not against enterovirus.

In contrast to autoimmune thyroiditis, subacute thyroiditis has no increased occurrence of antibodies against thyroperoxidase, thyroglobulin or TSH receptors. Interestingly, over-representation of one tissue type, HLA-Bw35, has been found among patients with subacute thyroiditis, which indicates that a genetic predisposition may be involved.

26.2 Symptoms

Clinically, subacute thyroiditis is characterized by a relatively rapid development over a few days to a few weeks. Typically, there is general tenderness over the neck. The thyroid is often slightly to moderately enlarged with a characteristic, firm consistency at palpation. In typical cases, the tenderness is considerable, often over the entire thyroid, but it can also be localized in one lobe. In the latter case, the inflammatory process can later occur in the entire thyroid or move to other areas.

The patient often presents with pain over the neck, and may also have pain when swallowing. Quite frequently, the pain radiates from the thyroid up under the chin, up to the ears or sometimes down towards the chest.

E. Nyström, G.E.B. Berg, S.K.G. Jansson, O. Tørring, S.V. Valdemarsson (Eds.),
Thyroid Disease in Adults,
DOI: 10.1007/978-3-642-13262-9_26, © Springer-Verlag Berlin Heidelberg 2011

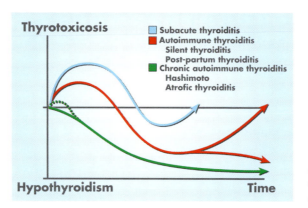

Fig. 26.1 Progression of subacute thyroiditis compared to various forms of autoimmune thyroiditis

Muscular pain, headaches and a general feeling of being unwell are typical. Fever is intermittent, often with a normal temperature in the morning and an increase to 38–39°C in the afternoon. Because of the extensive inflammation in the thyroid, stored hormone can leak out of the follicles and cause thyrotoxic symptoms.

The local symptoms in the neck may be more or less pronounced in subacute thyroiditis, or may even be absent. Some patients can therefore present with thyrotoxic symptoms or only with fever of unknown origin.

26.3 Progression

The course of this disease is quite characteristic (Fig. 26.1). The initial phase lasts a few weeks or months. In rare cases, the inflammatory process can continue for a longer period, often with exacerbation in different areas of the thyroid. In milder cases, the acute phase of the disease disappears spontaneously within a few weeks and both inflammatory and thyrotoxic symptoms cease. In other cases, the disease picture becomes more aggressive and can require anti-inflammatory treatment for a short while. Some patients can experience a phase with mild hypothyroidism before the integrity of the follicle is recovered. Most patients regain normal thyroid function. A few are affected by persistent hypothyroidism.

The size and consistency of the thyroid normalize in the large majority of cases, but occasionally persistent irregularities can be noted in the thyroid at palpation.

26.4 Diagnosis

Diagnosis is based on clinical findings: frequently elevated sedimentation rate, C-reactive protein and leucocytosis. Due to hormone leakage from the thyroid, elevated T4 is often seen with a decrease in TSH. T3 can also increase, but often less pronounced than T4.

26.4 Diagnosis

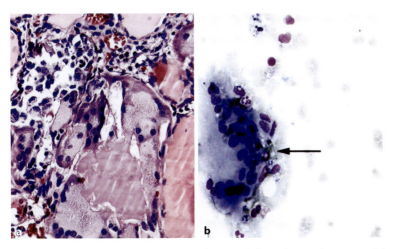

Fig. 26.2 a, b a Image of subacute (granulomatous) thyroiditis. In the centre of the image giant cells can be seen which phagocyte the colloid. **b** Cytology reveals a few multinucleated giant cells (*arrow*) and lightly reactive changed epithelial cells, but few inflammatory cells

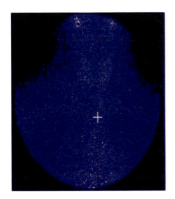

Fig. 26.3 Scintigraphy showing inhibited uptake compatible with thyroiditis

If additional support for the diagnosis is required, investigations can be supplemented with fine-needle biopsy for cytology. Occasionally it is difficult to obtain an aspirate, but in typical cases, polynuclear cells and granulomatous epitheloid cells are a pathogenic finding. Initially in the progression of the disease, polynuclear giant cells are present (Fig. 26.2). Later, lymphocytes and macrophages dominate the picture. If the clinical picture and laboratory tests are typical, a cytological examination is not necessary.

If the diagnosis is uncertain, iodine (I-131) uptake or scintigraphy can be performed, both of which reveal very low uptake in the acute phase with thyrotoxicosis (Fig. 26.3). Serum TPOAb are not elevated.

Important differential diagnoses are acute bacterial thyroiditis (see Chap. 25) and haemorrhage in the thyroid. The latter gives acute localized pain and tenderness at palpation. The patient has normal thyroid function and no reaction in the inflammation markers. A cytologic investigation will show blood or blood residues.

26.5 Treatment

There is no causal treatment. If the patient has symptoms, the inflammatory component can be alleviated using anti-inflammatory agents, acetylsalicylic acid or NSAID. In more severe cases, glucocorticoids can be administered, for example 30 mg prednisolone daily. Typically, the symptoms disappear rapidly within 24–48 h. The dose is tapered so that the daily dose is reduced by 5 mg each week, giving a treatment period of around 5–6 weeks. In cases with pronounced disease activity, the symptoms return if the cortisone dose is dropped below a certain level. In these cases, the dose should be increased slightly and then reduced again at a slower rate.

Beta blockers can be used temporarily against symptomatic thyrotoxicosis. Antithyroid drugs have no place in the treatment of this condition. If the patient develops hypothyroid symptoms, thyroxine should be started at a recommended dose of 50 µg. The requirement for thyroxine should be reconsidered after 3–6 months because the thyroid frequently regains its function completely. A simple way is to reduce the dose of thyroxine by half and check the TSH after about 6 weeks.

Elevated concentrations of thyroglobulin indicate that the follicle integrity is disturbed, and can be seen several months after the inflammatory symptoms have disappeared. This demonstrates that restitution of the thyroid can take a long time. Patients who have had subacute thyroiditis should therefore be checked using measurements of TSH during a period of 6 months after disappearance of the toxic symptoms.

Subacute Thyroiditis

- Slightly enlarged thyroid with focal or general tenderness
- Hormone leakage gives temporary thyrotoxicosis
- Pronounced increase in sedimentation rate, CRP and subfebrility in typical cases
- Polynuclear giant cells and granulomatous epitheloid cells at cytology
- Initially low uptake of iodine (I-131) and of isotope in scintigraphy
- Symptomatic anti-inflammatory treatment with NSAID or glucocorticosteroids
- Beta blockers will reduce thyrotoxic symptoms
- Can be followed by temporary hypothyroidism (seldom persistent)
- Occasionally progress over several months affecting different parts of the gland
- Long-term follow-up is not necessary after complete recovery

27 Other Causes of Thyrotoxicosis

The most common causes of thyrotoxicosis are toxic diffuse goitre and toxic multi- or uninodular goitre (see Chaps. 18, 20 and 21). Thyroiditis, with an initial hormone leakage phase from the thyroid gland, is another common cause of thyrotoxicosis (see Chaps. 9, 25 and 26). This chapter deals with thyrotoxicosis due to diseases that directly or indirectly affect thyroid function, but are uncommon and not always easy to diagnose and treat.

27.1 Central (Secondary) Hyperthyroidism/ TSH-Producing Pituitary Adenoma

TSH producing pituitary adenoma is a very rare cause of hyperthyroidism. Here, the patient has elevated concentrations of T4 and T3 while TSH is not suppressed. Instead, TSH lies within the reference range or is slightly to moderately elevated.

This unusual constellation of test results for TSH, T4 and T3 often makes interpretation difficult. Probably, the most common cause for normal TSH in combination with high values of free T4 and/or free T3 is analytical interference, primarily relating to free T4 and free T3 and more seldom TSH. If analytical interference can be excluded by the laboratory, the two major diagnoses that may explain the laboratory findings are TSH producing pituitary adenoma and thyroid hormone resistance, a genetically caused insensitivity to thyroid hormone described in Chap. 34.

For further evaluation, some indication can be obtained from the TRH stimulation test. In thyroid hormone resistance, increasing TSH values can be expected after stimulation with TRH. On the other hand secretion of TSH in TSH-producing pituitary adenoma is autonomous. Consequently, no TSH reaction is to be expected after TRH in TSH-producing pituitary adenomas.

A TSH producing pituitary tumour can have isolated release of TSH, but it is not uncommon that TSH release is combined with a release of growth hormone or prolactin, for example. Some of these tumours can also release excessive amounts of the alpha subunit glucoprotein of some of the pituitary hormones (common to TSH, LH and FSH). Determination of the alpha subunit glucoprotein in serum, as a marker for a TSH producing pituitary tumour, is normally included in the investigation of TSH producing adenoma.

Morphological investigation of the sella turcica using MR, as well as investigations of other pituitary function, must be performed if a TSH producing pituitary adenoma is suspected.

A patient with a TSH producing adenoma should primarily be referred to pituitary surgery. Beta blockers and antithyroid drugs can be given preoperatively so that the patient is euthyroid before pituitary surgery. TSH can be expected to rise when T4/

E. Nyström, G.E.B. Berg, S.K.G. Jansson, O. Torring, S.V. Valdemarsson (Eds.),
Thyroid Disease in Adults,
DOI: 10.1007/978-3-642-13262-9_27, © Springer-Verlag Berlin Heidelberg 2011

T3 levels are normalized during medical treatment. This may lead to an increase in tumour size and surgery should therefore not be delayed.

> The effect of surgery can be determined by daily postoperative analyses of TSH, which should decrease immediately after surgery, while T4, due to its longer half-life, drops more slowly. Administration of thyroxine in the days following surgery can therefore be postponed a few days, which facilitates early postoperative assessment by repeated measurement of TSH for 1 week after surgery.
> Pharmacological treatment of a TSH producing pituitary adenoma with somatostatin analogues has been demonstrated to have a good effect on overproduction of TSH, and may be used if the pituitary tumour is large and can not be removed by radical resection.
>
> In cases when the patient is primarily incorrectly treated with radioiodine or thyroid surgery, an increase in the size of the pituitary tumour can be expected. This underpins the importance of a correct diagnosis and that treatment must primarily target the pituitary tumour.

27.2 hCG-Dependent Hyperthyroidism

hCG-dependent stimulation of the thyroid occurs in the early stages of pregnancy. In some cases, the stimulating effect of hCG is so strong that it results in elevated T4 and T3 concentrations and low TSH, along with symptoms, and is called gestational hyperthyroidism. This form of thyroid hyperfunction may be especially pronounced in pregnant women suffering from severe nausea and vomiting, so called hyperemesis gravidarum.

When hCG falls as the pregnancy progresses, the hyperthyroidism and associated symptoms normally recede around weeks 12–15 of pregnancy.

The thyroid related symptoms rarely require treatment. Beta blockers can be used in milder cases. Antithyroid drugs, primarily propylthiouracil, can be considered in severe cases, but should only be given for a short period of time until the condition spontaneously resolves when the hCG concentration falls. In contrast to Graves' disease, there are no increases in TRAb in hCG-dependent hyperthyroidism.

If trophoblastic tumour (mole) develops during pregnancy, hCG levels can reach extremely high levels. In these uncommon cases, pronounced hyperthyroidism can develop. Antithyroid drugs can be administered so that the tumour can be removed by radical surgery, which cures the condition.

27.3 Ectopic Production of Thyroid Hormones

Metastases from differentiated thyroid cancer can have the capacity to take up iodine and synthesize hormone. These tumours can be demonstrated using scintigraphy and can be treated with surgery or radioiodine.

In rare cases, thyroid follicles can be found in the ovaries as a result of intrauterine developmental disturbances. Tumours containing such follicles may have retained the ability to synthesize and release thyroid hormone, which is called struma ovarii. This results in inhibition of TSH secretion, and thus inhibition of thyroid gland function and radionuclide uptake at scintigraphy or iodine (I-131) uptake test. Here, scintigraphy with images of the lower part of the abdomen can be helpful in diagnosis.

27.4 Thyrotoxicosis Factitia

A conscious and deliberate intake of high doses of thyroxine, factitia, results primarily in a dose-dependent increase in T4, while an increase in conversion of T4 to reverse T3 will lead to a more moderate increase in T3. Intake of triiodothyronine is reflected immediately in the elevated free T3 values and gives more pronounced symptoms.

Secretion of TSH is inhibited, and thereby the synthesis and release of hormone from the thyroid. This is reflected by low uptake at scintigraphy or measurement of I-131 uptake. Consequently, release of thyroglobulin also drops. Determination of thyroglobulin is therefore valuable if exogenous intake of thyroid hormone is suspected.

It is often difficult to verify the correct cause of abnormal hormone values in these cases. When the patient admits misuse of thyroid hormone, a gradual reduction in the intake of hormone can be attempted in order to avoid symptoms that are perceived by the patient as arising from low intake of hormone.

A similar situation may occur in patients who use weight reducing agents containing thyroid hormone or analogues such as 3,5,3'-triiodo thyroacetic acid (TRIAC). Use of TRIAC can be disclosed since it may be codetermined during analysis of T3.

Unintentional intake of thyroid hormone has occurred in people who have eaten meat products containing thyroid gland. An example is the epidemic of thyrotoxicosis that occurred in the USA after consuming hamburgers containing beef thyroid, so-called "hamburger toxicosis".

27.5 Iodine-Induced Hyperthyroidism

Administration of large amounts of iodine can result in various forms of thyrotoxicosis and can cause particular diagnostic and therapeutic problems (see Chaps. 6, 21 and 33).

27.5.1 Exacerbation of Latent Graves´ Disease

Iodine supplementation can trigger hyperthyroidism in patients with latent Graves' disease. In these cases, the thyroid has lost its normal protective autoregulatory mechanism against increased iodine exposure. Treatment follows the same principles as in patients with spontaneous disease, except that the radioiodine therapy may not be possible.

27.5.2 Progress in Patients with Autonomous Adenoma

A larger and more common risk group are patients with multinodular goitre (or with autonomous adenoma). Because autonomous areas are not considered to have normal protective and regulatory mechanisms against excess iodine, hormone production can increase in these patients after iodine exposure, for example, during X-ray investigation using iodine-containing contrast agents. Often, a down-regulation of NIS occurs with the result that the uptake is low in scintigraphy and after administration of I-131. Since multinodular goitre is more prevalent in the elderly, the risk for iodine-induced hyperthyroidism is greater among this patient group.

Iodine-induced hyperthyroidism often regresses spontaneously within weeks to months. If treatment with beta blockers is not sufficient, antithyroid drugs may be used until recovery occurs. Because of the low uptake of iodide, I-131 therapy is not possible.

27.5.3 Iodine-Induced Thyroiditis

Iodine can also induce thyroiditis through cell damage (see Chap. 7). Here, a transient thyrotoxicosis occurs. During the toxic phase, NIS is inactivated and uptake of iodine is therefore low. Alleviation of symptoms during the toxic phase is provided by beta blockers.

> An increased use of iodine-containing contrast agents for X-ray examinations, including computed tomography, have further highlighted the problem of iodine-induced hyperthyroidism.
> Antithyroid drugs are sometimes used to block the synthesis of the hormones, which thereby modifies any effects of increased exposure of iodide after iodine contrast examination.
> In patients with ongoing hyperthyroidism, potassium perchlorate is another option before administration of contrast agents in certain cases, for example before coronary angiography in patients with acute coronary disease and known or recently diagnosed hyperthyroidism.

Iodine blocking prior to medical investigations is discussed in Chap. 6.

Other Causes of Thyrotoxicosis

- TSH-producing pituitary adenoma causes hyperthyroidism as a consequence of autonomous secretion of TSH. TSH levels will be within or higher than the reference range
- In pregnancy hCG from the placenta can cause hyperthyroidism via stimulation of the TSH receptors. This explains why TSH can be lowered during the first part of pregnancy in a woman with an otherwise healthy thyroid and why hyperthyroidism can occur in connection with hydatidiform mole
- Additional supplementation of iodine can induce hyperthyroidism in patients with multinodular toxic goitre or autonomous adenoma. In Graves´ disease, iodine supplementation can exacerbate the degree of hyperthyroidism
- Iodine from iodine-containing contrast media or from certain medicines are common causes for iodine-induced hyperthyroidism

28 Nontoxic Goitre

28.1 Goitre and Its Causes

The term goitre describes an enlargement of the thyroid gland. However, the concept of goitre does not in any way describe the underlying pathophysiological mechanism that causes the goitre. Neither does it describe the hormonal activity of the thyroid gland.

This chapter focuses solely on nontoxic benign goitre. For functional disturbances in the thyroid, refer to the chapters on hypothyroidism (Chaps. 10–13) and hyperthyroidism (Chaps. 18, 20, 21). For further information on palpable lumps in the thyroid and thyroid cancer, refer to Chaps. 29 and 30, respectively.

Both diffuse and the nodular goitres are benign conditions that are very common. The term endemic goitre is used when goitre occurs in more than 10% of the population within a defined geographic area. A hypothetical model for development of nodular goitre independent of iodine is given in Chap. 21. The types of goitre and their causes are:

- *Diffuse goitre*
  - Thyroiditis
  - Hyperplasia of follicle epithelium
  - Iodine deficiency (endemic)
- *Multinodular goitre*
  - Sporadic colloid goitre
  - Iodine deficiency (endemic)
- *Unilateral goitre/uninodular goitre*
  - Sporadic colloid goitre
  - Solitary adenoma/neoplasia

28.2 Goitre Due to Iodine Deficiency

Iodine deficiency is a common cause of endemic goitre. Recently, WHO calculated that about 740 million people, equivalent to 13% of the world's population, have goitre due to an excessively low intake of iodine.

Biochemically, mild iodine deficiency is characterized by a modest decrease in T4 values and a reciprocal mild rise in TSH. In pronounced iodine deficiency, low T4 and elevated TSH is observed. Because of the iodine deficiency, the follicle cells often synthesize relatively more T3 than T4. Serum concentrations of T3 can therefore be normal (or even slightly raised) in spite of low T4.

Iodine deficiency leads to hyperplasia of the thyroid epithelium. Over time, some follicles will become inactive and distended with colloid. This will lead to focal nodular hyperplasia and nodular changes that can assume grotesque proportions and be associated with a risk for hypothyroidism.

28.3 Colloid-Rich Multinodular Goitre

Even in countries without iodine deficiency, goitre is a very common condition. One study in Northeast England revealed that nodular thyroid changes could be demonstrated in 0.8% of adult men and in 5.3% of adult women. The majority of patients with goitre have a multinodular nontoxic benign goitre (Fig. 28.1). In some cases, a local change in thyroid follicles dominates so that the goitre behaves like a unilateral goitre or even as a palpable solitary lump (Chap. 29).

28.3.1 Pathogenesis

Goitre occurs because of focal follicle cell hyperplasia at one or more sites in the thyroid gland. There is a positive correlation between total DNA content of the goitre and goitre weight. This indicates hyperplasia of the follicular epithelium, while interstitial

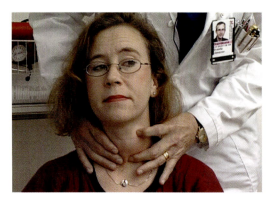

Fig. 28.1 Palpation of patient with goitre

tissue and colloid have relatively little significance for goitre growth. Both extrathyroidal and intrathyroidal growth factors control and modulate goitre growth. TSH is one growth factor with significant impact on the growth and function of the thyroid. As previously mentioned, several other growth factors also play important roles, either independently or together with TSH.

A goitre is often initially diffuse, but develops nodular areas with time. Depending on the varying sensitivities for growth factors in subpopulations of thyrocytes, larger or smaller nodular areas can develop. If such nodular areas retain their capacity to take up and accumulate iodine, these areas may become autonomously active with a consequent increase in hormone production (Chap. 21). In certain autonomously active nodules, TSH receptor mutations have been demonstrated.

28.3.2 Clinical Course

The clinical course of sporadic nodular goitre is highly varied. As a rule, younger or middle-aged individuals in the early phase of the pathophysiological process present with diffuse goitre, while the tendency with increasing age is a gradual development towards the characteristics of multinodular goitre. In adults and the elderly, a slow but continuous further growth of the goitre is often observed. The rate of growth varies greatly from person to person. About 10% of cases with euthyroid multinodular goitre progress to toxic multinodular goitre (Chap. 21).

28.3.3 Clinical Examination

Taking the medical history of a patient presenting with an enlarged thyroid will often provide the cause of benign nodular nontoxic goitre. This can normally be related back to the patient or someone close, noticing a lump in the neck on herself/himself, or the patient experiencing discomfort in the area of the neck. Occasionally, goitre is diagnosed as a secondary finding in connection with an X-ray of the chest when a mass in the upper mediastinum is noted, with or without effects on the trachea. Because a slow gradual growth of a multinodular nontoxic goitre is a common phenomenon, it is not uncommon for the patient to live with a swelling in the neck for a long time, not seeking medical care until the swelling becomes large and obvious.

A sudden growth or increase in growth can be caused by bleeding in a cystic process in a multinodular goitre. This can suddenly cause acute symptoms in the neck. These cases can be clinically difficult to distinguish from fast growing tumours.

If the goitre grows substernally into the upper mediastinum, the upper thorax aperture can gradually become constricted by the goitre, which may cause mechanical symptoms from the trachea, the oesophagus, blood vessels and recurrent nerves.

Compression of the trachea is not uncommon, but often gives quite mild symptoms until about 75% of the cross-sectional area is occluded. Minimal effort may in such cases make the patient dyspnoic (short of breath) due to inspiratory distress, a condition that may be misinterpreted as cardiac or respiratory problems. Sometimes the symptoms progress in connection with a respiratory infection, with swelling of the mucous membranes in the airways.

Patients with effects on the trachea frequently experience the most problems at night because of the difficulty to sleep on their back in a supine position. These patients commonly prefer to sleep on their side with the head raised or tilted.

In pronounced cases, the venous flow can be so obstructed that the patient experiences stasis of the neck veins (called superior vena cava syndrome) with dilated veins visible on the neck. The symptoms are exacerbated if the patient elevates the arms above and behind the head (Pemberton test).

A feeling of having a lump in the neck when swallowing and dysphagia occur if the goitre extends backwards and affects the oesophagus and pharynx. Mechanical stretching of the recurrent nerve due to a large goitre can cause hoarseness because of dysfunction of the vocal cords. Such symptoms highlight the important differentiation towards a malignant thyroid tumour.

In the physical examination of a patient with goitre it is important to verify the lower limit of a large goitre. If the goitre can not be delimited caudally, this suggests that the goitre stretches down intrathoracic. In this case, mapping should be done using CT, preferably without iodine-containing contrast media, or MR.

Another important reason why a patient with a goitre/lump seeks medical advise is concern for cancer. An accurate medical history is therefore invaluable in assessing patients with goitre and the concerns of the patient should be taken seriously.

28.3.4 Investigative Methods

28.3.4.1 Hormones

TSH is a reliable marker for determining whether the patient is euthyroid and if the goitre is nontoxic. The concentration of TSH may be low/normal, indicating an early stage of autonomous thyroid hormone production in a so far nontoxic goitre (Chap. 21). In addition, T4 and preferably T3 are measured. Autonomous nodules have a tendency for a relative increase in T3 synthesis and release. Determination of T3 is a sensitive marker for autonomous hormone production in a multinodular goitre. T4 might even be in the lower range, in connection with normal/high T3 and low TSH.

28.3.4.2 Scintigraphy

Radionuclear investigation using technetium scintigraphy is a valuable tool for determining whether autonomous areas are present in the thyroid. In general, a thyroid scintigraphy is not routinely indicated if TSH is normal. However, if a patient with a suspected nodular goitre/adenoma has symptoms and a TSH that is low/normal, a scintigraphy can still be performed and give valuable information on goitre size, extension, and of slight autonomicity of clinical importance.

28.3.4.3 Ultrasound Investigations

Ultrasound of the thyroid has increasingly taken over as the preferred investigative method of the thyroid if the question relates to size, morphology (cysts, solitary palpable lump, nodular changes, etc.) and relationship to surrounding tissues when the goitre is limited to the neck and TSH is normal. Ultrasound is also useful as a guided cytological aspiration diagnostic tool.

28.3.4.4 Radiological Investigation

A radiological examination of the thyroid and its relationship to adjacent structures often provides valuable information when deciding whether to treat or not. Previously, an X-ray of the soft tissues of the neck, sometimes with contrast media in the oesophagus, was performed. This investigation has today been replaced for the most part by more modern techniques such as ultrasound, CT or MR. Iodine-containing contrast media should be used with caution for investigation of goitre because large quantities of iodine can trigger dysfunction of the thyroid. This risk should be weighed against the additional diagnostic information that can be obtained with contrast media. A dialogue between the clinician and radiologist is therefore recommended.

Pulmonary X-ray is sometimes used to investigate goitre with intrathoracic expansion.

CT and MR investigations are increasingly replacing pulmonary X-ray exams, primarily for diagnosis of intrathoracic goitre. These techniques provide a far more exact picture of the relationship between the goitre and the surrounding blood vessels, larynx and other tissues. Even enlarged lymph nodes can be demonstrated.

28.3.4.5 Cytological Investigation

As previously pointed out and as presented in Chaps. 29 and 30, all patients with goitre should be considered for fine-needle aspiration for cytological diagnosis. In experienced hands, cytology can discriminate between malignant and benign conditions with relatively high probability. Information regarding rapid growth and consistency of the gland must also be included in the assessment.

28.3.5 Treatment

Symptoms are crucial to the decision whether to actively treat or just observe. In asymptomatic patients, for whom an investigation reveals a benign nontoxic goitre, only observation is necessary. Because of the risk of future dysfunction, follow-up of the patient is recommended. For new clinical assessments, biochemical tests (free) T4, (free) T3, TSH are performed. If further increase in size or local symptoms appears, fine-needle biopsy is repeated.

The most important reason for therapeutic intervention in patients with nontoxic multinodular goitre is compression of the trachea and oesophagus, or effects on the venous flow. Other indications may be intrathoracic growth, or the fact that a malignancy can not be ruled out (cytological finding, rapid growth). Discomfort in the neck and cosmetic problems are also factors that should be considered.

The therapeutic options for nontoxic goitre are:
- Surgery
- Treatment with radioactive iodine
- Treatment of iodine deficiency
- Thyroxine

28.3.5.1 Surgery

Surgery is the most established and effective treatment for a goitre that causes mechanical symptoms (Fig. 28.2). It also permits histological examination. Surgery entails rapid elimination of the symptoms of the patient. The extent of the goitre determines the extent of resection:
- Lobectomy
- Subtotal bilateral resection
- Lobectomy and contralateral lobe resection
- Total thyroidectomy

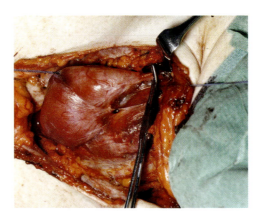

Fig. 28.2 Surgery of nontoxic goitre

After a unilateral lobectomy, most patients can manage without thyroxine, but after larger resections, lifelong thyroxine replacement therapy is often necessary. With limited intervention, the risk of progression of the goitre persists because often the entire thyroid is or will be involved in the pathological process. These consequences decrease with more radical surgery, which, on the other hand, involves an increased risk of surgical complications. Overall, however, the risk of complications is low provided surgery is performed by an experienced thyroid surgeon.

Indications for surgery of nontoxic goitre are:
- Large goitre with partial obstruction of trachea and/or oesophagus
- Symptom-producing intrathoracic expansion
- Large nodules (>4 cm), cytological investigation difficult
- Discomfort or cosmetic problems that lower the quality of life of the patient
- Genetic predisposition for thyroid cancer or exposure to ionizing radiation to the neck

28.3.5.2 Medical Treatment

Thyroxine treatment can reduce the size of the goitre in patients with manifest or subclinical hypothyroidism. An effect can also be seen in iodine-deficiency goitre. In euthyroid goitre with normal TSH levels, the effect of thyroxine treatment is, however, controversial. The effect may be beneficial in some individuals with a relatively small goitre. In patients with large goitres, the effect is doubtful. In these cases, progression of goitre size often appears even if TSH is low or suppressed. There is no data available supporting the supposition that long-term treatment with thyroxine will alter the natural progression with respect to development and growth of multinodular goitre.

The disadvantage of thyroxine treatment is the risk of exacerbating latent thyrotoxicosis. This applies in particular if autonomous areas are present and if TSH already lies in the lower area of the reference range, as often is the case.

28.3.5.3 Radioiodine Treatment

Radioiodine treatment is not a generally established method for treating nontoxic goitre. Studies have been reported in which radioiodine treatment results in a reduction of goitre size by up to 50% within a few years of observation. Many nodular goitres have low radioiodine uptake, which reduces the possibility of achieving adequate tissue effects from the radiation. In these cases, attempts have been made to increase radioiodine uptake by administering recombinant human TSH. The disadvantages of radioiodine treatment is the uncertain and slow effect.

The risks associated with radioiodine treatment of nontoxic goitre are:
- Radiation-induced thyroiditis
- Induction of antibody formation (TRAb) and development of Graves' disease
- Risk of acute swelling with increased compression symptoms in patients with a very large goitre
- Transient hyperthyroidism that may be deleterious in the elderly
- Development of hypothyroidism over time

In summary, radioiodine treatment can still be classified as a not fully established method in which long-term data for treatment and side effects are currently not yet available. However, it can be worth considering as an option in cases with only moderately enlarged but still symptomatic goitre where surgery may be too risky.

28.4 Intrathoracic Goitre

Expansion of multinodular goitre down into the mediastinum is not uncommon. In these cases, parts of the thyroid can be palpated below the larynx but no lower border can be detected beneath the jugulum. A solitary intrathoracic goitre can also occur.

28.4.1 Clinical Presentation
Intrathoracic goitre most commonly affects older patients. In patients with a short neck or thoracic kyphosis, the thyroid may be very difficult to examine. In these cases, diagnosis is often incidental on an X-ray or CT conducted for a totally different reason, or upon investigation of respiratory symptoms caused by the goitre.

28.4.2 Investigative Methods
The problem with an intrathoracic goitre is the lack of opportunity to adequately palpate, and the difficulty of obtaining biopsy material for exclusion of malignancy. Fine-needle biopsy is however often possible if the patient lies on their back with the neck extended. The extent to which the sample is representative, is however limited, because it is only possible to reach some areas of the goitre. One alternative worth considering is parasternal puncture using radiological guidance, but there is a risk of bleeding, which is difficult to treat.

28.4.3 Mapping
Normal chest X-rays can provide information on whether the goitre is intrathoracic by demonstrating a soft tissue swelling in the upper mediastinum with effects on the trachea.

For better mapping and determination of the relationship to the trachea, CT or MR are recommended. With regard to large multinodular goitres, it should be remembered that examination using iodine contrast can trigger thyrotoxicosis due to the high iodine exposure. Ultrasound and scintigraphy investigations have limited value in investigation of intrathoracic goitre.

28.4.4 Assessment

Operation of intrathoracic goitre should be considered if there is difficulty in making an adequate clinical and cytological assessment. Other causes are the risk of developing thyrotoxicosis and the risk of progressive compression of the airways or blood vessels in the upper thorax.

When assessing X-ray findings, the size of the goitre and its relationship to surrounding tissues should be examined. Any tracheal compression must be assessed. The caudal expansion in the thorax should also be noted. A lower limit above or below the aortic arch is often used as a guide in surgical intervention.

28.4.5 Surgery

Surgery is the method of choice for intrathoracic goitre. A patient with intrathoracic goitre should be considered for referral to a surgeon for assessment.

During surgery, the positioning of the patient on the operating table is very important. The surgeon must ensure that the patient has adequate extension of the neck, which will automatically result in the goitre being pulled up somewhat from its intrathoracic location.

The operation starts with exploration from the neck, which the surgeon uses to achieve control of the blood vessels supplying the thyroid, and thereafter a gradual mobilization of the intrathoracic component. This technique enables mobilization of about 90% of all intrathoracic goitres from a cervical incision. Sternotomy/thoracotomy becomes unnecessary.

If the goitre stretches below the aortic arch and/or mobilization of the intrathoracic component is not successful via a cervical exploration, sternotomy is recommended to safely mobilize the goitre from the thorax. Resecting the cervical component and leaving an intrathoracic component is not recommended, because it entails a risk of uncontrolled bleeding in the mediastinum or recurrence.

> **Intrathoracic Goitre**
>
> - Should be considered for referral to surgical assessment
> - Liberal indications for surgery if the patient has symptoms
> - Accurate preoperative mapping of the expansion
> - If sternotomy is necessary, the convalescence time is slightly longer

29 Thyroid Lumps

29.1 Incidence/Prevalence

Lumps occur frequently in the thyroid. In countries without iodine deficiency, it is estimated that palpable lumps in the thyroid occur in 4–7% of the population. Using sensitive examination methods such as ultrasound, changes in the thyroid can be demonstrated in more than one third of people. In countries with moderate or pronounced iodine deficiency, where goitre is endemic, the prevalence of palpable lumps in the thyroid is considerably higher.

Most lumps in the thyroid are benign. Only about 5% of all palpable lumps in the thyroid are malignant. The challenge for the doctor meeting a patient with a palpable lump in the thyroid gland is to diagnose in a reliable and cost-effective manner those few patients who have thyroid cancer and need immediate care. It is neither meaningful nor possible to surgically remove all lumps in the thyroid.

29.2 Classification of Palpable Thyroid Lumps

Lumps in the thyroid do not comprise a pathological entity in themselves, but are clinical manifestations of a wide range of thyroid diseases. Lumps can be classified as multiple or solitary lumps (Table 29.1). The most common lump in the thyroid comprises a dominant part of a multinodular goitre. Lumps can be subdivided into *neoplastic* and *non-neoplastic* changes. The neoplastic lumps can be subdivided into *benign* and *malignant* neoplasms.

29.3 Diagnosis of Thyroid Lumps

The basic investigation of a lump in the thyroid includes a medical history, clinical examination, analysis of thyroid hormones and cytology. Ultrasound, thyroid scintigraphy and radiological imaging also are useful in the diagnostic work-up.

29.3.1 Medical History and Clinical Examination

Accurate medical history and clinical examination are important because they provide information that can indicate whether the changes are malignant or not. The following medical history details and clinical observations *indicate a low risk* of thyroid malignancy:
- Familial occurrence of Hashimoto's thyroiditis or other autoimmune thyroid disease
- Goitre and benign thyroid conditions in close relatives
- Hypo- or hyperthyroidism

E. Nyström, G.E.B. Berg, S.K.G. Jansson, O. Törring, S.V. Valdemarsson (Eds.), *Thyroid Disease in Adults*, DOI: 10.1007/978-3-642-13262-9_29, © Springer-Verlag Berlin Heidelberg 2011

- Tenderness associated with palpable thyroid lump
- Soft, smooth and moveable lump
- Multiple changes without any dominant palpable lump

The following findings and medical history details *increase the probability* of malignant thyroid disease:
- Hard, irregular lump attached to surroundings
- Enlarged cervical lymph nodes
- Lump associated with dysphagia or hoarseness
- <16 or >60 years
- Male gender
- History of exposure to radiation to the neck, particularly in childhood or adolescence

Table 29.1 Clinical and histopathological classification of thyroid lumps

Non-neoplastic palpable lumps	
Hyperplastic conditions	Colloid nodule/nodules
Inflammatory conditions	Acute bacterial thyroiditis (abscess)
	Subacute thyroiditis
	Hashimoto's thyroiditis
	Riedel's thyroiditis
Neoplastic palpable lumps	
Benign neoplasms	Adenoma
	Cysts
Malignant neoplasms	
Primary carcinoma	Papillary thyroid cancer
	Follicular thyroid cancer
	Hürthle cell (oxyphilic) cancer
	Poorly differentiated thyroid cancer
	Anaplastic thyroid cancer
	Medullary thyroid cancer
Secondary malignancies (not arising in thyroid cells)	Lymphoma
	Metastases

It is important that the examiner uses an accurate and systematic technique at palpation of the thyroid and surrounding lymph nodes (see Chap. 5). Lumps in the thyroid are best described accurately with dimensions given in centimetres, by consistency, and with limits described in relation to surrounding muscles, skin and tracheal wall.

29.3.2 Biochemical Work-Up

Analysis of thyroid hormones and TSH can not differentiate between benign and malignant conditions. However, analysis can provide valuable information on the occurrence of hypoactivity, which could indicate that the local process is part of a chronic lymphocytic thyroiditis (Hashimoto's thyroiditis), or hyperactivity, as in autonomous functioning adenoma. Overproduction of thyroid hormone is very uncommon in malignant thyroid diseases.

Analysis of TPOAb can be valuable in diagnosing chronic lymphocytic thyroiditis, particularly in those cases in which the TSH concentration is elevated. It should nevertheless be pointed out that occurrence of Hashimoto's thyroiditis does not rule out a concomitant malignancy in the thyroid.

Determination of Tg is not indicated in the primary investigation of lumps in the thyroid because Tg can be elevated in various conditions in addition to cancer, such as nodular goitre, thyroiditis and hyperthyroidism. Determination of Tg is on the other hand a valuable tumour marker in follow-up of differentiated thyroid cancer after surgery.

> In patients with a family medical history of medullary thyroid cancer, determination of serum calcitonin should be performed and, if available, genetic screening for point mutations in the RET proto-oncogene (by specialists). In some centres, analysis of calcitonin is routinely performed in all patients with thyroid nodules in order to detect medullary thyroid cancer. In other centres this routine is not considered cost effective in the investigation of lumps in the thyroid, unless there is a family medical history or other findings that indicate MEN 2 syndrome.

29.3.3 Imaging Investigations

The basic investigative methods used for lumps in the thyroid are ultrasound and, in certain cases, scintigraphy (see diagnostic methods described in Chap. 4). CT and MR are considered supplementary investigations that can give important additional information if a thyroid cancer has been confirmed and includes information regarding the relation of the tumour to airways, oesophagus, blood vessels, etc.

A chest X-ray is a basic method for investigation of the thorax and lungs, but CT is a far more sensitive method for detecting metastases in lung parenchyma and for investigating mediastinal involvement such as intrathoracic expansion of a goitre. X-ray of the soft tissues of the neck provides information on the indirect impact on the trachea/oesophagus. This investigation thus has a relatively low diagnostic value and has mostly been replaced by CT/MR.

29.3.4 Morphological Diagnostics: Fine-Needle Aspiration Cytology

In contrast to the above diagnostic procedures, *only* fine-needle biopsy can determine whether a thyroid lump is benign or malignant. Cytological investigation must therefore always be an integral part of the investigation of thyroid lumps. Using fine-needle biopsy, an experienced cytologist can determine with high probability whether a lump is benign or malignant (see Chap. 4).

In larger international studies, the sensitivity of fine-needle biopsy for thyroid malignancy was reported to vary from 68–98% and the specificity was between 72 and 100%. Using ultrasound guided biopsy, even difficult-to-palpate lumps in the thyroid can be examined cytologically, thus contributing to increasing diagnostic certainty.

The following diagnoses can be determined with high probability using fine-needle biopsy:
- Hashimoto's thyroiditis
- Colloid nodule (nodular goitre)
- Subacute (granulomatous) thyroiditis
- Cysts, intrathyroidal hemorraghe
- Primary thyroid carcinoma (Table 29.1)
- Malignant lymphoma in the thyroid
- Metastases in the thyroid from other primary tumour

Intermediate or premalignant suspicious cytological findings include:
- Follicular neoplasia: A relatively large group of lumps in the thyroid can be designated as follicular neoplasias. In these cases it is not possible to cytologically definitively differentiate a follicular adenoma (benign lump) from follicular thyroid carcinoma that is characterized by invasive growth through the tumour capsule and/or by intravascular growth. Differential diagnosis between these two conditions therefore requires surgical removal of the lump and accurate histopathological investigation with examination of several sections.
- Lumps with suspected or typical papillary formations are highly indicative for papillary cancer and should always be removed for final diagnosis.
- Hürthle cell or oxyphile neoplasms are considered as a subgroup of follicular tumours, but malignancy is difficult to determine using cytology.

29.4 Treatment of Palpable Thyroid Lumps

29.4.1 Palpable Lumps with Benign Cytology

Because fine-needle cytology has a high diagnostic reliability, surgical excision of benign lumps in the thyroid is often unnecessary for diagnostic purposes (with the exception of follicular neoplasia as above). After adequate investigation, including accurate clinical investigation, thyroid function tests and representative fine-needle cytological diagnosis, many patients can be informed that they have a benign condition and that treatment is not necessary. Often, follow-up is recommended after 6–12 months, and may include a second fine-needle biopsy, at least if enlargement or other focal signs are noted.

Surgical treatment can be indicated for benign lumps if the lump is large and causing local pressure symptoms on the trachea, oesophagus or soft tissues in the neck. For lumps that demonstrate continuous growth, surgical excision should be considered.

Surgery for unilateral lumps should involve a total lobectomy on the affected side. In multinodular goitre, bilateral thyroid resection or total thyroidectomy may be proposed.

29.4.2 Lumps with Follicular Neoplasia, Unclear Cytology or Nondiagnostic Samples After Fine-Needle Biopsy

In general, lumps with unclear or suspect cytological diagnosis are removed surgically in order to obtain a satisfactory histopathological diagnosis. It has been reported that some 10–30% of follicular lesions in the thyroid turn out to be malignant at histopathological examination.

In cases with insufficient samples at fine-needle cytology, reaspiration is recommended, preferably with ultrasound guidance.

29.4.3 Thyroid Cysts

Cystic changes in the thyroid are quite common, and are mostly due to multinodular goitre. Such processes comprise 10–15% of all thyroid lumps. The occurrence of malignancy in cysts is lower than in solid lumps. However, malignant tumours in the thyroid can undergo cystic degeneration so that the tumour seems to be limited to tumour vegetation in the cyst wall (see Sect. 4.4). It is therefore necessary to investigate the fluids from cystic thyroid lumps. It is important to be aware of recurrent cysts with the property of refilling with fluid after emptying. If ultrasound reveals solid components in the cyst wall, fine-needle biopsy guided by ultrasound to this area should be tried, and surgical extirpation considered.

29.4.4 Autonomously Functioning Lumps

See Chap. 20.

29.4.5 Suppressive Treatment with Thyroxine

Suppressive treatment with thyroxine for reducing the growth in benign lumps in the thyroid is controversial. Proponents of this treatment claim that it can reduce the size of lumps while others claim that TSH suppression has no effect. There is no definitive evidence to support TSH suppressive treatment.

Routine thyroxine treatment after hemithyroidectomy for benign lumps in the thyroid has also been discussed for a long time. In this case, there is also no reliable data to support that this reduces the risk of new lumps in the thyroid. On the contrary, thyroxine treatment might be hazardous, because overdosing increases the risk of cardiac problems (arrhythmia). At present the recommendation is that thyroxine treatment is only indicated if TSH is elevated.

Chapter 29: Thyroid Lumps

29.5 Investigation Algorithm

Figure 29.1 provides an algorithm for investigating thyroid lumps.

If TSH is elevated, primary hypothyroidism is diagnosed. Autoimmune/lymphocytic thyroiditis may be suspected as the cause of the palpatory finding. Further investigations includes determination of TPOAb and fine needle biopsy.

If TSH is normal, i.e. the patient is euthyroid, the most important question is whether the palpable lump is benign or malignant. These patients must be investigated using fine needle biopsy before intervention.

If TSH is suppressed or non detectable, this indicates an increased hormone production in the thyroid, i.e. the palpable lump could be autonomously producing hormone and comprise a solitary autonomous adenoma, or be a dominant nodule in a multinodular goitre. In these cases, there is indication for scintigraphy to confirm the diagnosis and prepare treatment with radioactive iodine or surgical extirpation.

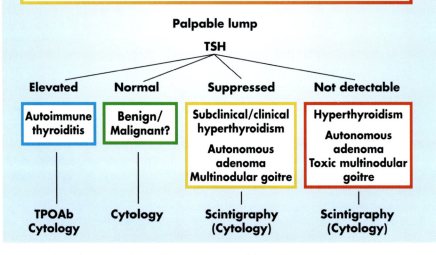

Fig. 29.1 Algorithm using TSH for the investigation of thyroid lumps

Thyroid Cancer

Thyroid cancer is one of the most common malignant endocrine tumours, with an annual incidence in Sweden of about 4/100,000 inhabitants (about twice as many women as men). Mortality is low at only 1/100,000 inhabitants annually according to Swedish cancer statistics. Worldwide incidence varies, however.

Normally, the patient seeks medical attention when she or he notices a lump in the neck. Palpable lumps in the thyroid occur relatively frequently and the patient is often worried that they have cancer. Prompt and appropriate investigations are therefore mandatory.

30.1 Classification of Thyroid Tumours

The thyroid contains two types of hormonally active cells: follicle cells and C cells, which lie adjacent to follicle cells in the connective tissue. C cells constitute about 1–2% of the parenchyma of the gland. A thyroid tumour is normally derived from one of these two cell types. Rarely, the tumour is a lymphoma or a metastasis from an extrathyroidal primary tumour. The classification of thyroid tumours is based on the following subdivisions:

1. *Epithelial tumours* (originating in the follicular epithelium)
- Follicular adenoma
- Follicular cancer
- Papillary cancer
- Poorly differentiated cancer
- Anaplastic cancer

2. *Variants of epithelial tumours* (originating in the follicular epithelium)
- Oncocytic adenoma (Hürthle cell adenoma)
- Oncocytic cancer (Hürthle cell cancer)
- Clear cell, mucinous and squamous differentiated cancer

3. *Epithelial tumours* (originating in the C cells)
- Medullary thyroid cancer

4. *Nonepithelial tumours*
- Sarcoma
- Lymphoma
- Metastases

E. Nyström, G.E.B. Berg, S.K.G. Jansson, O. Tørring, S.V. Valdemarsson (Eds.),
Thyroid Disease in Adults,
DOI: 10.1007/978-3-642-13262-9_30, © Springer-Verlag Berlin Heidelberg 2011

30.2 Characteristics of Common Thyroid Tumours

- *Follicular thyroid adenoma* is a benign tumour arising in the follicle epithelium which is built up of distinct follicle formations. The tumour is encapsulated. The follicle structures can vary in size and can also demonstrate a trabecular pattern at histopathological investigation. It can be difficult to distinguish between a follicular adenoma and a hyperplastic nodule in a nodular colloid goitre. The follicular adenoma, however, normally demonstrates a different histology compared to the surrounding glandular tissue.

- *Oncocytic adenoma* (Hürthle cell adenoma) is a follicular thyroid adenoma in which the cells display a rich eosinophilic cytoplasm (mitochondria-rich) or oncocytic differentiation (see also Fig. 4.17a,b).

- *Follicular thyroid cancer* is a malignant epithelial tumour originating from the thyroid follicular epithelium. The tumour is encapsulated and often grows like follicles, but can also demonstrate trabecular formations and solid areas. A prerequisite for diagnosis of invasive cancer is that the tumour grows through the capsule and/or invades the blood vessels. Those cancers for which histology only reveals invasion of the tumour into the capsule are known as minimally invasive cancers. It should be pointed out that during cytological investigation, distinction can not be made between follicular adenoma and follicular cancer. This is because it is not possible to evaluate the relationship of the cell to the surroundings. Therefore it is not possible from cytology to decide if the tumour is behaving aggressively towards or has grown through the capsule. Cytologists often use the term follicular neoplasia for these conditions. Consequently, follicular neoplasia should therefore be treated by surgical excision to obtain a correct histopathological diagnosis (Fig. 4.16a,b).

- *Oncocytic cancer* (Hürthle cell cancer) is a follicular thyroid cancer in which a majority of tumour cells (>90%) demonstrate oncocytic differentiation with eosinophilic (mitochondria-rich) cytoplasm. This type of tumour has a higher recurrence risk and thus poorer prognosis than the common follicular thyroid cancer (Fig. 4.17c,d).

- *Papillary thyroid cancer* is a malignant epithelial tumour originating in the thyroid follicular epithelium. The tumour reveals areas with papillary structure and/or characteristic nuclear change (ground-glass nuclei and nuclear grooving). Papillary thyroid cancer exhibits several growth patterns that can have prognostic importance. Occasionally, there is a dominant follicular growth pattern in papillary cancer. The prognosis of these follicular growing tumours is the same as for the other papillary tumours (Fig. 4.16c,d). Papillary thyroid cancer is the most common form and has the best prognosis of tumours in the thyroid.

- *Poorly differentiated cancer* is a malignant epithelial tumour that originates from the follicular epithelium, in which the tumour is characterized by a solid growth pattern and scarce or absent thyroglobulin content. Sometimes, poorly differentiated cancer occurs as a subcomponent of a well-differentiated thyroid cancer.

- *Anaplastic cancer* is a highly malignant and undifferentiated tumour that originates from the thyroid follicular epithelium. The tumour often grows throughout the entire thyroid gland and contains highly atypical tumour cells that grow in an irregular formation. The tumour cells do not synthesize thyroglobulin. The cells show a pronounced variation and differential diagnosis can pose problems in distinguishing anaplastic thyroid cancer from sarcoma and lymphoma. Immunohistochemical investigations and characterization of the tumour can facilitate diagnosis.

- *Medullary thyroid cancer* is a malignant epithelial tumour that originates in the thyroid C cells. The tumour grows in solid formations with spindle-shaped or polygonal tumour cells. Frequently, amyloid deposits are observed in the tumour. Immunohistochemically, medullary thyroid cancer typically contains calcitonin. Medullary thyroid cancer can occur in a sporadic (75%) or genetically transferred form. In the latter case, it is often an integrated part of the inherited syndrome multiple endocrine neoplasia type 2 (MEN2). Medullary thyroid cancer then occurs in conjunction with pheochromocytoma and sometimes parathyroid hyperplasia (MEN2A). In another very rare variant of the MEN2 syndrome, medullary thyroid cancer and pheochromocytoma are associated with a typical marphanoid-like appearance and multiple mucosal neurinoma (MEN2B). Hereditary forms of medullary thyroid cancer often display multiple primary tumours and hyperplasia of the C cells throughout the thyroid. The inherited variant is caused by an autosomal dominant transferred mutation in the RET proto-oncogene. Mutations in this gene have also been demonstrated in the tumour cells in about 30% of the sporadic cases. In these cases, the consequence of the mutation is limited to the thyroid.

30.3 Epidemiology

Thyroid cancer is 2–4 times more common in women than in men. However, the probability that a solitary palpable lump in the thyroid is malignant is higher in men.

Papillary thyroid cancer is the most common form, comprising about 70–80% of all thyroid cancer cases in Sweden. The reported annual incidence of thyroid cancer varies from country to country. Particularly high numbers are reported in Iceland and Hawaii, where there is a relatively high iodine intake in food. In countries with high iodine intake, papillary thyroid cancer comprises more than 85% of all cases. Countries with low iodine intake have reported a higher incidence of follicular and poorly differentiated or anaplastic cancer. Therefore, iodine availability may be important for the prevalence and type of thyroid cancer, but the precise causal relationship remains to be explained.

The clinical significance of small "occult" tumour changes (less than 1 cm) is uncertain. From a critical point of view (Sect. 30.9.2), the outcome of an ultrasound investigation may be helpful when deciding if fine-needle biopsy should be performed (Fig. 30.1). Postmortem examinations have reported a very high frequency of small foci of thyroid cancer, which in many cases can be considered to be in situ cancer.

The annual mortality in thyroid cancer varies from country to country. Overall, mortality from thyroid cancer only comprises about 1% of deaths from malignant diseases.

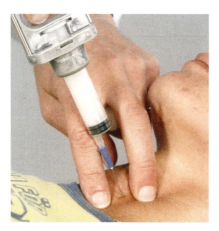

Fig. 30.1 Fine-needle aspiration biopsy from a thyroid lump

Thyroid cancer occurs at all ages, but is rare below 16 years of age. Nevertheless, an increased occurrence has been observed in children younger than 10 years old who have been exposed to radiation. There is an age-related increase in incidence and the risk increases with advancing age. The median age at diagnosis is 45–50 years. However, among those with a genetic disposition for medullary thyroid cancer, this type of malignancy may develop during early childhood.

30.4 Risk Factors

A number of risk factors for thyroid cancer have been studied:

1. Well-documented risk factors
- Heredity
- Exposure to radiation

2. Less well-documented risk factors
- Iodine intake
- Graves' disease
- Thyroiditis
- Pregnancy and other hormonal conditions

30.4.1 Hereditary Factors
It is estimated that about 5% of papillary cancer may have a genetic cause.

> Several unusual syndromes are linked to an increased occurrence of thyroid cancer, usually papillary cancer. In the majority of these, it has been possible to demonstrate the underlying genetically transferred mutation. Examples of such familial syndromes are Familial adenomatous polyposis (Gardner´s syndrome), Turcot´s syndrome, Cowden´s disease and Carny´s complex. Another syndrome, familial nonmedullary thyroid carcinoma, has also been described, but the genetic cause is not known.

With regard to medullary thyroid cancer, genetic factors are common and 25% are inherited via a mutation in the RET proto-oncogene. A number of different point mutations have been demonstrated. Three different conditions with inherited medullary thyroid cancer have been described: multiple endocrine neoplasia type 2A, multiple endocrine neoplasia type 2B and familial medullary thyroid cancer (FMTC). Genetic screening of families has enabled demonstration of gene carriers. Early prophylactic thyroidectomy can be offered to young individuals in whom the mutation has been demonstrated in order to avoid development of medullary thyroid cancer.

30.4.2 Oncogenes and Tumour Suppressor Genes

A number of oncogenes and tumour suppressor genes have been studied in human thyroid tumours. Activating point mutations in the RAS gene have been demonstrated at a high frequency in various histological types of thyroid tumours. Altered tyrosine kinase receptors have also been demonstrated, primarily in papillary thyroid cancer. A high prevalence of RET/PTC rearrangements has been demonstrated in radiation-induced papillary thyroid cancer. TSH receptor mutations occur and can be demonstrated in about 60% of hyperactive adenomas. These, however, do not result in malignant changes in the thyroid. P53 mutations are often expressed in poorly differentiated and anaplastic thyroid cancers and are presumably a stage in dedifferentiation of a previously differentiated thyroid cancer that results in failing control of apoptosis. The interaction between the various mutations is not fully understood (see Chap. 8).

30.4.3 Radiation

A connection between exposure to radiation in childhood and thyroid cancer has been known since the 1950s. Extensive epidemiological studies have analysed the increased risk associated with external radiation, nuclear weapon testing and nuclear power plant accidents. The thyroid gland is one of the organs in the body that is sensitive to induction of cancer after radiation, in particular if exposure occurs at a young age. External radiation of the neck is thus a risk factor in the development of thyroid cancer. A dose-dependent relationship is likely to exist.

After the nuclear power plant accident at Chernobyl in 1986, large quantities of radioactive isotopes were released. A rapid and dramatic increase in the occurrence of papillary thyroid cancer was demonstrated after the accident. This was an aggressive type of papillary thyroid cancer that affected children in the regions around Chernobyl, primarily in and around Belarus. The incidence was 75 times higher during a 10-year period among people younger than 10 years of age at exposure. This increase in incidence was also found in those subjected to intrauterine exposure. A similar increase in incidence has so far not been demonstrated in adults in Belarus. The most common genetic changes in radiation-induced papillary thyroid cancer consist of a mutation within the RET/PTC gene (see Chap. 8). This gene is likely sensitive to the effects of radiation in children and in growing adolescents.

The significance of iodine deficiency, both at exposure and later, has been shown in Belarus, where the population in general had a very low iodine intake. In nearby Poland, where iodine prophylaxis was started within a few days of the nuclear power plant accident, a similar increase in the incidence of thyroid cancer in children exposed to equivalent doses was not observed.

30.4.4 Treatment with I-131

Based on the fact that radiation in certain situations has been shown to increase the risk for developing thyroid cancer, the incidence in patients receiving I-131 for hyperthyroidism has been investigated. Several series of patients from as early as the 1940s were studied. These studies have not supported the fear that radioiodine treatment increases the risk for thyroid cancer, neither in children nor in adults. This has been interpreted to be due to the fact that the highly absorbed dose in the scheduled treatment results in cell death and a reduction in the capacity for cell division.

30.4.5 Iodine

Several centres throughout the world have noted an increasing incidence of thyroid cancer and it has been speculated as to whether this increase in prevalence could be linked to the increased availability of iodine as a result of the ongoing extensive global program to control iodine deficiency. In the USA, an increase in prevalence of about 4% annually has been noted in the last 4 years.

A study in southern Germany, in an area that was previously iodine deficient but is now iodine sufficient, has not been able to demonstrate any difference in the incidence of thyroid cancer between 1981 and 1995. However, a different distribution of tumour types has been observed. Papillary cancer has become more common, and follicular and anaplastic cancer more uncommon after introduction of the program to control iodine deficiency. The prognosis for patients with papillary cancer is better than for follicular and anaplastic cancer, and is the reason the expected survival rate for patients with thyroid cancer as a group has increased.

30.5 Diagnostic Investigation

When investigating a suspected thyroid cancer, suspicion of which is founded on medical history or clinical findings (hard, fixed nodule), the most important diagnostic tool is fine-needle aspiration biopsy of the palpable lump. For other investigations of lumps in the thyroid, please refer to Chap. 29.

Ultrasound investigation is used increasingly for mapping tumours in the thyroid. MR or CT are sometimes used for preoperative mapping of thyroid cancer and as guidance for planning surgical intervention. For preoperative mapping of metastases in the lungs, a pulmonary X-ray or, preferably, CT *without* iodine contrast is performed. Note that CT with iodine contrast should be avoided so as not to interfere with subsequent investigation or treatment with I-131.

Ultrasound characteristics suggestive for malignancy are:
- Hypoechogenic
- Microcalcifications
- Diffuse demarcation
- Absence of halo
- High vascularity

As a rule, thyroid function is not affected by the presence of malignant tumours in the thyroid. Basic investigations of a lump in the neck should, however, include analysis of TSH and free T4. In cases of suspected medullary thyroid cancer, determination of calcitonin should be performed as this is a highly sensitive biochemical marker. Determination of thyroglobulin and antibodies against thyroglobulin are routine investigations at follow-up after treatment (i.e. total thyroidectomy with or without adjuvant radioiodine treatment) for papillary and follicular thyroid cancer, but have no role as a primary diagnostic tool.

Thyroid scintigraphy is not used routinely for investigation of suspected thyroid cancer. Sometimes investigations performed for another reason reveal a cold area, which gives rise to tumour suspicion. Such findings should be investigated further using cytology. Genetic examination is now routine in medullary thyroid cancer and also in family members to verify or rule out genetic disposition.

30.6 Prognostic Factors

The overall prognosis for thyroid cancer is good after treatment. In differentiated thyroid cancer, there is a 5-year overall survival rate above 90%. It is desirable to identify prognostic variables that can identify patients with an expected poorer prognosis and try to intensify the treatment of this group.

Factors in thyroid cancer that can result in poorer survival rates include:

1. Patient characteristics
- High age
- Male gender

2. Tumour characteristics
- Papillary cancer of the tall-cell or columnar type, or the sclerosing form
- Poorly differentiated follicular or anaplastic cancer
- Aneuploidy
- High proliferation and mitotic rate

3. Tumour expansion
- Large tumour
- Infiltrative growth outside the thyroid capsule
- Lymph node metastases in the neck and mediastinum
- Multifocality
- Distant metastases

4. Treatment-related factors
- Nonradical resection
- Elevated and increasing thyroglobulin more than 3 months after surgery
- Noniodine accumulating metastases

30.6.1 Age

Age at diagnosis is an important prognostic factor with respect to differentiated (papillary and follicular) tumours. In adults, recurrence and mortality risk increase with age.

Patients who develop the disease in old age tend to have more locally aggressive tumours and more often distant metastases at diagnosis. The fact that these patients are more often affected by aggressive tumour types, can not, however, be the only explanation for the poorer prognosis, because younger patients with a similar histological picture have a more benign clinical course.

Thyroid cancer is rare in children, but does occur. It has been noted that small children in particular (younger than 10 years of age) often have a more advanced disease at presentation, with more distant metastases and aggressive tumour types. These children have a more grave prognosis than older children and adolescents.

30.6.2 Gender

The question of whether gender has importance for the prognosis is controversial. Several studies have, however, reported that men often have a more advanced tumour than women at diagnosis.

30.6.3 Lymph Node Metastases

Lymph node metastases often occur in papillary thyroid cancer. In certain studies, metastases in the lymph nodes have been demonstrated in 65% of cases and in studies in which the lymph nodes have been examined in detail, even higher numbers have been reported (Fig. 30.2). These nodes are often localized in the neck in the proximity of the thyroid. The prognostic significance of the occurrence of lymph node metastases has been the subject of discussion for many years. The most common viewpoint is that lymph node metastases are associated with a higher risk of recurrence and cancer-related mortality.

Medullary thyroid cancer patients often have lymph node metastases, a finding that is associated with a distinctly poorer prognosis. Also, follicular thyroid cancer may

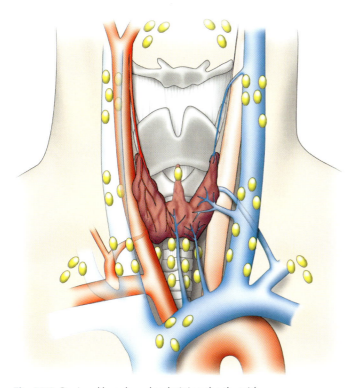

Fig. 30.2 Regional lymph nodes draining the thyroid

disseminate the lymphatic vessels giving rise to metastases, both locally and distally. Follicular cancers are, however, more prone to give distal metastasis. Follicular cancer of a widely invasive type, which involves not only the tumour capsule but also blood vessels, thus give rise to blood-borne distant metastases.

30.7 Prognostic Classification System

There are several different prognostic classification systems for grading thyroid cancers. In recent years, guidelines in both Europe and the USA recommend the tumour–nodes–metastasis (TNM) classification system compiled by the American Joint Committee on Cancer (see below). This classification system was last updated and revised in 2002.

For medullary thyroid cancer, the size of the primary tumour is important, as is the occurrence of lymph node and distant metastases. For classification in prognostic risk groups for papillary and follicular cancer, whether the patient's age is above or below 45 years is considered to be the most important factor. The classification characterizes the tumour in accordance with four prognosis stages (I–IV). Stage I indicates the best and Stage IV indicates the worst prognosis.

TNM Classification

T Primary tumour
- Tx= Primary tumour can not be assessed
- T0 = No evidence of primary tumour
- T1 = ≤2 cm
  In supplement to the 6th edition:
  T1a= ≤1 cm
  T1b =>1 cm ≤2 cm
- T2 = >2 cm ≤4 cm limited to the thyroid
- T3 = >4 cm and limited to the thyroid or any tumour with minimal extrathyroidal extension
- T4 = Tumour of any size extending in various degrees (a–b) beyond the thyroid capsule, invading surrounding tissue

N Regional lymph node metastases
- Nx= Regional lymph nodes can not be assessed
- N0 = No metastases in at least 6 examined lymph nodes
- N1 =Regional lymph node metastases
  – N1a = Lymph node metastases in pretracheal nodes
  – N1b= Lymph node metastases in jugular or mediastinal lymph nodes

M Distant metastases
- Mx = Distant metastasis can not be assessed
- M0 = No distant metastasis
- M1 = Distant metastasis

Prognostic Stage in Accordance with TNM
- Papillary and follicular thyroid cancer
  (a) Patients <45 years
  Stage I: All T, All N, M0
  Stage II: All T, All N, M1
  (b) Patients ≥45 years
  Stage I: T1, N0, M0
  Stage II: T2, N0, M0
  Stage III: T3, N0, M0
             T1–3, N1a, M0
  Stage IV: T4 or N1b or M1

- Medullary thyroid cancer
  Stage I: T1, N0, M0
  Stage II: T2–4, N0, M0
  Stage III: All T, N1, M0
  Stage IV: All T, All N, M1

- Anaplastic thyroid cancer
  Always designated as Stage IV

30.8 Treatment

Treatment of thyroid cancer usually involves surgery as the primary treatment. In certain cases of papillary and follicular cancer with a high risk for relapse, adjuvant treatment with radioiodine should be given. For other patient groups (in more favourable prognostic stages), surgery is the only form of treatment.

30.8.1 Surgical Treatment

Surgical treatment of palpable thyroid cancer involves total thyroidectomy (Fig. 30.3). The purpose of the operation is to remove all thyroid tissue. Often, complete removal of lymph nodes of the nearest lymph node stations that drain the thyroid is also recommended. The pretracheal lymph nodes are excised in front of the trachea down towards the upper thymus horn. In certain cases the lymph nodes laterally along the jugular vein and the carotid artery are also removed.

In differentiated (papillary, follicular) cancer limited to one thyroid lobe and with a favourable prognostic histology, some surgeons advocate hemithyroidectomy as sufficient surgical intervention. There is a lack of studies that convincingly demonstrate that total thyroidectomy is superior to the more limited lobectomy in these cases.

Advocates of routine total thyroidectomy claim that surgery eliminates the problem of multiple microscopic tumour sites in addition to one dominant site, which normally occurs in the thyroid. In some studies, total thyroidectomy results in a lower risk for tumour recurrence and improved survival rates. Perhaps the greatest advantage, however, is that by removing the entire thyroid (together with lymph node metastases, if necessary) all thyroglobulin producing tissue is removed. Biochemical analysis of thyroglobulin in blood can thereby later be used as a sensitive marker at follow-up for detecting recurrence. In addition, radioiodine treatment of distant metastases is facilitated if there is no significant accumulation of isotope in residual thyroid tissue.

If the operation is performed by an experienced surgeon, the risk of complication is small after total thyroidectomy (i.e. vocal cord paresis due to injury of the recurrent laryngeal nerve and hypoparathyroidism).

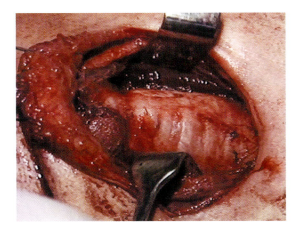

Fig. 30.3 Surgical view after total thyroidectomy

30.8.2 Treatment with I-131

Radioiodine treatment can be given both as an adjuvant treatment in addition to the primary thyroidectomy and as treatment of metastasing disease. Treatment of distant metastases with I-131 can provide palliation of painful skeletal metastases and cure or inhibit growth of lung metastases. Imaging is performed using a gamma camera after administration of isotope.

The purpose of adjuvant radioiodine therapy is:
- To ablate thyroid remnants to facilitate follow-up using thyroglobulin analysis
- To reduce the risk of relapse by ablating microscopic sites of tumour
- To detect and treat metastases

30.8.2.1 Iodine Uptake

Iodine is taken up at the basal membrane of the thyrocytes using the iodide pump (NIS), transported to the apical membrane and bound to thyroglobulin, which is stored in the follicle (see Chap. 2). Highly differentiated thyroid cancers can take up radioiodine using the same mechanism. Eventually, tumour cells may lose the ability to concentrate iodine.

In cancer tissue, the various stages of iodination are often less effective than in normal thyroid tissue due to:
- Down regulation of NIS protein
- Inactive NIS due to internalization
- Dedifferentiation – with fewer functionally developed follicles

The effect of the administered radioactivity can therefore be 10–100 times lower than at radioiodine treatment of normal thyroid tissue. The best possibility of achieving the desired effect by radioiodine treatment is if the treatment can be given early in the course of the disease, i.e. before the cells dedifferentiate further.

30.8.2.2 Importance of TSH in I-131 Treatment

TSH stimulates the uptake of iodide by the thyroid cells (including thyroid cancer cells) by increasing the genetic expression and function of NIS. TSH stimulation of the cells should be high in order to achieve a high uptake of radioactive iodide into the cell and follicle.

Elevated TSH values prior to radioiodine treatment can be achieved in two ways:
- Withdrawal of thyroxine substitution for a period of time, whereupon the patient develops endogenous hypothyroidism with high TSH. Often, this is achieved by treating the patient with triiodothyronine instead of thyroxine for at least 4 weeks. Next, the patient does not take any thyroid hormone at all for 2 weeks before isotope investigation or treatment. This results in a period with pronounced hypothyroidism, which may be very strainful, particularly for elderly and weak patients.
- The patient is given human recombinant TSH as an injection. This results in high concentrations of TSH with an increase in iodine uptake, even though the patients receive their normal thyroxine dose. Thus the patient does not need to undergo a period with hypothyroidism in order to achieve elevated TSH.

30.8.2.3 Significance of Low Iodine Intake

The tumour cells should be emptied of excess iodine prior to treatment in order to optimize radioiodine uptake. This means that the patient must avoid iodine-containing contrast media about 3 months before therapy. The patient must also follow a diet low in iodine 1–2 weeks before treatment.

30.8.2.4 Administered Radioiodine Activity

A relatively high amount of radioactivity is given (2,000–8,000 MBq), compared to treatment of hyperthyroidism (100–600 MBq), in order to achieve satisfactorily high radiation of the tumour cells. In adjuvant treatment, the aim is to give about 300 Gy to the remaining thyroid tissue. In the treatment of metastases, the aim is to give an absorbed dose as high as possible to the tumour, at least 80 Gy, in order to have an effect on the tumour.

In practice, the patient drinks or swallows a capsule with an aqueous solution of I-131. Because of the high radioactivity, the patient then has to stay in a radiation shielded room for a few days until the radioactivity tapers. Investigation with a gamma camera is performed after 3–5 days. In connection with the treatment, the patient is given lemon juice to stimulate emptying of the salivary glands and thus prevent accumulation of activity there. Reduced saliva production is a known long-term side effect in thyroid cancer patients who undergo repeated radioiodine therapies.

It is becoming more and more accepted to give radioiodine treatment without prior diagnostic radioiodine investigation for two reasons. Firstly, it has been found that a test dose of 50–100 MBq affects the uptake of subsequent therapeutic radioactivity (3,000–4,000 MBq), which means that the absorbed dose to the thyroid cancer cells is lower than anticipated, so-called stunning. Secondly, it has been shown that even a test radioactivity dose of 75–100 MBq is not always enough to detect tumour tissue.

Adjuvant treatment using up to 4,000 MBq has not been shown to have any undesired effect on a subsequent pregnancy and the treatment does not preclude later pregnancy. It is known however that sperm production is poorer for a short length of time after treatment probably due to temporary hypothyroidism. It is recommended to wait about 6 months after radioiodine treatment before pregnancy.

30.8.2.5 Radioiodine Treatment After Surgery

Even though treatment with I-131 is given postoperatively throughout the world as part of the primary treatment, a randomized prospective study has never been conducted to prove the efficacy of such treatment. In retrospective studies it has, however, been shown that the recurrence frequency is lower in patients with thyroid cancer in prognostic unfavourable stages who received ablative treatment with radioactive iodine. The possibility to follow the patient with thyroglobulin also increases when all normal thyroid tissue has been ablated.

Treatment principles vary between centres. Some centres routinely give radioiodine treatment as an adjuvant to surgery in thyroid cancer while other centres have a more conservative attitude. The European and American Thyroid Associations (ETA and ATA) have compiled treatment recommendations proposing that patients who are assessed to be in a favourable prognostic risk group do not routinely need radioiodine treatment. According to European consensus recommendations radioiodine should be offered to patients in low and high risk groups.

The risk group classifications according to the European Consensus Statement from 2006 are:
- *Extreme low risk*   Unifocal T1a (≤ 1 cm) N0M0 without growth through the thyroid capsule
- *Low risk*   T1b (> 1cm) N0M0 or T2 N0M0 or multifocal T1N0M0
- *High risk*   T3, T4 or N1 or M1

30.9 Follow-Up

Follow-up after surgery includes medical history, palpation of the neck and lymph node stations, biochemical assessment and ultrasound, if required.

30.9.1 Biochemical Assessment

As part of the follow-up of patients treated for thyroid cancer, determination of tumour markers for the various types of cancer is of great importance. For follicular and papillary thyroid cancer, determination of concentrations of serum thyroglobulin is the most important. Thyroglobulin analysis is more sensitive at TSH stimulation. Analysis of thyroglobulin antibodies should be carried out, since these antibodies affect the thyroglobulin analysis. Occasionally, the analysis of thyroglobulin antibodies per se has been shown to be useful at follow-up (falling TgAb concentrations may reflect absence of tumour tissue).

Calcitonin is a sensitive tumour marker for medullary thyroid cancer. Carcinoembryonic antigen (CEA) is also occasionally used. Using these analyses, it is possible to demonstrate recurrence or metastases at an early stage.

In a patient who has undergone total thyroidectomy and perhaps radioiodine treatment for papillary or follicular thyroid cancer and does not have any known metastases, it would be expected that the thyroglobulin value lies at or below the lower detection limit for the biochemical analysis. If values are elevated or increasing, metastases should be suspected and investigations initiated.

30.9.2 Ultrasound

The most common site of recurrence, primarily from papillary thyroid cancer, is lymph node metastases in the neck. Ultrasound investigations are increasingly used in the follow-up of these patients (Fig. 30.4).

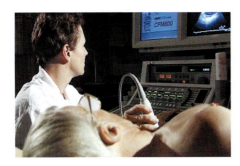

Fig. 30.4 Follow-up by ultrasound investigation

30.9.3 PET

PET is a new technique with promising results in difficult cases with persistent thyroglobulin secretion with no otherwise visible tumour. Often, PET is run in conjunction with CT. Positive PET scans are seen specifically in low differentiated tumour tissue, with low or no uptake of iodine.

30.9.4 TSH Suppression with Thyroxine

Thyroid cancer is in many cases an extremely slow-growing tumour. The risk of recurrence decreases gradually but can persist for many years, and tumours can recur up to 15–20 years after the primary operation. Patients who have undergone surgery for thyroid cancer are therefore followed-up regularly for many years.

It has been proposed that elevated TSH can stimulate any remaining thyroid cancer cells to grow and contributes to development of metastases. Patients who have been operated for differentiated thyroid cancer (papillary and follicular) should be given thyroxine in a dose that results in TSH suppression to levels <0.1 mIU/L. Personalized treatment based on individual prognosis factors should be managed by a specialist. The thyroxine dose should however not be so high that the patient experiences side effects such as cardiac problems. In cases with low risk, the thyroxine dose may be reduced gradually and TSH allowed to reach the lower normal reference range. Free T4 should lie around the upper normal limit. A decision to lower TSH suppressive thyroxine substitution should always be discussed with a physician with special experience in the field.

Chapter 30: Thyroid Cancer

Thyroid Cancer

- A solitary lump in the neck is the most common onset symptom
- The most commonly occurring tumour forms have the best prognosis
- High age at diagnosis is an important negative prognostic parameter
- For the majority of patients affected by thyroid cancer, the prognosis for long-term survival is good (90–95%)
- Risk factors for developing thyroid cancer include exposure to radiation and certain hereditary factors
- Surgery combined with radioiodine treatment constitute the cornerstones of treatment
- Lifelong thyroxine treatment with careful observation of TSH concentrations and follow-up with determination of biochemical tumour markers is recommended
- Discussions regarding what level of TSH the thyroxine administration should be aimed at in different categories of thyroid cancer patients are ongoing

31 The Thyroid and Pregnancy

31.1 Maternal Physiology During Pregnancy

Pregnancy results in physiological changes that affect thyroid function. The management of thyroid disease in a pregnant woman sets particular challenges because diagnosis, treatment and follow-up can vary from that for a nonpregnant patient. It is very important that these patients are cared for correctly right from the start of pregnancy, because the development of the foetus may otherwise be negatively affected. This applies not least to the central nervous system.

During pregnancy, there is an immunosuppression with a reduction of helper T cells (CD4) and an increase in the number of suppressor T cells (CD8). These changes relate to the lowered rejection tendency following the course of pregnancy. At the same time, lowered activity is noted in immune-mediated diseases such as rheumatoid arthritis, myasthenia gravis and thyroid diseases such as Graves' disease. Autoimmune diseases often arise after parturition or existing conditions can be reactivated with a transient or long-term period of increased disease activity following pregnancy.

During pregnancy there is a hormonal interaction between the mother, the placenta and the foetus. Beginning early in pregnancy, the concentration of chorionic gonadotropin (hCG) in serum rises (Figs. 31.1, 31.2). The hormone hCG is a placental glycoprotein with a weak TSH receptor-stimulating capability. Additional physiological changes during pregnancy include a gradual increase in the blood volume of the mother by 40%, which results in lowered plasma albumin concentrations, and an increase in cardiac output. Renal blood flow and GFR increase by up to 50%.

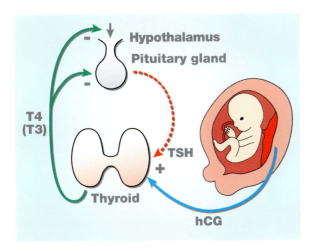

Fig. 31.1 Hormonal interactions between the mother, the placenta and the foetus

E. Nyström, G.E.B. Berg, S.K.G. Jansson, O. Törring, S.V. Valdemarsson (Eds.),
Thyroid Disease in Adults,
DOI: 10.1007/978-3-642-13262-9_31, © Springer-Verlag Berlin Heidelberg 2011

Chapter 31: The Thyroid and Pregnancy

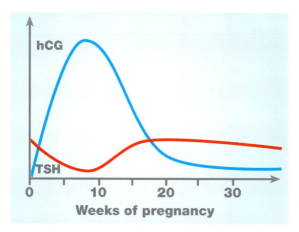

Fig. 31.2 The concentration of hCG rises early in pregnancy

A physiological, reversible increase of thyroid size is often seen during pregnancy. There are several causes for these changes. An increased renal clearance of iodide and increased supply of iodine to the foetus result in a lowered maternal iodine reserve. To compensate for this, there is an increased uptake of iodine into the thyroid of the mother. According to WHO, the daily total intake of iodine for pregnant women should be 175–200 µg/day to meet these demands. In iodine deficiency, the thyroid increases more in size. In countries such as Iceland, USA and Sweden, where iodine supplementation is adequate, only a limited (5–10%) increase in thyroid size is observed during pregnancy. In countries with low iodine intake, the thyroid volume can increase by up to 30%. It is therefore probable that a relative iodine deficiency can contribute to the occurrence of goitre during pregnancy.

Another factor contributing to the occurrence of goitre during the early stages of pregnancy may be the increased hCG level that stimulates growth. Indirect evidence that hCG exerts stimulating effects on the TSH receptor, and thus the thyroid, is provided by the small decrease (within the normal range) of TSH in serum that occurs during the first trimester (Fig. 31.2). Furthermore, there is a positive correlation between free T4 and hCG levels.

31.2 TSH, T4 and T3 During Pregnancy

The concentrations of total T4 and T3 increase due to an increased TBG concentration, which is a consequence of increased hepatic synthesis of TBG caused by raised oestrogen levels. This can be observed as early as a few months into pregnancy (Fig. 31.3). The highest TBG concentration is attained in weeks 20–24, and this elevation persists until a few weeks before parturition. Because of these changes, total T4 and total T3 rises from weeks 6–9 and reach an average of around 150–160 nmol/L (total T4) or 3.6 nmol/L (total T3) around gestational week 18.

However, during the second and third trimester, the concentrations of free T4 and free T3 drop continuously, by up to 20–30% for free T4 (Fig. 31.4). The outcome of

31.2 TSH, T4 and T3 During Pregnancy

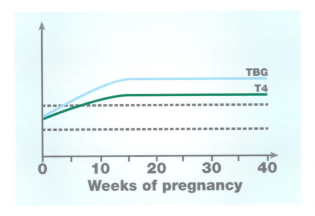

Fig. 31.3 Variation of TBG and total T4. The *dashed area* denotes reference ranges for nonpregnant women

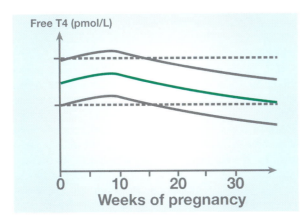

Fig. 31.4 Variation of free T4 during pregnancy (mean value ±2SD). The *dashed area* denotes reference ranges for nonpregnant women

analysis of free thyroid hormones during pregnancy seems to be dependent on the method applied. Free T4 values immediately below or in the lower part of the normal reference range without an increase in TSH are therefore normal findings.

The changes in free thyroid hormone levels noted for pregnant women are probably due, in the majority of cases, to interference in the biochemical analysis by the increased concentrations of thyroid hormone binding protein (TBG). The guidelines for laboratory values presented above are approximate. Preferably, the laboratory should be able to give information on the reference ranges for thyroid-associated hormone analyses for the three trimesters separately, since the divergences from nonpregnancy will change along the progress of pregnancy. The reference range should be determined using the methods of the laboratory on a representative regional population. Unfortunately, this information is so far lacking at many institutions.

Most often, TSH is found to lie within the reference range throughout the entire pregnancy. A reduction may be seen in the first trimester (hCG-dependent). In normal pregnancies, a decreased TSH is thus seen in 10% of first trimester pregnancies, in in 5 % of second and in 1 % of third trimester pregnancies.

> **Immunological/Physiological Changes During Pregnancy Result In:**
>
> - Lowered TSH, related to high hCG concentrations, during the first trimester
> - Elevated serum concentrations of total T4 and total T3 due to an increase in thyroid hormone binding protein, TBG
> - Modification of the immune system during pregnancy and with an increased risk for developing autoimmune thyroid diseases during the postpartum period

31.3 Maternal/Placental Interaction

T4 can to some extent cross the placenta. This mechanism is particularly important during the period when the foetal thyroid itself is not capable of synthesizing T4 and T3. In addition, the placenta contains a deiodinase (D3), which catalyses the conversion of T4 to rT3, and also of T3 to T2. This deiodinase thus protects the foetus against excessively high thyroid hormone concentrations.

TSH does not cross the placenta. Iodide crosses the placenta freely, and concentrates in the foetal thyroid from week 10. Large excessive intake of iodine by the mother can transfer to and block the foetal immature thyroid and cause hypothyroidism and goitre in the foetus.

TSH receptor antibodies (TRAb) belong to the IgG class. They cross the placenta to a limited extent and have a relatively short half-life. If TRAb levels are detectable in maternal circulation, there is a risk that the antibody will cross the placenta in the second half of pregnancy. Transplacental passage of TSH receptor-stimulating or blocking antibodies can thereby cause thyroid function disorders in the later foetal stages, or more commonly, for one or a few months after delivery. If the mother has Graves' disease, stimulating TRAb will be present. Signs of thyrotoxicosis may then be observed in the foetus, or the newborn child. In the extremely rare case that the mother has hypothyroidism due to blocking TRAb, there may instead be signs of hypothyroidism intrauterinely or in the newborn child. If a suppressed maternal TSH is detected during the second and third trimester of pregnancy in a female with known thyroid disease, determination of TRAb should be performed to exclude or confirm underlying Graves' disease.

31.4 Thyroid Function in Mother and Foetus

The foetus is able to synthesize TRH and TSH from week 10 of pregnancy. The foetal thyroid is also formed around week 10. From about gestational week 16 (i.e. 14 weeks of pregnancy) it synthesizes increasing amounts of thyroid hormone and from week 19 in more adequate extent. The interaction between the pituitary and thyroid is, however, not considered to be mature before the middle of pregnancy. Foetal conversion of T4 to T3 becomes active from about week 30.

As is apparent from Fig. 31.5, several important structures of the CNS are already formed during the first trimester. These include structures related to intellectual and cognitive abilities, and require an adequate concentration of thyroid hormone for normal development. The CNS continues to develop including myelinization and continued formation of the hippocampus, not least in the first year after birth, and this development is also dependent on thyroid hormone.

Thus the mother, the foetus and the newborn child are all dependent on a sufficient iodine supply for the production of thyroid hormone. After birth, the child receives iodine in breast milk. There are, however, still countries with pronounced iodine deficiency, where each year many children are born with neurological developmental retardation due to iodine deficiency in the mother and the newborn child (Fig. 31.6). Particularly badly affected are children born to mothers who do not have a high enough iodine intake during the first trimester. Concomitant deficiency of iodine and selenium further exacerbate the condition. The mother should therefore already have adequate iodine intake at conception.

It is important that the newborn child also has adequate iodine intake. It should be noted that the concentration of iodine in breast milk is affected in mothers who smoke. Tobacco smoke contains thiocyanate, which inhibits uptake of iodine in the mammary glands, where the NIS pump is expressed during lactation. This decreases the iodine content of breast milk. It is therefore very important to stop smoking when breastfeeding. If not, the mother must receive additional iodine, for example in a multivitamin preparation containing 150 μg iodine.

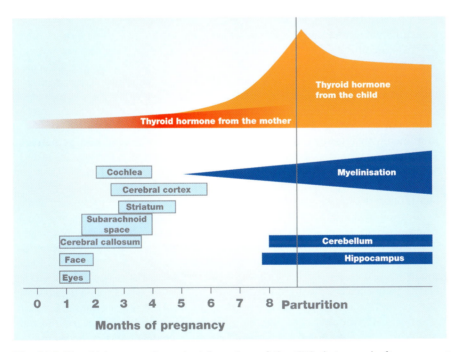

Fig. 31.5 Thyroid hormone-dependent formation of the CNS during and after pregnancy (schematic representation modified from Morreale de Escobar G, Obrego MJ and Escobar del Rey F (2004) Eur J Endocrinol 151:U25–37)

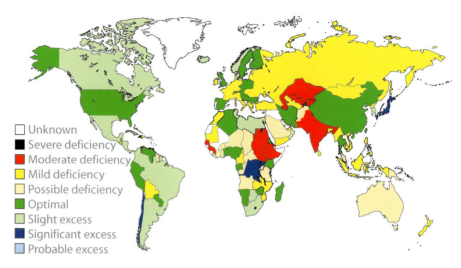

Fig. 31.6 Global iodine availability (natural availability and iodine consumed as food additives)

31.5 The Thyroid and Fertility

Thyroid function is important for female fertility. Among the 10–15% of fertile women who wish to become pregnant but are unsuccessful after 1 year, it is more common that TSH is high but within the normal range, or elevated in combination with detectable TPOAb. Therefore, thyroid function should be checked, including determination of TPOAb, in infertility investigations. TPOAb are more frequently present in women who have had repeated spontaneous abortions, and thyroid function should also be checked in this patient group.

In women with fertility problems, thyroxine is given on wider indications than normal. Thus, thyroxine should be initiated if the TSH concentration is above 2.5 mIU/L. Presence of TPOAb strengthens the indication. Furthermore, detectable TPOAb and TSH >3.5 mIU/L entails an increased risk for prematurity.

Substitution is recommended to be initiated cautiously with 25 µg thyroxine/day. Depending on the initial level of TSH, the dose is then increased by 25 µg. The goal is to achieve a TSH value of 0.4–2.0 mIU/L. It is also important that this patient category has adequate iodine intake. In many European countries today, an iodine supplement of 150 µg is recommended for women who are pregnant or who are planning to get pregnant.

Fertility is normal or only slightly reduced in moderately hyperthyroid females. The risk of miscarriage and foetal injury is, however, increased. It is important to be aware that women of reproductive age with either hypo- or hyperthyroidism may become pregnant in spite of abnormal hormone levels and symptoms of disease. Women of reproductive age with thyroid dysfunction must therefore always be informed of the importance of using contraceptives until their thyroid function is stabilised/cured or adequate substitution secured.

31.6 Hypothyroidism and Pregnancy

Studies have demonstrated the presence of TPOAb in 10–20% of women of reproductive age and elevated TSH in around 2%. These are divergences that comprise a risk factor for abnormalities in the foetus. Mild hypothyroidism may also progress to more pronounced hypothyroidism at the beginning or later in pregnancy.

31.6.1 Women with Previously Undiagnosed Hypothyroidism

It is important that thyroid hormone levels are normal already at the start of pregnancy and remain so until delivery. There is currently no general consensus for screening for hypothyroidism of all women before or during pregnancy. It is, however, generally accepted that TSH must always be checked promptly when pregnancy is confirmed in women who may have an increased risk for autoimmune thyroiditis or hypothyroidism. Included here are women who themselves have, or have a familiar predisposition for autoimmune thyroiditis, or have other manifestations of autoimmune disease such as insulin-dependent diabetes, atrophic gastritis and coeliac disease.

There is agreement that the reference range for TSH in pregnant women is lower than for nonpregnant. This applies primarily to the first trimester, in which the upper reference limit for TSH is 2.5 mIU/L. A slightly higher value may be acceptable later in pregnancy.

If TSH >2.5 mIU/L is found and confirmed at follow-up of TSH during the first trimester, thyroxine substitution should be initiated. The occurrence of TPOAb strengthens the indication. Dosage is individual and dependent on the TSH level. Normal dosage can be 25–50 µg thyroxine daily at TSH levels 2.5–10 mIU/L, 50–100 µg daily at TSH levels 10–20 mIU/L and 100 µg or more at TSH levels >20 mIU/L. The thyroxine dose is adjusted so that TSH lies between 0.4 and 2.0 mIU/L.

Substitution with thyroxine is given at a dose that is estimated to be equivalent to the total anticipated daily requirement right from the start, without increments.

In certain cases, more pronounced hypothyroidism may be diagnosed in a woman who is already pregnant, either because a previously unknown hypothyroidism is detected or because substitution with thyroxine is unintentionally interrupted, or is affected by medicines that affect resorption of thyroxine. In these cases of pronounced hypothyroidism, a specialist should be consulted. Treatment with thyroxine at a dose expected for that stage of pregnancy is initiated/reinitiated without delay and without gradual increments. Follow-up of TSH and free T4 is performed as early as 2 weeks later, and thereafter regularly until TSH attains the target values of 0.4–2.0 mIU/L.

> **Hypothyroidism and Pregnancy**
>
> *Previously Unknown Hypothyroidism*
>
> - At TSH levels 2.5–10 mIU/L: Repeated analysis supplemented with TPOAb
>   If TSH levels ≥2.5 mIU/L: Thyroxine in individualized dosage Recommended: 25–50 µg/day. Presence of TPOAb strengthens treatment indication
> - Pronounced rise in TSH (>10 mIU/L): Repeated analysis supplemented with TPOAb. Treatment with thyroxine started immediately. Individualized dosage recommended.
>   TSH 10–20 mIU/L: 50–100 µg/day
>   TSH >20 mIU/L: 100 µg/day
>   Contact with specialist in thyroid disease with regard to therapy/follow-up
> - Target value after initiation of thyroxine: TSH 0.4–2.0 mIU/L
> - Consider contact with obstetrics and gynecology

31.6.2 Women Already Receiving Thyroxine Substitution

Around 1–2% of pregnant women receive substitution with thyroxine because of a previously known thyroid disease. In these women, who are already on thyroxine substitution, it is almost always necessary to increase the dose to compile with the increased thyroid hormone requirements during pregnancy. This applies in particular to women who are totally without thyroid function, for example after long-term primary hypothyroidism or ablative treatment with surgery or radioiodine.

On average, women with primary hypothyroidism need to increase their daily thyroxine dose by 25 µg. Ablatively treated patients may require an increase of up to 50 µg. In these patient groups, the thyroxine dose needs to be raised as early as week 5 of pregnancy. Women being treated for infertility with assisted conception (and in connection with this, oestrogen administration) constitute a special case. At conception, they should immediately increase their thyroxine dose because the administered oestrogen has already stimulated a TBG increase with increased binding of thyroid hormone. The thyroxine dose must be adjusted so that the TSH level is 0.4–2.0 mIU/L.

Because a pregnant woman may need to increase her thyroxine dose at a very early stage of pregnancy, all thyroxine-treated women of reproductive age must be informed as soon as a pregnancy is confirmed, that they must continue thyroxine substitution and have their thyroid hormone concentration checked as soon as possible. Subsequently, function tests must be checked every 4–6 weeks and the dose adjusted as indicated above. Under no circumstances should thyroxine treatment be discontinued. Note that concomitant treatment with iron supplementation (and multivitamin tablets containing iron), calcium preparations and fibre-rich food will affect resorption of thyroxine, and therefore the patient should take the thyroxine dose 4–6 h before or after these preparations and fibre-rich food (see Chap. 12).

In most cases, thyroxine-treated women who become pregnant can be cared for within the primary health care services and contact a thyroid disease specialist if necessary.

> *Previously Known Disease with Thyroxine Substitution*
>
> - Check of TSH and free T4 as soon as pregnancy is confirmed and subsequently every 4–6 weeks. TSH target 0.4–2.0 mIU/L
> - The woman should be instructed to increase her intake of thyroxine (25–50 µg) if she can not contact her doctor as soon as her pregnancy is confirmed
> - If TSH is elevated (>2.0 mIU/L), the dose is further increased, often by about 30% (25–50 µg)
> - Thyroxine treatment must not be discontinued for any reason
> - Most cases managed by primary health care services
> - The woman can resume her regular dose of thyroxine after delivery

31.7 Hyperthyroidism and Pregnancy

The incidence of hyperthyroidism among pregnant women is about 0.1% and most patients have the disease at the time of conception. As pointed out above, hyperthyroidism does not necessarily affect fertility unless the condition is severe. The risk of malformation is increased in hyperthyroidism. For most women of reproductive age, hyperthyroidism is caused by Graves' disease, and rarely by toxic nodular goitre or adenoma. The possibility that a pregnant woman can develop subacute thyroiditis or, in rare cases, a trophoblastic tumour that causes hyperthyroidism via hCG, should not be disregarded.

One particular transient form of a hyperthyroid-like condition, gestational hyperthyroidism, is occasionally seen as a solitary phenomenon, but has been seen in 2/3 of patients with hyperemesis gravidarum. This condition can most probably be ascribed to a pronounced increase in hCG production causing an enforced stimulation of the TSH receptor.

The clinical diagnosis of thyrotoxicosis during pregnancy is often difficult because symptoms such as tachycardia, palpitations, sensations of heat, and moist warm skin are often seen in healthy pregnant women. Tachycardia, weight loss or lack of weight gain in spite of a good appetite, can be signs of thyrotoxicosis as are nail changes (onycholysis). The occurrence of eye symptoms (TAO), which can often be mild, as well as goitre, skin changes and proximal muscle weakness indicate Graves' disease. Cardiac symptoms can be severe with arrhythmia and cardiac failure in seriously affected women.

The diagnosis is confirmed by elevated free T4 and suppressed TSH. Normal TSH excludes thyrotoxicosis with few exceptions. Note that total T3 and T4 are slightly elevated in the thyroid of a pregnant healthy woman due to the oestrogen-induced TBG increase. The presence of TRAb in blood tests confirms the diagnosis Graves' disease.

Administration of radioactive isotopes for investigation or treatment is contraindicated in pregnancy.

31.7.1 Treatment of Hyperthyroidism

Treatment is essential to prevent maternal, foetal and neonatal complications. Treatment and follow-up of the patient should be managed by a physician with appropriate experience in thyroid disease.

Complications of thyrotoxicosis in pregnancy are normally only seen in poorly managed patients. In the mother, complications include hypertension and pre-eclampsia, cardiac insufficiency, miscarriages, premature birth, premature ablation of the placenta and thyrotoxic crisis (thyroid storm). For the foetus, there is the risk of intrauterine growth retardation, prematurity and neonatal death, as well as thyrotoxicosis in exceptional cases. It is important to underline that if the disease is well-controlled, there is a high probability that the pregnancy will progress uneventfully.

31.7.1.1 Medical Treatment

Patients are treated with propylthiouracil as monotherapy without concomitant thyroxine treatment. Combination treatment with antithyroid drugs and thyroxine should be avoided as this involves unnecessary high doses of antithyroid drugs. In addition, T4 does not cross the placenta in sufficient quantities to substitute for decreased thyroid function in the foetus induced by transplacental passage of high dose antithyroid drugs.

The objective of the antithyroid drug therapy is to achieve euthyroidism as quickly as possible and at the lowest possible dose, after which the mother must be maintained euthyroid. Current studies indicate that thiamazol carries higher risk of adverse effects on the foetus than propylthiouracil, and the latter drug should therefore be selected when treating the pregnant patient. Further advantages of propylthiouracil are the shorter half-life of the compound and the inhibitory effect on the peripheral conversion of T4 to T3. The initial dose is normally 150 mg per day administered over three doses.

If palpitations are problematic, beta blockers may be given during pregnancy, and doses of propranolol up to 20–40 mg four times daily may be required. Alternatively, metoprolol 25–50 mg two times daily can be given. In most cases, beta blockers can be discontinued after a few weeks. Long-term treatment with beta blockers should be avoided. Patients should initially be followed-up every 2–3 weeks, using free T4 and TSH (initially, TSH is usually not detectable). Free T4 should be kept within the upper half of the assumed reference range for pregnancy. Overtreatment with antithyroid drugs can increase the risk of thyroxine deficiency in the foetus.

Progression of Graves' disease is generally milder in pregnant than nonpregnant women. Down-regulation of the immune system activity is one contributing factor, and the lowered TRAb levels generally results in a reduction in the requirement for antithyroid drugs later during pregnancy. Therefore the dose of propylthiouracil may be relatively quickly tapered to 50 mg two times daily, and then further reduced, guided by free T4 and TSH. If the foetus displays poor growth, this can indicate inadequate control of maternal hyperthyroidism.

If the patient has been euthyroid on 50 mg propylthiouracil daily for 2–4 weeks, treatment can probably be discontinued but with medical follow-up throughout the entire pregnancy and, in particular, in the months following the delivery. The risk of recurrence after giving birth is very high.

If the patient has goitre, ophthalmopathy or a long-term medical history, treatment may need to be continued throughout the pregnancy. If the diagnosis is made after week 28, and the patient has severe symptoms, consideration should be given to initiate treatment in a hospital ward, as the risk for complications for both the mother and child is very high.

Breastfeeding Consideration should be given to the fact that after the delivery, antithyroid drugs pass into the milk (Fig. 31.7). Mostly, it is preferred to give propylthiouracil to breastfeeding women, as it is probably secreted to breast milk to a lesser extent than thiamazol although in general only minor amounts are transferred with the milk. The dose of propylthiouracil should preferably be kept as low as possible. Doses below 150–200 mg/24 h, and in special cases up to 300 mg/24 h, can be considered safe. If thiamazol is given, the dose should also be kept low (below 10–20 mg/24 h). The pediatrician should preferably be notified that the mother is breastfeeding and receiving antithyroid drugs.

31.7.1.2 Surgical Treatment

Generally, medical treatment is successful, but surgery can be an alternative that involves few risks for the mother and child. Surgery should preferably be performed in the second trimester. Surgery is relevant if the disease can not be controlled with antithyroid drugs at the doses indicated above or antithyroid drugs are not tolerated. Preoperative treatment should be antithyroid drugs at such a dose that the clinical symptoms are under control. After surgery, thyroxine substitution is given to ensure there is no transient hypothyroidism.

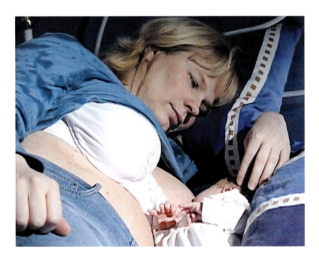

Fig. 31.7 A breastfeeding mother with thyroid disease

> **Hyperthyroidism and Pregnancy**
>
> - Previously known and newly diagnosed disease: should be managed by a specialist in thyroid disorders
> - Treated only with antithyroid drugs, not in combination with thyroxine
> - Managed by analysis of TSH and free T4. Concentration of free T4 within the upper half of the normal range
> - The dose of antithyroid drugs can normally be tapered gradually during the pregnancy and in many instances withdrawn in the second trimester
> - The patient should be given the lowest possible dose, 50–150 mg propylthiouracil per 24 h. In the event of therapeutic failure, surgery may be considered in the second trimester
> - High risk of recurrence in the postpartum period after medical treatment
> - If breastfeeding, the patient can receive antithyroid drugs (maximum dose propylthiouracil: 50 mg x 3, or in special cases up to 300 mg per 24 h)

31.8 Goitre and Palpable Lumps in the Thyroid

Second to autoimmune thyroiditis and Graves' disease, the early phase of multinodular nontoxic goitre is probably the most common cause of goitre in women of reproductive age. In areas with iodine deficiency this is a more common cause of goitre in pregnant women.

Palpable lumps in the thyroid occur somewhat more frequently in pregnant women. The frequency increases with age. In addition to unilateral nontoxic goitre, other processes should be considered including nonneoplastic conditions (cysts, inflammatory changes including autoimmune thyroiditis) and neoplasms (benign adenomas, malignant tumours).

Analysis of TSH and T4/T3 is always performed. If normal or increased TSH, TPOAb are analysed, if lowered TSH, TRAb are analysed as well.

Morphological investigation includes ultrasound, and fine-needle biopsy for cytological diagnosis. As in nonpregnant women, fine-needle biopsy for cytological diagnosis is the most important tool for solitary palpable lump in the thyroid and must always be considered at unclear findings. As pointed out earlier in this chapter, scintigraphy is contraindicated in pregnant women.

If the findings are benign, status is monitored by clinical follow-up during pregnancy. In nontoxic colloid goitre without pressure symptoms, action is rarely necessary. Thyroxine is given if TSH is increased, but not with the single aim of reducing volume. If pressure symptoms are severe, surgery can be considered.

31.9 Development of Thyroid Diseases During the Postnatal Period

If malignancy is suspected and is supported by cytology at the beginning of pregnancy, surgery can be considered in the second trimester before week 24, particularly if ultrasound reveals progress in size. In case of differentiated thyroid cancer, thyroxine is given after surgery to lower TSH levels (0.1–0.3 mIU/L), but not below the detection limits, during the remaining stages of pregnancy. If thyroid malignancy occurs later in pregnancy, surgery might be postponed until after delivery.

All cases of goitre or palpable lumps in the thyroid that are detected during pregnancy, must be followed-up after the delivery.

31.9 Development of Thyroid Diseases During the Postnatal Period

As previously presented, immunosuppression occurs during pregnancy, with an activation/reactivation of autoimmune diseases after parturition.

If a woman develops thyrotoxicosis postnatally, this could be new or recurrent Graves' disease. A very common cause of mild thyrotoxicosis after delivery is, however, postpartum thyroiditis, a condition similar to silent thyroiditis and can be considered another expression of autoimmune thyroiditis. As in silent thyroiditis, postpartum thyroiditis exhibits a biphasic progression, with an initial toxic phase followed by a hypothyroid phase.

31.9.1 Diagnosis of Thyroid Dysfunction Postnatally

In addition to routine thyroid tests, TRAb and TPOAb should also be analyzed at the first consultation. Elevated TRAb values indicates Graves' disease.

Diagnosis using radioactive iodine isotopes is contraindicated when the mother is breastfeeding. Tc-scintigraphy can be performed but in this case, the mother must not breastfeed for 24 h, and the milk during this time should be pumped and discarded.

31.9.2 Graves´ Disease

Among women of reproductive age with Graves' disease, one in two developed the disease after giving birth. In many women who had Graves' disease early in pregnancy, the disease recurs a few months after giving birth.

In contrast to postpartum thyroiditis, the toxic symptoms subsequently progress over some weeks. If the eye symptoms typical of TAO occur, the diagnosis is quite likely. The diagnosis of Graves' disease is confirmed by elevated TRAb values and treatment is started with antithyroid drugs. As previously mentioned, breastfeeding women should be treated with antithyroid drugs in accordance with the same guidelines as pregnant women with Graves' disease, i.e. monotherapy with propylthiouracil. If the patient does not breastfeed, treatment is given as for regular patients with Graves' disease.

31.9.3 Postpartum Thyroiditis and Primary Hypothyroidism

This autoimmune disease has biphasic progression (see Chaps. 10 and 26). The first toxic phase, which often only gives mild or no symptoms, occurs 2–4 months after parturition, and lasts 2–6 weeks.

The subsequent hypothyroid phase is generally slightly more pronounced. This occurs about 3–8 months after parturition and lasts 4–10 weeks, if it does not become permanent. As in silent thyroiditis, the patient with postpartum thyroiditis often presents with a slightly enlarged thyroid with ultrasound characteristics indicating thyroiditis and the same cytological picture at fine-needle biopsy (lymphocytic infiltration) and the presence of TPOAb. Occasionally, the patient does not have detectable TPOAb. Changes in thyroid function in conjunction with postpartum thyroiditis have been observed in epidemiological studies in 3–16% of women after giving birth.

Depending on the general situation of the woman in the year after giving birth, it can often be difficult to associate symptoms such as sensations of heat, palpitations, tiredness and sensations of cold with thyroid disease. Most certainly, many women go through a period with symptoms of thyroid dysfunction after giving birth without this being diagnosed. Thyroid tests should therefore be analysed on liberal indications postpartum.

If elevated concentrations of thyroid hormone and suppressed TSH are found within some months after delivery in a woman with mild thyrotoxic symptoms, the diagnosis is probably postpartum thyroiditis. The possibility that the patient can have Graves' disease must always be considered, in particular if the symptoms have been pronounced for more than 4–5 weeks.

Until the diagnosis is confirmed, the patient should be monitored with check-up of thyroid function, which will spontaneously normalize within a few weeks if postpartum thyroiditis is present. If the patient has problems with palpitations, beta blockers can be given in low doses, even if breastfeeding.

If TSH is found to be elevated in the postnatal period, and the woman has symptoms of hypothyroidism, thyroxine substitution must be given, with a recommended dose of 50–100 µg, monitored after 1–2 months. In many cases, thyroxine substitution can be tapered down after 3–6 months. In 30% of affected women hypothyroidism becomes permanent. Those who recover should be informed of the risk of recurrence during and after subsequent pregnancies.

Because the symptoms of postpartum thyroiditis are very often diffuse and difficult to recognize, screening for the disease has been discussed, but has so far not been established. One possibility is to analyse TPOAb during the later stages of pregnancy. High concentrations in late pregnancy have been shown to predict the risk of developing postpartum thyroiditis. Screening can also be performed postpartum with routine diagnostic methods.

Postpartum Thyroiditis

- Autoimmune disease; TPOAb nearly always detectable
- Affects about 1 in 20 women in the year after delivery
- Initially mild, short thyrotoxic phase that affects the patient 2–4 months after delivery
- A subsequent hypothyroid phase occurs 2–8 months after giving birth, with more pronounced symptoms
- Risk of permanent hypothyroidism or later recurrence
- The clinical symptoms during hypothyroidism can be misinterpreted because they often occur during a time of particular stress for the mother
- Thyroxine substitution on wide indications
- Graves´ disease: important differential diagnosis during the toxic phase

32 Thyroid Disease in Adolescents

32.1 Goitre

A transient diffuse enlargement of the thyroid can occur during puberty. In countries with sufficient availability of iodine, a diffuse enlargement of the thyroid can otherwise be caused by autoimmune thyroiditis. From a global perspective, iodine deficiency is the most common cause of goitre in adolescents.

Enlargement that affects only part of the thyroid should arouse suspicion of tumour.

Rarely occurring defects in enzymatic processes for synthesis of thyroid hormone or in the TSH receptor function can also cause dysfunction and/or increased size of the thyroid.

Investigation of goitre follows the same principles as in adults. Thyroid function is checked by analysis of TSH, T4 and T3. TPOAb may indicate autoimmune thyroiditis. Fine-needle biopsy for cytological diagnosis is used more rarely in children and adolescents, but is always indicated for the investigation of a palpable lump in the thyroid. A fine-needle biopsy should preferably be combined with and guided by ultrasound investigation.

If autoimmune thyroiditis is diagnosed, treatment with thyroxine should be initiated if the patient has hypothyroidism or subclinical hypothyroidism. If the patient is euthyroid, treatment should also be considered.

If a low intake of iodine is suspected/detected, it is simplest to advise a daily supplement with a common vitamin/mineral supplement with 150 µg of iodine. High doses of iodine should be avoided because they may inhibit thyroid function, especially in the immature gland. Iodine intake is discussed in detail in Chap. 6.

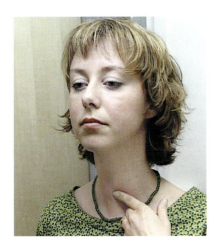

Fig. 32.1 Thyroid disease in adolescents

32.2 Autoimmune Thyroiditis and Hypothyroidism

32.2.1 Causes and Occurrence
In younger people, hypothyroidism requiring treatment is reported to occur in about 1–1.5/1,000 individuals. Hypothyroidism can be congenital, due to disturbed formation and development of the thyroid gland. Autoimmune thyroiditis is the most common cause of hypothyroidism. This disease is more uncommon in children and adolescents than in adults. The disease can be diagnosed in small children but is uncommon before puberty and increases thereafter with age. Autoimmune thyroiditis is more common in girls than boys but the gender difference is less pronounced than in adults. Furthermore, autoimmune thyroid disease is more frequent in children with Down's syndrome.

If hypothyroidism is associated with loss of hearing, Pendred's syndrome can be suspected. This is caused by a mutation in the gene for one of the proteins, pendrin, which is thought to take part in transport of iodine across the apical cell membrane in the follicle cell.

Central hypothyroidism, with low T4 and without concomitant increase in TSH, occurs in tumours and after surgery or radiation therapy of the pituitary. Isolated deficiency of TSH is rare.

32.2.2 Symptoms
Goitre is the most common symptom and results in the diagnosis of autoimmune thyroiditis. It is found in approximately two thirds of autoimmune thyroiditis cases. As in adults, goitre involves a diffusely enlarged thyroid without tenderness.

In other cases, the symptoms of hypothyroidism lead to its diagnosis. Tiredness, difficulty to keep up in school, loss of appetite, general weakness, constipation, dryness of the skin and feeling cold are common symptoms. It is important to be aware that inadequate longitudinal growth can be due to hypothyroidism.

Hypothyroidism may also lead to disturbances of pubertal development: in children it can lead to precocious puberty and in adolescents to delayed puberty.

Deficiency of thyroid hormone in newborns up until 2–3 years of age can have major negative consequences for mental and neurological development. Thyroid hormone is also important for growth and organ maturation during childhood and puberty.

32.2.3 Diagnosis
The diagnosis is commonly made by determination of TSH, thyroid hormones and TPOAb. Ultrasound investigation reveals a characteristic pattern with low echogenicity compared to normal thyroid tissue. Fine-needle biopsy for cytological diagnosis (Fig. 32.2) must always be made when the child presents with a lump.

Frequently, there is a delay before hypothyroidism is diagnosed in adolescents. It is highly important to map the function of the thyroid if there are any disturbances in growth or other development, or if goitre is present in adolescents. Particular attention must be paid if the patient has another autoimmune disease such as insulin-dependent diabetes or coeliac disease or other diseases in this group of disorders.

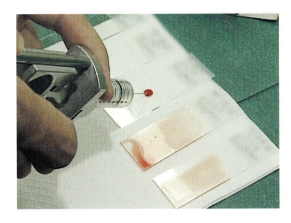
Fig. 32.2 Cytologic smear

32.2.4 Progression
Progression of autoimmune thyroiditis in adolescents is less well mapped than in adults. However, there are indications that 20–30% recover, while the remainder will develop hypothyroidism.

In 5–10% of adolescents, autoimmune thyroiditis can initially result in a release of stored hormone secondary to the inflammatory process with disruption of the follicles. In these cases, transient and sometimes relapsing thyrotoxic symptoms may occur over 1–2 months and may be followed by hypothyroidism.

32.2.5 Treatment
In hypothyroidism, patients are substituted with thyroxine, and it is assumed that the need for treatment is permanent. Dosage is managed as in adults by following TSH. It can be assumed that the goitre, which is often found in adolescents with hypothyroidism, may recede during treatment with thyroxine. Substitution should also be given in subclinical hypothyroidism. Here, however, the possibility of spontaneous remission is greater and treatment may be tapered out and re-evaluated.

Treatment with thyroxine is not generally established as a method to reduce goitre size in adolescents with TSH within the reference range. Some data indicates, however, that a reduction can be achieved in an enlarged thyroid, not only in hypothyroidism, but also in subclinical hypothyroidism and in adolescents with normal TSH, especially if TPOAb levels are elevated.

32.3 Hyperthyroidism/Thyrotoxicosis

32.3.1 Causes and Occurrence
In adolescents, Graves' disease is the most common cause of hyperthyroidism. The initial phase of autoimmune thyroiditis, as in subacute thyroiditis, can also sometimes cause thyrotoxicosis.

More uncommon etiologies include congenital or later-occurring mutations in the gene for the protein that comprises the TSH receptor. In the first case, the consequence is overactivity, which affects the entire thyroid and therefore the scintigraphy appears similar to that in Graves' disease even if TSH-receptor antibodies are absent. In the latter case, with an acquired mutation in the gene for the protein in the TSH receptor, the mutation can result in an occurrence of autonomous adenoma (Chap. 20), which is another, although uncommon, cause of hyperthyroidism in young people.

Symptoms of thyrotoxicosis can occur in genetically dependent disturbances in the receptor for triiodothyronine, known as thyroid hormone resistance (Chap. 34).

The incidence of Graves' disease has been calculated to be around 1–3/100,000 children and adolescents, but is affected by the availability of iodine in the population. As in adults, the disease is 6–8 times more common in girls than in boys. Thyroid autoimmune disease in other family members is not uncommon. The patient may also have other concomitant autoimmune diseases, such as insulin-dependent diabetes.

32.3.2 Symptoms

According to European studies, goitre is found in nearly all adolescents with Graves' disease. Other common symptoms are tachycardia, nervousness, restlessness, concentration disturbances and hypertension. Loss of appetite and weight loss have been reported in about half of the affected children and adolescents. Increased longitudinal growth can occur. Cardiac murmurs are not uncommon. In smaller children, weight loss and rapid intestinal movement is more predominant than in adolescents.

Retraction of the upper eyelid is relatively frequent and results in a staring gaze. Thyroid-associated ophthalmopathy occurs in more than half of the children and adolescents with Graves' disease. Progression is often described as milder with the possibility of remission. With increasing age, the eye disease increasingly acquires the adult characteristics.

32.3.3 Diagnosis

Diagnostic methods are the same as for adults. Because the disease is so uncommon and the symptoms so varied, it is easy to miss the diagnosis if the symptoms can be explained by other conditions. TSH in combination with T4 and/or T3 provides guidance. Detectable TRAb reveals that Graves' disease is the cause. Scintigraphy and ultrasound provide supplementary information.

32.3.4 Treatment

Treatment of Graves' disease in children and adolescents varies from region to region. In Europe, the preferred treatment at most clinics is antithyroid drugs followed by surgery. Development of Graves' disease at young age is often associated with a lower probability of persistent remission after medical treatment compared to adults. Treatment with antithyroid drugs, preferably thiamazol, is often given for a fairly long period, and in repeated periods but without achieving persistent remission. Surgery then becomes relevant, particularly if the goitre is large. The alternative is I-131 treatment, which is increasingly used in some clinics in the world, also as primary treatment.

32.4 Palpable Thyroid Lumps

The finding of a palpable lump in the thyroid in young people should always be treated as a suspicious malignancy. A concomitant thyroid lump and enlarged lymph node further underline this. In contrast to adults, multinodular colloid goitre in adolescents is unusual as a cause of solitary palpable lump in the thyroid.

Solitary lumps should always be investigated carefully. If TSH values are low, the lump may have autonomous hormone production. In these cases, scintigraphy is performed, which can demonstrate an autonomous adenoma, solitary or as part of a multinodular goitre.

If the patient is euthyroid, the first step is ultrasound investigation and fine-needle biopsy.

Determination of TPOAb should be done to determine whether autoimmune thyroiditis is the cause of the finding. In these cases, cytological investigation reveals the picture of lymphocytic thyroiditis.

If cytology reveals a follicular pattern or papillary formations, malignancy must be suspected and surgery performed for a definitive diagnosis.

Of the various forms of malignant primary tumours in the thyroid, papillary thyroid cancer is the most common in adolescents and can sometimes initially manifest as a regionally enlarged lymph node. If investigation or microscopic examination reveals medullary cancer in the thyroid the tumour can be sporadic or comprise part of a genetically dependent syndrome, multiple endocrine neoplasia type 2 (MEN 2), which must always be suspected if occurring at young age. An investigation must therefore be made with respect to genetics and any other manifestations of the syndrome. Determination of calcitonin in blood samples is used as a tumour marker in medullary thyroid cancer (see Chap. 30).

Previous external radiation treatment is a general risk factor for occurrence of malignant tumours in the thyroid. An increased incidence of thyroid cancer in children and adolescents exposed to radiation in the neighbouring areas after nuclear power plant incidents (e.g. Chernobyl) has been noted, with greater risk being associated with lower age. A concomitant iodine deficiency in the affected children is believed to be a contributing factor.

As previously mentioned, follow-up studies have not shown any increased risk of tumour development after I-131 treatment of hyperthyroidism in adults. To what extent this applies to radioiodine treatment in adolescents is still under discussion. Long term follow-up after radioiodine treatment of children and adolescents in the USA has not shown any negative effects.

Chapter 32: Thyroid Disease in Adolescents

Thyroid Disease in Adolescents

- Thyroid hormones are of extreme importance in organ development and growth
- The symptoms of both hypothyroidism and hyperthyroidism can easily be misinterpreted to have other explanations in adolescents
- Hypothyroidism can be congenital but is more often caused by autoimmune thyroiditis if presenting later in childhood
- Diffuse toxic goitre is the most common cause of thyrotoxicosis in adolescents
- Goitre in children and adolescents must always be investigated with respect to thyroid function and for the underlying cause
- Solitary lumps should generate suspicion of thyroid cancer/tumour
- Pronounced TAO is uncommon in adolescents

33 Medicines and Other Medical Preparations

33.1 General

Regulation and metabolism of thyroid hormones is dealt with in detail in Chap. 2. Some medicines can affect regulation and metabolism of thyroid hormones. Medicines such as dopamine and corticosteroids in high doses can impair TSH and thereby the release of thyroid hormones at the hypothalamic level. Conversion of T4 to T3 can be affected by compounds such as corticosteroids and propranolol, a nonselective beta blocker.

33.2 Iodine

Iodine, as discussed in several earlier chapters, has a central role in the thyroid and thyroid hormone production. Iodine may be administered to a patient in order to rapidly block the synthesis and release of hormones from the thyroid prior to surgery. When iodine is used as a disinfectant, for example in obstetrics, or for treatment of dermatological conditions, the function of the thyroid may be affected through locally absorbed iodine.

33.3 Amiodarone

Amiodarone is an antiarrhythmic drug that may induce both hypothyroidism and thyrotoxicosis. It is particularly important to be aware of amiodarone-triggered thyrotoxicosis because the condition is difficult to recognize and to treat. The condition can appear a long time (6–12 months) after amiodarone treatment has been concluded.

Amiodarone is a class III antiarrhythmic drug that primarily blocks the potassium channels in the myocytes, but also has beta-blocking properties. The substance has a structure resembling thyroid hormone and each molecule contains two iodine atoms, which is equivalent to 37% iodine by weight.

The side effects are numerous, one of which is that patients treated with amiodarone may be affected by thyroid dysfunction. The effects on the thyroid can be caused directly by the pharmacological properties of the substance, but also by a direct toxic effect on thyroid cells and the high iodine content.

33.3.1 Pharmacology

Patients with arrhythmia are normally prescribed 200 mg amiodarone daily, which is equivalent to 75 mg iodine, and liberates about 6 mg free iodine into the circulation after metabolic deiodination. This corresponds to an iodine load that is about 40 times higher than the recommended daily 150 μg intake. The half-life is very long, 20–100 days, because amiodarone is stored in the body, primarily in fat-containing tissue.

33.3.2 Pathophysiology

The pharmacological effects of the amiodarone molecule on the metabolism and function of thyroid hormone is complicated and is thought to be exerted through several mechanisms:

- Decreased deiodination of thyroid hormones T4 to T3 giving a high T4 with normal T3
- Reduced binding of T3 to nuclear receptors giving a transient TSH increase after starting amiodarone treatment
- Cytotoxicity, triggering thyroiditis
- Beta receptor blocking effects (masking some thyrotoxic symptoms)
- Pharmacological effects of high iodine exposure

> A high iodine uptake can trigger hypothyroidism, primarily in patients with underlying autoimmune thyroiditis. This probably occurs because of disturbances in the autoregulatory mechanism that controls the iodine handling of the cells. This results in persistent inhibition of oxidation and organification of iodide and hormone synthesis.
> A high iodine supply can also exacerbate thyrotoxicosis in patients with predisposing factors (subclinical Graves´ disease or autonomous thyroid function due to nodular goitre or autonomous adenoma, see Chap. 31).

33.3.3 The Prevalence of Thyroid Function Disturbances in Amiodarone Treatment

The effects on deiodination and T3 nuclear receptors described above affect thyroid hormone levels in as many as 50% of patients treated with amiodarone. Effects on the peripheral metabolism of T4/T3 do not, however, always result in a clinically significant disturbance of thyroid function. We estimate that at most 15% of amiodarone-treated patients in Sweden are affected by clinically significant alterations of thyroid hormone secretion and metabolism.

Both thyrotoxicosis and hypothyroidism thus occur frequently with amiodarone treatment. Development of hypothyroidism often occurs early in treatment, while onset of thyrotoxicosis may occur a long time after treatment is initiated and even as late as 6–12 months after discontinuation of the drug.

33.3.4 Early Effects

As presented above, many of the patients show an effect on thyroid hormone levels in the first months of treatment. TSH and T4 increases, while the levels of T3 drops. In spite of these changes, the patient is generally euthyroid. The level of TSH tends to normalize after a few months, but other changes may persist.

33.3.5 Hypothyroidism

In most cases with hypothyroidism, the patient develops the condition 6–12 months after initiation of amiodarone treatment. Patients with TPOAb run a risk of developing this condition, as do patients with elevated TSH prior to treatment. The symptoms of hypothyroidism are the same as those seen in spontaneous autoimmune hypothyroidism. Because this category of patient often suffers from tiredness and is affected by cardiac problems and other medicines, it can be very difficult to make a clinical diagnosis. The higher the TSH value the more likely the patient has symptomatic hypothyroidism. At values above 10–20 mIU/L, thyroxine treatment is indicated in most cases. If the patient has cardiac problems, thyroxine treatment should be introduced cautiously, with an initial dose of 25 μg every other day and then slowly increased.

Development of hypothyroidism does not constitute a contraindication for continued amiodarone treatment. If treatment is continued, the patient can require higher doses of thyroxine to normalize TSH than ordinary patients. If amiodarone treatment is discontinued, the treatment with thyroxine can be reassessed after 12 months.

33.3.6 Amiodarone-Induced Thyrotoxicosis

Thyrotoxicosis associated with amiodarone treatment is a problematic and sometimes difficult-to-treat condition. The patient can develop the condition several years after amiodarone treatment was initiated and up to a year or more after it finished. The association can therefore easily be overlooked.

Two different mechanisms are considered to cause thyrotoxicosis during treatment with amiodarone: type 1 and type 2.

Thyrotoxicosis type 1 is probably caused by the high iodine content of the preparation and results in iodine-triggered hyperthyroidism. This is generally seen in patients with (subclinical) Graves' disease, multinodular goitre and autonomous adenoma as predisposing factors or in patients with iodine deficiency. This type of amiodarone-induced thyrotoxicosis may be treated with high doses of antithyroid drugs and in severe cases by further adding potassium perchlorate.

Thyrotoxicosis type 2 reveals a picture similar to that of thyroiditis with hormone leakage and thereby elevated serum concentrations of thyroid hormones. Radioiodine uptake is blocked, while IL-6 and CRP can be elevated. This type of amiodarone-induced thyrotoxicosis might respond to treatment with steroids.

Types 1 and 2 present a very similar clinical picture and a hybrid form probably frequently occurs as well. Because type 1 and 2 are treated in different ways, it is desirable to be able to easily decide which type of thyrotoxicosis the patient has. In practice, determination of radioiodine uptake, IL-6 and CRP has been shown in most cases to have poor clinical significance in this respect. Ultrasound investigations with colour doppler can be of value. Blood flow is increased in type 1 and reduced in type 2.

Development is generally rapid and the patient is often diagnosed through routine checks of thyroid function, which should be performed regularly in amiodarone-treated patients. Elevated T3 and suppressed TSH is considered to provide the best basis from which to confirm amiodarone-induced thyrotoxicosis. The patient, who in many cases previously had normal values, may have recently felt more tired, lost weight and often displayed impaired arrhythmia control. Because amiodarone has beta-blocking properties, the patient is often not affected by tachycardia or tremor.

If possible, treatment with amiodarone should be discontinued. If not, it is recommended that the dose be reduced to 200 mg every third day or 100 mg every day if this is possible with regard to the arrhythmia.

33.3.7 Treatment
Treatment of drug-related thyrotoxicosis should preferably take place in consultation with thyroid specialists. Due to high iodine exposure leading to low iodine uptake, radioiodine treatment is rarely an alternative.

As pointed out above, it is unfortunately difficult in practice to distinguish between type 1 and 2, and hybrid forms are probably common. Rarely does the clinical picture support type 2 so strongly that the first step is to initiate treatment only with prednisolone. A realistic treatment regimen in overt thyrotoxicosis can therefore be to start immediately with thiamazol 20 mg + 20 mg. Supplementation with potassium perchlorate is often indicated. The recommended dose is 1 g daily (equivalent to 100 mL per day of a 1% aqueous solution). A treatment effect is seen at the earliest after 3 weeks and most often the treatment continues for 2 months. Initially, thyroid hormone concentration should be monitored every week. Because treatment with perchlorate has been reported to affect bone marrow function (it may cause severe blood dyscrasias), this should be checked every 14 days. The length of treatment should be limited to 8 weeks. In case of persistent hyperthyroidism, surgery should be considered (see below).

When T4 falls and approaches the upper limit of the reference range, treatment with potassium perchlorate should be discontinued. The patient must continue with thiamazol at lower doses until the concentration of T4 reaches the mean value of the reference range or TSH levels starts to rise.

If the concentration of free T4 does not fall after 2–4 weeks of treatment, daily 40–60 mg prednisolone doses are also initiated. In very difficult cases, it can be appropriate to start immediately with prednisolone at the same time as thiamazol/perchlorate, especially if colour doppler has not shown high thyroid tissue blood flow.

In cases where the patient is therapy resistant, it may be necessary to operate. Thyroidectomy can also be a reasonable option in those patients who, after medical therapy, have become euthyroid but who have to continue with amiodarone treatment, at least in type I cases.

Surgery for well-controlled amiodarone-induced thyrotoxicosis is normally a relatively uncomplicated procedure, but the cardiac problems of the patient and continuing thyrotoxicosis will comprise risk factors in emergency cases. Surgery should constitute total thyroidectomy to secure relief from thyrotoxicosis and make future amiodarone therapy possible. Successful intervention has also been reported with surgical treatment in very ill patients requiring intensive care.

33.3.8 Amiodarone and the Thyroid – General Aspects
A patient who starts treatment with amiodarone should, if possible, undergo thyroid investigation before starting. A low or suppressed TSH level might indicate autonomous thyroid function due to, for example, multinodular goitre or an autonomous adenoma, both typical risk factors for the development of hyperthyroidism type 1. Assessment by an endocrinologist/thyroid specialist is recommended in cases that are difficult to interpret. If a patient with autoimmune or, most importantly, uni/multi-

nodular thyroid disease with autonomous thyroid function is to be treated with amiodarone, careful consideration must be given to the increased risk of thyrotoxicosis.

If there is a strong indication for treatment with amiodarone, it is probably greatly advantageous with respect to autonomous nodules to administer a preventative treatment, such as radioiodine, before amiodarone treatment is started. Amiodarone-treated patients must be followed-up regularly with respect to thyroid function. Even a minor degree of hyperthyroidism may be beneficial to treat with regard to cardiac arrytmias.

33.4 Other Iodine-Containing Preparations

Administration of an iodine-containing contrast medium can trigger clinical/subclinical hyperthyroidism. Most iodine contrast media contain about 300 mg iodide/mL, which is equivalent to 30 µg free iodide/mL, or 7,000 µg free iodide/investigation. It can be necessary to postpone nuclear medical investigations or treatment of the thyroid with isotopes for several months after contrast administration. This indicates that untreated manifest hyperthyroidism as well as suspected thyroid cancer, in which radioiodine investigation/treatment is planned, constitute a relative contraindication for investigations with iodine contrast. Patients with autonomous thyroid function run a relatively high risk of developing hyperthyroidism after investigation with iodine contrast media.

> **Amiodarone and the Thyroid**
>
> - Thyroid function must always be investigated before treatment with amiodarone and regular follow-up is recommended
> - About half of patients demonstrate abnormal hormone concentrations (TSH, T4 and/or T3) without having hypothyroidism or thyrotoxicosis
> - Risk of iodine-induced hypothyroidism if signs of autoimmune thyroiditis
> - Risk of iodine-induced hyperthyroidism and/or thyroiditis (transient) in patients with autoimmune thyroid disease, multinodular goitre or autonomous nodule
> - Symptoms of thyrotoxicosis can be masked by the beta-receptor blocking effect of amiodarone
> - Thyrotoxicosis can develop during treatment but also up to 1 year – or even longer – after discontinuation of amiodarone
> - Substitution with thyroxine is given in confirmed hypothyroidism
> - Antithyroid drugs (at high dose) in type 1 cases
> - Potassium perchlorate in severe type 1 cases
> - Steroids are tried if thyroiditis is a reasonable cause (type 2)
> - Thyroidectomy can be a valuable option in difficult-to-treat cases
> - Radioiodine treatment is not normally applicable because of the iodine-blocking effect of amiodarone

> **Iodine Contrast Media**
>
> Care should be exercised at:
> - Manifest hyperthyroidism
> - Autonomous thyroid function/subclinical thyrotoxicosis (multinodular/uninodular goitre; Graves' disease)
>
> Avoid at:
> - Suspected thyroid cancer with planned isotope investigation/radioiodine treatment

Note that iodine contrast media is often administered routinely, for example at CT. If a previously unknown nodular enlarged thyroid is discovered at investigation with iodine contrast media, it is recommended that the patient is followed-up with testing (TSH, T4, T3) at 6 and 12 weeks after the investigation.

If iodine contrast investigation is still considered, iodine uptake by the thyroid gland can be blocked with perchlorate in selected cases.

33.5 Antithyroid Drugs

Both thiamazol and propylthiouracil affect several stages in the synthesis of thyroid hormones (see Chap. 2). Propylthiouracil also inhibits the peripheral conversion of T4 to T3. As described in Chap. 18, these preparations can give rise to various side effects, of which the most serious is neutropenia/agranulocytosis. Patients treated with thiamazol/propylthiouracil must be given written information on the risk of these adverse effects. For more harmless side effects, for example rash, it is generally possible to switch between preparations.

33.6 Lithium

Lithium can inhibit release of thyroid hormone and thus cause hypothyroidism. The mechanism has not been completely determined. An increase in the amount of iodine in the thyroid has been proposed as a possibility. Another possibility is that lithium counteracts TSH-stimulated hormone release. Treatment with lithium can result in as many as every second patient experiencing an enlarged thyroid and every fifth patient can be affected by a more or less pronounced hypothyroidism. This development is more common among patients who have TPOAb, but may also occur in other cases. Lithium has also been associated with hyperthyroidism.

> **Lithium Treatment and the Thyroid**
>
> - Free T4, TSH and TPOAb are determined when treatment is initiated
> - Individuals with TPOAb run an increased risk of developing hypothyroidism
> - Thyroid function should be followed-up regularily

33.7 Oestrogen

Oestrogen causes an increase in the concentration of the thyroid binding protein (TBG). Women with thyroxine-substituted hypothyroidism who start oestrogen therapy, may need a higher dose thyroxine to compensate for the increased thyroxine binding capacity of TBG and to keep adequate free T4/T3 concentrations. Thyroid function must therefore be monitored on several occasions during the first months after oestrogen therapy is started in women with treated hypothyroidism. This only applies to peroral therapy, because transdermal administration of oestrogen does not involve the liver or affect TBG levels. A reduction in the need of thyroxine may follow the drop in oestrogen after menopause.

33.8 Interferon

Treatment with interferon has been shown to induce TPOAb or result in an increase of previously detectable TPOAb, as well as cause a thyroiditis that is clinically similar to silent autoimmune thyroiditis. TPOAb positive patients run a greater risk. Interferon is thereby thought to be able to unmask an autoimmune thyroiditis in predisposed patients.

In other cases, treatment with interferon results in a form of thyroiditis that clinically resembles subacute thyroiditis in which TPOAb can not be detected. There are even cases with Graves' type hyperthyroidism. For differential diagnosis of these two conditions, iodine uptake test or scintigraphy can be performed, which reveal an increased uptake in hyperthyroidism but a reduced uptake in interferon-induced thyroiditis.

33.9 Carbamazepine/Fenantoin

The effects of anticonvulsant medicines on the thyroid are complex. Effects include elevated degradation of thyroid hormone, elevated conversion of T4 to T3 and reduced binding of thyroid hormone to TBG. Generally, lowered levels of free T4 and normal TSH are observed. The patient is considered to be euthyroid when the TSH concentration lies within the reference range. The effects depends on various analytical methods used.

33.10 Miscellaneous

Additional data on the effects of medicines on thyroid hormone regulation and metabolism will most certainly come to light. Even though pharmacological interactions with thyroxine are remarkably few and mild, care should always be exercised when a thyroxine-substituted patient takes new medicines. Thyroid-associated diseases such as TAO can also be affected negatively by medicines, as has been reported for preparations in the glitazone family.

Dietary elements can also have pharmacological effects. The cassava root contains thiocyanate, which blocks iodine uptake. People who eat food containing incorrectly prepared cassava root can develop goitre and hypothyroidism. Intake of large amounts of soy protein is thought to affect the thyroid in several ways. Soy contains phytooestrogens with oestrogenic effects. In addition, a component called genistein, can inhibit synthesis of thyroid hormone. Soy protein can also reduce the absorption of perorally administered thyroxine.

Data have been published confirming that tyrosine kinase inhibitors can affect thyroid function and thyroid function tests.

33.11 Medicines that Can Inhibit Thyroxine Absorption

There are a number of medicines that, to some extent, can affect the absorption of thyroxine. Particular attention should be paid to iron and calcium preparations, as well as aluminium based antacids. The most important patient group with respect to this are thyroxine-substituted pregnant women who receive iron supplements. Other medications known to reduce absorption of thyroxine are sucralfate, ion exchangers (for bile acid reflux, hyperlipidaemia), raloxifene, tamoxifen, rifampicin and ciprofloxacin. There must be an interval of at least 4 h between taking the absorption-affecting medicine and thyroxine. Fibre-rich food and bulk-forming laxatives can also affect uptake. For more details, see Chap. 13.

34 Thyroid Hormone Resistance

Thyroid hormone resistance is defined as a dominant hereditary condition in which the gene for the thyroid hormone receptor protein has mutated so that the normal binding of thyroid hormone on the T3 receptors in the cell nuclei of different organs is reduced. The condition is extremely rare, but important to be familiar with, because a missed diagnosis may result in incorrect treatment of the patient for proposed thyrotoxicosis due to high T4 and T3 concentrations.

A number of mutations have been associated to this condition. All affect the beta thyroid hormone receptor subunits and all affect amino acids that are associated with the groove in the receptor where T3 binds. The condition results in reduced binding of T3 to the receptor or inhibition of its interaction with the co-activators that participate in the complex process resulting in gene transcription and synthesis of hormones, peptides and proteins. Commonly, the transcription process is partly inhibited in thyroid hormone resistance. In those tissues/cells in which thyroid hormone normally has an inhibitory effect on the transcription process (e.g. on production of TSH), this inhibition is lowered in thyroid hormone resistance. There are no known instances of mutations in the thyroid hormone receptor alpha subunits.

Individuals with thyroid hormone resistance show elevated concentrations of thyroid hormones and normal or elevated TSH (Fig. 34.1). In most cases, there is an effect on T3 receptor sensitivity in all cells (general thyroid hormone resistance). A form with selective resistance for thyroid hormone in the pituitary has also been discussed. While patients with the general form often appear euthyroid and do not necessarily show any symptoms due to high concentrations of T4 and T3, the patient with presumed selective resistance in the pituitary shows symptoms of thyrotoxicosis, because cells in the body other than the pituitary are thought to have normal sensitivity for the high T4 and T3 levels. Because only the beta subunit of the T3 receptor has mutated and is insensitive to T3, organs whose T3 receptors are dominated by the alpha subunit (e.g. heart) can be affected by high T4 and T3 in the general form of thyroid hormone resistance. This explains why such a patient may have problems with tachycardia or atrial fibrillation without other general signs of thyrotoxicosis.

It is not rare to find that a patient with thyroid hormone resistance who has been symptom-free for many years, passes into a state with palpitations and nervousness and then becomes symptom-free once again. Similarly, people within the same family and with the same mutation can exhibit different symptoms. Thus it appears that the two variants of thyroid hormone resistance are not different diseases. The reason for the variation in phenotype over time and between individuals, even though they have the same mutation, has not been explained.

Thyroid hormone resistance may be suspected if elevated T4 and T3 (total and free) are found in a patient with normal or elevated TSH (Fig. 34.1). When investigating these cases, it must be ensured that abnormal laboratory results are not due to analytical interference.

E. Nyström, G.E.B. Berg, S.K.G. Jansson, O. Tørring, S.V. Valdemarsson (Eds.),
Thyroid Disease in Adults,
DOI: 10.1007/978-3-642-13262-9_34, © Springer-Verlag Berlin Heidelberg 2011

Chapter 34: Thyroid Hormone Resistance

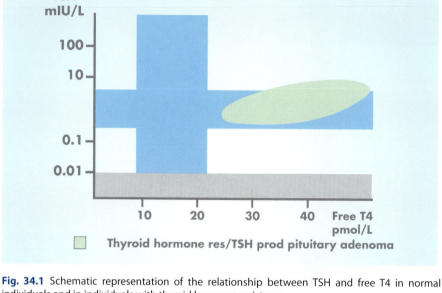

Fig. 34.1 Schematic representation of the relationship between TSH and free T4 in normal individuals and in individuals with thyroid hormone resistance

Differential diagnosis is a TSH-producing pituitary tumour. Specialist investigations for this type of pituitary tumour will normally show elevated concentrations of the TSH alpha subunit (normal concentration in thyroid hormone resistance). In these instances the pituitary is investigated using MR. An important element in investigation for thyroid hormone resistance is investigation of family members. Finding other members of the family with the same abnormal laboratory test results supports the diagnosis of thyroid hormone resistance.

If thyroid hormone resistance is suspected, the laboratory should be contacted for further investigations. Only a limited number of laboratories have facilities to identify and characterize mutations in the gene for the thyroid hormone receptor.

If thyroid hormone resistance is found in a person where this has not been previously known, the patient must always be informed of the finding. There is no specific treatment for hormone resistance. However, thyrotoxic symptoms can be treated with beta blockers or other antiarrhythmic drugs. Use of the thyroid hormone analogue TRIAC has been reported to be of value in these cases to suppress TSH. Before this unusual condition was identified, people with thyroid hormone resistance were often incorrectly treated for presumed hyperthyroidism (surgery and/or radioiodine). These patients require high substitution doses of thyroxine when the thyroid gland has been removed. They should be under the care of an endocrinologist.

Thyroid Hormone Resistance

- Elevated levels of T3 and T4, of both total and free fractions, in combination with normal or elevated TSH
- Often surprising findings in clinically euthyroid patients
- Caused by mutation of the gene for the beta receptor protein for thyroid hormone (T3)
- Many are symptom-free, others can have problems with tachycardia
- If several members of one family have the same abnormal laboratory finding, the diagnosis is likely
- Investigation (at specialist level) demonstrates mutation in the beta receptor in the region which binds T3

Index

A
acropachy, *see* Graves' disease
Addison's disease 43, 87, 120, 121, 217
adenoma XVII, 12, 181
 see also autonomous nodulus
- antithyroid drugs 146, 184, 199, 263, 276
- autonomous 94, 135, 181, 195
- follicular 94, 232, 235, 236
- Hürthle cells 64, 235, 236
- scintigraphy 53
- solitary 221
- subclinical thyrotoxicosis 196
- toxic 145, 181, 199
- TSH-R mutation 12, 182
adolescents 267
- goitre 267
- hypothyroidism 268
- hyperthyroidism 269
- tumour 270
algae capsule 52, 67, 74, 109
amiodarone 14, 74, 199, 273
- antithyroid drugs 276
- breastfeeding 251
- hyperthyroidism 199, 257, 275
- hypothyroidism 257, 257
- isotope investigation 52
- iodine intake 255
- potassium perchlorate 276
- thyroiditis 106, 275
- thyrotoxicosis type 1 and 2 195, 275
- thyrotoxicosis 219, 273
- thyroxine 196
- treatment 193
- ultrasound investigation 55
analytical interference 26, 35, 44

analytical strategy 40
anaplastic cancer of the thyroid 94, 235, 237
antibody XX, 34, 36, 42, 87
- analytical interference 31, 35, 44, 215, 281
- diagnostic information 42
- Graves' disease 37, 87, 155, 162
- Hashimoto 87, 98
- heterophilic 31, 34, 44
- iodothyronine 34, 44
- pregnancy 102, 254
- subclinical hypothyroidism 112, 128
- thyroglobulin (TgAb) 38, 42, 84, 88, 98, 248
- thyroiditis 88, 98, 99
- thyronine 34, 44, 45
- thyroperoxidase *see* TPOAb
- thyrotoxicosis 37, 87, 88
- TRAb 37, 88, 89, 99, 151, 155, 162
- TSH-receptor antibody *see* TRAb
- TPOAb 36, 88, 99, 102, 111
antithyroid drugs 3, 14, 84, 109, 146, 159
- agranulocytosis 148
- adverse effects 148
- drugs, dose 146
- hyperthyroidism 146, 159
- hypothyroidism 109
- mode of action
  see also – propylthiouracil or methimazole 14, 146
- monotherapy of Graves'
- radionuclide test (24 h 131I-uptake test) 53
- preoperative treatment 163
- treatment of Graves' disease 158

atrial fibrillation 141, 197, 199, 200, 201
Astwood, Edwin Bennett 3
autoimmune polyglandular syndrome (APS) 21, 120, 214
autoimmune thyroiditis 98, 106, 268
- atrophic 101, 206
- encephalopathy 103
- focal 103, 207
- Hashimoto 98, 101, 102, 205, 268
- juvenile 102, 207
- lymphocytic 98
- myxoedema 101, 113, 115, 131
- ophthalmopathy 177
- painless 99, 102, 206
- postpartum 99, 101, 206, 264
- silent 99, 101, 206
autoimmunity 79
- cytokine 87
- Graves' disease 88, 155
- interpherone 87
- iodine 86
- lymphocyte, -T, -B 80
- ophthalmopathy 89
- smoking 86
- thyroiditis 98, 106, 107, 111
autonomous hormone production 181, 188, 224
autonomous nodule 181
- diagnosis 183
- radioiodine 50, 136, 185
- scintigraphy 53, 183
- subclinical hyperthyroidism 195
- surgery 184
- symptoms 182
- treatment 184
  see also adenoma

285

Index

B
basal metabolic rate (BMR) 22, 24
Basedow, Carl Wilhelm 3
Basedow´s disease XVII
see also Graves´ disease
Baumann, Eugen 1
beta blockers 14, 146, 163, 193, 197, 209, 260
beta radiation 47
biochemical investigations, overview 42

C
calcitonin 39, 44, 231
calcium preparations 280
carbamazepine 279
cassava 280
Cassen, Ben 4
central 31, 116, 215
- hyperthyroidism 135, 136, 215
- hypothyroidism 31, 145, 109, 126
- thyroid hormone resistance 281
Chapman, Earl 4
chemosis 169, 174, 175, 225
choriongonadotrophin (hCG) 12, 135, 136, 251, 257
Ci (Curie) XXI
clinical activity score (CAS) 175
cold adenoma 182, 239
colloid goitre 59
combination therapy 160
congenital TBG insufficiency 34
corneal lesion 170, 177
Cordarone, *see* amiodarone 273
Courtois, Bernard 1, 9
cretinism 71
CTLA-4 82
Curie (Ci) XXI
cysts 57, 230, 233
cytology 59, 61, 99, 213, 232, 236, 271

D
deiodinases (I, II, III) XVII

de Quervain´s thyroiditis 59, 100, 104, 211
see also subacute thyroiditis
destruction thyroiditis 15, 50, 97, 147, 158
diffuse toxic goitre XVII, 53, 61, 70, 136, 149, 151, 155, 191, 201, 217, 263, 270
see also Graves´ disease
- crisis 201
- crisis treatment 202
diiodothyronine 18
diiodotyrosine 13
Down´s syndrome 85, 268

E
ECG – low voltage 113
ectopic hormone production 135, 136, 216
elderly, thyrotoxicosis in 199
encephalopathy (steroid sensitive) 103
endocrine ophthalmopathy
see TAO
exophthalmos 3, 170, 172
- unilateral 174
euthyroid goitre
see nontoxic
eye symptoms
see TAO
- goitre, 221
- Evans, Robert, 3

F
factitia 136, 217
Fas/Fas-L 83
fasting 24, 26
fertility 115, 142, 256
fine-needle biopsy 55, 58
- cytological finding, *see* cytology
follicle cell 6, 12, 84, 94
follicular adenoma 94, 232, 235, 235
follicular thyroid cancer 93, 94, 235
follicular tumour 63, 94, 235
foetal development 71, 251
free T3 XIX, 12, 24, 26, 33, 35, 44, 117, 215, 217, 252
free T4 XIX, 12, 17, 29, 30, 33, 35, 41, 44, 111, 124, 132 , 215, 241, 252, 262

G
gamma camera XXI, 48, 51, 53
genetic diagnostics 39
gestational hyperthyroidism 216
giant-cell thyroiditis 59, 62
see subacute thyroiditis 213
glitazone 280
glucose metabolism 142
goitre XVIII, 61, 135, 187, 221, 228
- nontoxic 221
- cytology investigation 225, 232, 234
- intrathoracic 227
- unilateral 222
- tracheal compression 223
- ultrasound 55, 224
- superior vena cava syndrome 223
goitre ovarii 135, 217
Graefe´s sign, von 141, 167,
Graves, Robert 3
Graves´ ophthalmopathy
see TAO
Graves´ disease 155
- Addison´s disease 87
- acropachy 155
- antithyroid drug 146, 158
  - autoimmunity 87, 155
- dermopathy 141, 156
- diabetes mellitus 87, 142
- diagnose 157
- heredity 155
- histology 61
- immunological manifestations 155
- pregnancy 159, 257
- radioiodine uptake test 50, 158
- surgical treatment 163, 164
- clinical diagnose 158
- quality of life 165
- medical treatment 158
- myasthenia gravis 87
- ophthalmopathy
  see TAO
- pathophysiology 89, 155
- pernicious anemia 87
- radioiodine treatment 108, 149, 161
- recurrence 147, 158, 161, 164

- smoking 86, 155, 161
- stress 155
- subclinical hyperthyroidism 195
- symptoms 139, 155
- thyroxine treatment 159, 162, 164
- TRAb 37, 88, 151, 162, 168, 176, 254
- treatment 145, 158
- treatment options 159

Graefe's sign 141
Gray (Gy) XXI, 185
Gross, Jack 3
growth factors 91
Gull, William 1
Gy (Gray) XXI, 150

H

H_2O_2 12, 13, 15, 17
hamburger thyrotoxicosis 217
Harrington, Charles 3
Hashimoto's encephalopathy 103
Hashimoto's thyroiditis 37, 59, 62, 83, 98, 99, 205
Hashitoxicosis 98
hCG (human chorionic gonadotropin) 135, 216, 251, 257
Hertel ophthalmometer 171, 175
Hertz, Saul 3
heterophil antibodies
  see antibodies
history 1
histology, thyroid 60
hot nodule 53, 181
hungry bone syndrome 164
Hürthle cells 64, 232
Hürthle cells adenoma 64, 236
Hürthle cells cancer 64, 230, 236
hypercalcemia 142
hyperthyroidism
see also thyrotoxicosis XVIII, 43, 59, 135, 145, 155, 181, 189
- antithyroid drugs 146
- apathetic 143
- -beta adrenergic blocker 146, 163, 193
- causes 135, 199, 269
- central (secondary) 31, 215
- crises 201

- diagnostics 157, 183, 189
- elderly 199
- Graves' disease 155
- history 3
- iodine therapy 148, 202, 203
- iodide-induced 74, 191, 217, 275
- laboratory check-up 154, 161
- Lugol's solution
  see iodine-potassium iodide 109
- medically induced 273
- neonatal 88, 254
- potassium perchlorate 148, 218, 276, 277
- radionuclide examination 47, 52, 158, 183, 189, 190, 213
- subclinical 195
- symptoms 139, 155, 182, 188
- treatment 145, 158, 183, 184
- -medical 146, 158, 193
- -radioiodine 149, 161, 185, 192
- -surgery 152, 163, 184, 192
hypocalcemia 23, 164
hypothyroidism
- Addison's disease 120, 121, 126
- autoimmunity 63, 83
- central, 109
- check-up 121
- after treatment for hyperthyroidism 108
- after external radiotherapy 104
- after surgery 109
- causes 107
- coma, myxoedema 131
- coronary sclerosis 114, 115, 121
- EKG (electrocardiogram – low voltage 113
- history 3
- iodine-induced 109
- medicine-induced 109
- myxoedema 113
- natural course 111
- organ related symptoms 113

- pregnancy 256
- prolactine rise in 114
- radioiodine treatment 144
- radionuclide examination 52
- subclinical 52
- symptom 111
- TAO 89, 168
- TPOAb (thyroid peroxidase antibodies) 36, 87
- thyroxine treatment 119
- treatment 119
Höjer, Axel 1, 73

I

I-123 65, 75
I-131 XX, 4, 50, 150, 161, 168, 185, 192
iatrogenic
  see factitia
imatinib 280
immunological processes 79
immunological examinations, overview 42
interferon 87, 99, 104, 207, 279
intrathoracic goitre 55, 225, 227
investigations 29, 47
- biochemical 29, 42
- clinical palpation 67
- cytology 55, 59, 61
- CT 54
- fine-needle aspiration biopsy 55
- free T3, free T4 42
- gamma camera 51
- MR, 54
- nuclear medicine 48
- perchlorate test 52
- PET 54
- radionuclide uptake test 49
- SPECT 49
- 24 h 131 I-uptake test 52
- thyroglobulin 38, 44
- thyroid hormones 32, 44
- thyroid scintigraphy 48, 50, 136
- TPOAb 36
- TRAb 37
- TSH 11
- ultrasound with Doppler technique 55, 58
- X-ray 85

iodine in urine 39, 72
iodide pump (NIS, sodium iodide symporter) XVII, 10, 47, 246
iodine availability 71
iodine content
– iodine, potassium iodide 75, 109, 148, 203
– food 72
– X-ray contrast agents 74, 201, 218, 224, 277
iodine intake 72
– global 72
– Sweden 72
– WHO recommendation 72, 73
iodine-potassium iodide 75, 109, 148, 203
iodine (I), iodide (I–) 14, 71, 148, 203
– allergy 53, 150
– blocking overload 52, 53, 75, 76, 203, 218
– deficiency 15, 52, 71, 221
– nuclear power plant accident 75
– pool 11
– prophylaxis 76
– transport 9
– uptake 49, 246
iodization programme 73
iron medication 280
isotopes XX, 48
isotope examination 47, 52
– pregnancy, breast feeding 52, 53, 259

K

Kendal, Edward Calvin 3
Krahn ophthalmometer 170, 175
Kocher, Theodor 3, 153

L

lactation
  see breastfeeding lagophthalmus 167
Lahey, Frank 199
lipids/lipoproteins 23, 114
lithium 110, 127, 278
low T3-syndrome in NTI 25

Lugol´s solution
  see also iodine-potassium iodide 109
lymphocytes (-B, -T) 80, 251

M

MacKenzie, C.G. 3
MacKenzie, Julia 3
maternal hyperthyroidism 146, 259
MBq (megabecquerel) XXI
medical treatment 146
– Graves´ disease 158
– nontoxic nodular goitre 226
Mendeleev, Dmitri XXI
The Merseburg triad 3
MHC 79, 80
microsomal antigen 87
Moebius sign 167
mola 216
monoiodine-tyrosine 13
monotherapy, antithyroid drugs 159, 260
multinodular goitre (nontoxic) XVII, 48, 54, 74, 108, 181, 188, 193, 233
– antihyroid drug 193
– autonomous 181
– clinical course 223
– clinical work-up 234
– differential diagnosis 191
– intrathoracic 227
– iodine deficiency 221
– risk groups 191
– scintigraphy 53
– symptom 223
– toxic 181
– treatment 225
– work-up 224
  see also adenoma
Murray, George 2
myxoedema 2, 113
– coma 131
– cretinism 71
– L-thyroxine for injection 133
– mucopolysaccharides 113
– pretibial 113, 155, 166

N

Na/I cotransporter
  see NIS

NIS XVII, 10, 14, 15, 47, 65, 73, 246
nodular goitre
  see multinodular goitre 221
nodule (benign, malignant) 229, 230
– classification, 230
– MEN 2* 231
– suppressive treatment 233
– thyroglobulin 231
– work-up flow chart 234
nodule nodular goitre 181, 187, 221
nodular toxic goitre 188
neonatal hypothyroidism 88, 254
nonthyroidal illness (NTI) XVII, 25, 35, 44, 199
– common disease 25, 27
– drugs 26, 26
– rT3 26
nontoxic nodular goitre 74, 188, 221
– investigation 223
– multinodular 188, 221
– natural course 238, 281
– pathogenesis 188, 222
– subclinical hyperthyroidism 189, 193
– treatment 225
– treatment with thyroxine 226
normal values 35
nuclear power plant accident 75, 240

O

oestrogen 34, 39, 86, 122, 279
oncogenes 93
onycholysis 142
ophthalmometer 170, 175
ophthalmopathy XVIII, 67, 89, 170, 175
  see also TAO

P

painless thyroiditis 99, 102, 206
papillary thyroid cancer 63, 94, 235
Pemberton´s test 224
Pendred´s syndrome 268

Index

perchlorate, potassium 147, 276
perchlorate test 52
pertechnetate 48
phenantoin 279
photofobia 170
phytooestrogen 280
Pitt-Rivers, Rosalind 3
placenta 19, 52, 88, 219, 251, 254, 260
Plummers disease 16, 136, 188
Polyglanddular autoimmune syndrome (Pas) XVII, 87,
postpartum thyroiditis 85, 97, 101, 102, 136, 206, 264
– isotope uptake 146
potassium iodide tablets 75
potassium perchlorate 52, 147 218, 275, 276
prealbumin (transthyretin) 33, 39, 44
pregnancy 251
– antithyroid drugs 147, 160, 216, 260
– assisted reproduction 258
– beta adrenergic blockers 260, 264
– fertility 115, 142, 256
– hCG 135, 216, 251, 259
– Graves´ disease 88, 159, 163, 259, 263
– goitre 252, 262
– hyperemesis 216
– hyperthyroidism 146, 259, 262
– hypothyroidism 257, 258, 264
– immune suppression 251
– isotope examination 259
– iodine uptake 255
– physiology 251
– postpartum thyroiditis 36, 85, 90, 97, 98, 101, 264
– radioiodine treatment 150, 260
– palpable lump 262
– surgery, 261
– TBG (thyroxine-binding globuline) 32, 252
– thyrotoxicosis 259
– TRAb (TSH receptor antibo-dies) 37, 88, 254, 257, 263

– trophoblastoma 216
– thyroid hormone TSH, 252
pretibialt myxoedema 113, 156, 166
propranolol
 see beta blockers
proptos
 see also exophthalmos 169, 175, 180
– unilateral 174
propylthiouracil (Tiotil) 3, 14, 19, 146, 159, 260
– breastfeeding 261
– mode of action 19, 147
– pregnancy 252
– side effects 147
– thyrotoxic crisis 202
psychiatric symptom 114, 139, 165
– RAD XXI
– quality of life 128, 165
– radioiodine treatment 149
– adolescents 270, 271
– autonomous nodule 184, 185
– breastfeeding 53
– consequences of 149, 151, 246
– Graves´ disease 161
– hyperthyroidism 149
– indications 152
– multinodular goitre (non-toxic) 226
– ophthalmopathy 151, 168
– pregnancy 52, 255
– polyclinic (limits for) 150
– radiation/radiation protection 149
– thyroiditis 151
– toxic 191
– TRAb 151, 162

R
radioiodine uptake test 49, 52, 65, 106, 150, 161, 192, 217
radionuclide investigations 47
raloxifene 280
receptors
– thyroid hormone (TR), 46, 281
– TSH (TSH-R) 36, 122, 126, 182

recurrent nerve paresis 152, 224
– thyroid hormone resistance 215, 281
– diagnosis 282
– symptom 281
– TR-mutation 281
– treatment 282
RET-gene 94, 231
reverse T3 (rT3) XIX, 18, 19, 25, 44
– 3,3´5´-triiodothyronine XIX, 19
rifampicine 280
Rutherford, Ernest 4

S
Sandell-Kolthoff reaction 39
scintigraphy 48, 51, 53, 136
secondary
 see central
selene 16
– deficiency 16, 17, 71, 107, 255
– pregnancy 77, 255
SHBG 22
Sievert (Sv) XXII
silent thyroiditis
 see thyroiditis 101, 135, 136, 206
smoking 86, 161, 177, 255
SPECT 49
radioiodine examination 49, 50, 65, 136
Stellwag's sign 167
steroid treatment 105, 162, 168, 179, 202, 214, 276
steroid-sensitive encephalopathy 103
subacute thyroiditis 51, 136, 208, 211
– diagnosis 65, 104, 213
– differential diagnos 213
– symptoms 211
– treatment 125, 214
– uptake of isotope (I-131) 53, 136, 213
subclinical hypothyroidism 127
– definition 127
– indication for thyroxine 128
– infertility 129, 256
– prevalence 127

289

Index

- screening 129
- symptom 128
subclinical thyrotoxicosis 183, 189, 193, 195
- causes 195
- definition 195
- treatment 198
sucralfat 280
surgical treatment 152
- autonomous adenoma 184
- Graves' disease 163
- nodular nontoxic goitre 225, 227
- sternotomy 228
- toxic nodular goitre 192
Sv (Sievert) XXII

T

T3-receptor 18, 281
- cellular effects 18
T3-thyrotoxicosis 189
TAO (thyroid-associated ophthalmopathy) 89, 167
- autoimmune thyroiditis 176
- ATA classification 176
- clinical activity score (CAS) 175
- euthyroid 176
- examination 169
- follow-up 180
- illustrations, thyroid-associated ophthalmopathy 172
- classification according to NOSPECS 176
- clinical findings 170
- corrective surgery of the
- upper eye muscle corrective surgery 178
- general symptom 167
- Graves' disease 167
- handling, trake care 174, 178
- long-term perspective 180
- NSAID 179
- ophthalmometer 171
- orbital decompressive surgery 178
- pathophysiology 168
- per eyelid muscle 177
- radioiodine treatment 151, 168
- retrobulbar radiation 179
- risk factors 168

- steroid treatment 179
- symptom, diagnosis 169
- tarsoraphi 227
- TRAb (TSH Receptor Antibody) 168
- treatment 177
TBG (thyroid hormone binding globuline) 32, 33, 39, 44
- congenital deficiency 34
technetium (Tc-99m) XX, 47, 48
thiamazol (Thacapzol) 14, 109, 146, 160
- adverse events 147, 148, 260
- amiodarone 276
- breast feeding 261
- drug effect 14, 147
- pregnancy 260
- hyperthyroidism 147, 159
- thyroid storm 202
thiocyanate 10, 86, 256, 280
thyroid storm 201
- iodine treatment 202, 203
Chernobyl 149, 240
TNM classification 244
toxic adenoma 41, 181
- antithyroid drugs 147, 184
- isotope uptake 49, 53
- radioiodine treatment 149, 185
  see also adenoma
toxic goitre
- adenoma, multinodular goitre 181, 187
  see also Graves' disease
toxic nodular goitre 187
- medical treatment 193
- radioiodine 192
- surgical treatment 192, 193
TRIAC 217
TPO, see thyroperoxidase,
TPOAb, see thyroperoxidase
- antibodies
TRAb
  see also Graves' disease 37, 42, 87, 88, 99
- multinodular goitre 190
- pregnancy 254
transthyretin 32, 39, 44
TRH (tyreoliberin) 17, 42
TRH-test 32, 42, 215

triiodothyronine (T3) XIX, 3, 12
- 3, 3′,5′-triiodothyronine, (rT3) 3, 26
- peripheral effects 22
- synthesis 12
- treatment with 123
  see also thyroid hormone
trophoblastic tumour 135, 216
TSH (thyroid stimulation hormone) 11, 17, 29, 34, 40, 42
- -adenoma 215
- analysis of 29, 34
- biological inactive 44
- detection limit 30, 34
- heterofil antibodies 31, 34
- nonthyroid illness (NTI) 25
- pregnancy 252
- receptor (TSH-R) 11, 92, 182
- recombinant 246
- reference range 30, 35
- regulation 16, 29
- regulation of growth 91
- suppressed 30, 34, 183, 188
TSH receptor 11, 88, 92, 94, 182
thyroid
- anatomy 5
- clinical examination 67
- growth regulation 91
- histology 61
- hyperplasia 92
- illustration, operation 152, 153
- mutation 93, 182, 281
- neoplasia 93, 230
- oncogenes 93, 239
- palpation 68, 69
thyroid cancer 235
- age, gender 24, 242
- anaplastic 235, 237
- C cells 235
- Chernobyl 149, 240
- calcitonin 39, 44, 231, 248
- classification 235
- CT 241
- evaluation using a radioactive isotope 241
- follicular 235, 236
- Hürthle cell- 236
- incidence 235

Index

- lymph node metastasis 242
- medullar 235, 243
- mortality 235
- MR 241
- NIS 246
- oncocytic 236
- p53 94, 239
- papillary 63, 235, 237, 244
- poorly differentiated 236
- prognostic factors 241, 242
- radioiodine treatment 240, 246
- radioiodine uptake 246
- recombinant TSH 246
- RET proto-oncogene 231, 239
- risk factors 238
- thyroglobulin analysis 38, 241, 248
- TNM classification 244
- TSH stimulation 246
- TSH suppressive therapy 30, 249
- ultrasonography 55

thyroid homeostasis 24, 241, 248
- age-dependent variation 24, 35
- diurnal/annual variation 24
- individual variation 35
- stress, environmental 24

thyroid hormone XIX, 12, 20, 21, 33, 44
- acute illness 25
- amiodarone 273
- analytical strategy 40
- antibodies 34, 36, 38
- antiepileptic drug, salicylic acid 33, 34, 279
- antithyroid drugs 146, 158, 159
- autonomous adenoma 183
- connective tissue 23
- deiodination 18, 19
- diagnostic sensitivity 35, 44
- effects 21
- feedback regulation 111
- foetal, hormone production 254
- free T3, free T4 33
- general illness 25
- genomic effect 21
- pregnancy 251

- half-life of T3, T4 22
- hyperthyroidism/thyrotoxi-cosis 41, 135, 139, 145, 189
- iodine treatment 163
- calorigenic effects 139
- nodular goitre 187, 189, 221
- mitochondrial effect 18
- multinodular goitre 187
  – nonthyroid illness (NTI) 25
- contraceptives, oestrogens 33, 122, 279
- metabolism 19, 20
- organ effects 18, 22, 23
- peripheral effects 18, 22, 23
- placenta 251, 254
- plasma protein binding 33
- psychiatric disease 103
- radioiodine treatment 149, 161, 185, 192
- receptors 18
- reference interval 35
- resistance 281
- synthesis, secretion 12-14
- thyroiditis 98, 205
- thyrotoxicosis factitia 136, 217
- TSH/free T4 relation 29-31
  see also propylthiouracil or PTU or methimazole
- mode of actions 19

thyroid hormone resistance 281
thyroid scintigraphy 48, 50, 53
thyroidectomy 164, 245
thyroiditis 97, 135, 205, 211, 264
- acute bacterial 105
- adolescents 207, 268
- amiodarone 275
- atrophic 85, 98, 206
- autoimmune 98, 107, 176, 286
- causes 99
- classification, overview 99
- chronic autoimmune (lym-phocytic)
  see Hashimoto 98, 205
- biphasic 97, 99
- destructive 97, 211
- de Quervain 97, 104, 211
- drug-induced 99, 273

- focal 207
- giant-cell 62, 211
- Hashimoto 37, 62, 84, 98, 99, 107, 112, 205
- histology 62
- interferon 87, 207
- iodine-induced 218, 277
- isotope uptake 50, 52
- juvenile 98, 102
- postpartum 101, 206, 265
- radiation-induced 104, 208
Riedel 105, 209
- silent, painless 99, 101, 206
- subacute (granulomatous) 97, 104, 208, 211
- thyrotoxicosis 97, 135, 136, 157, 275

thyrotropin-releasing hormone
- (TRH) 17, 42, 215
thyrotoxic periodic paralysis 140
thyroid peroxidase (TPO) 13, 14, 36
thyroid peroxidase antibodies (TPOAb) 36, 42, 87, 98, 101, 205
thyrotoxicosis
  see also hyper-
- thyroidism 135, 139, 145, 155, 181, 187, 195, 199, 201, 215, 268
- adolescents 268
- amiodarone 275
- bone tissue 23, 142
- cardiac symptoms 140
- causes 135, 268
- CNS 141
- collagen 23
- crisis 201
- dermopathy 142
- diabetes mellitus 142
- dietary causes 73–75
- drug-induced 273
- ectopic causes
  see goitre ovarii
- elderly 199
- energy metabolism 139
- fertility 142, 256
- Graves' disease 155
- hyperparathyroidism 104
- iodine-induced 74, 136, 217
- lipoproteins 23

291

Index

- muscular weakness 140
- nervous system 139, 140
- organ effects 139
- pregnancy 257, 259
- radionuclide uptake 50
- psychiatric problems 139, 165
- skin symptom 142, 156
- surgical treatment 152, 163, 183, 192
- symptoms 111
- thyroiditis 50, 97, 149, 158, 205, 275
- thyrotoxicosis factitia 14
- treatment regiments 145, 158, 183, 191, 201

thyrotoxic crisis 201
thyrotropin
 see TSH
thyroxine (T4)
- 3,5,3′5′ tetraiodothyronine 12, 19
- compliance 125
- drug-induced 122
- intolerance 162
- parenteral treatment 124, 132
- resorption 122
- temporary treatment 125
- overdosing 124, 196, 217
- treatment of central hypothyroidism 126
 see also thyroid hormone
- thyroxine treatment 157
- Wolff-Chaikoff effect 14, 16, 73

U

ultrasound, thyroid gland 55
urinary iodine secretion 11, 39, 73

Printing and Binding: Stürtz GmbH, Würzburg